MW00611308

HISTORIES OF SUICIDE:
INTERNATIONAL PERSPECTIVES ON SELF-DESTRUCTION
IN THE MODERN WORLD

Suicide is one of the leading causes of death worldwide, with more than one million fatalities each year. During the postwar period, the rate of completed suicides has risen dramatically, especially among young men and Aboriginal peoples living in the Western world. While this has naturally led to growing concern amongst health-care practitioners and policy experts, relatively little is known about the history of attempted and completed suicide. *Histories of Suicide* is the first book to examine the history of suicide in diverse national contexts, including Japan, Scotland, Australia, Soviet Russia, Peru, United States, France, South Africa, and Canada, to reveal the different social, political, economic, and cultural factors that inform our understanding of suicide.

This interdisciplinary collection of essays assembles historians, health economists, anthropologists, and sociologists, who examine the history of suicide from a variety of approaches to provide crucial insight into how suicide differs across nations, cultures, and time periods. Focusing on developments from the eighteenth century to the present, the contributors examine vitally important topics such as the medicalization of suicide, representations of mental illness, psychiatric disputes, and the frequency of suicide amongst soldiers.

JOHN WEAVER is Distinguished University Professor of History at McMaster University.

DAVID WRIGHT is the Hannah Chair in the History of Medicine at McMaster University.

EDITED BY JOHN WEAVER
AND DAVID WRIGHT

Histories of Suicide

International Perspectives on Self-Destruction in the Modern World

UNIVERSITY OF TORONTO PRESS
Toronto Buffalo London

© University of Toronto Press Incorporated 2009
Toronto Buffalo London
www.utppublishing.com
Printed in Canada

ISBN 978-0-8020-9360-8 (cloth)
ISBN 978-0-8020-9632-6 (paper)

Printed on acid-free paper

Library and Archives Canada Cataloguing in Publication

Histories of suicide : international perspectives on self-destruction in
the modern world / edited by John Weaver and David Wright.

Includes bibliographical references and index.
ISBN 978-0-8020-9360-8 (bound)   ISBN 978-0-8020-9632-6 (pbk.)

1. Suicide – History.   2. Suicide.   3. Suicide – Sociological aspects.
I. Weaver, John   II. Wright, David, 1965–

HV6543.H586 2009   362.2809   C2008-904897-0

University of Toronto Press acknowledges the financial assistance to its
publishing program of the Canada Council for the Arts and the Ontario Arts
Council.

University of Toronto Press acknowledges the financial support for its
publishing activities of the Government of Canada through the
Book Publishing Industry Development Program (BPIDP).

Contents

Acknowledgments

The editors acknowledge, with gratitude, support for this publication and the conference from whence it arose. The book was directly supported by a publication subvention from the Social Sciences and Humanities Research Council of Canada, through its Aid to Research Workshops and Conferences program. Administrative and typesetting assistance was provided by Barbara-Ann Bartlett and Shawn Day of the History of Medicine Unit, McMaster University. The history of suicide conference, where most of these papers were read, was held at McMaster University in August 2006. It received generous funding from several organizations, centres, and departments, including The Wilson Centre for Canadian History, under the directorship of Professor Viv Nelles; the Office of the Provost of McMaster University; and both the Department of Psychiatry and Behavioural Neurosciences and the Department of History, McMaster University. The conference also received, in the form of graduate travel bursaries, financial support from the Society for the Social History of Medicine (GB). Additional administrative assistance was provided by McMaster's History of Medicine Unit, which is supported by the Hannah Chair Endowment, a joint endowment funded by McMaster University and Associated Medical Servies Toronto, Inc.

Four of the thirteen chapters have appeared elsewhere in whole or in part. Julie Parle's chapter was derived from her book *States of Mind: Searching for Mental Health in Natal and Zululand, 1868–1918* (2007), permission granted by the University of KwaZulu-Natal Press; Paulo Drinot's chapter appeared originally in the *Latin American Research Review*, permission granted by the University of Texas Press; Kenneth Pinnow's chapter was originally published in the journal *Kritika* and is reprinted with permission of the editors; and the chapter by Howard

Kushner was originally published in the *Journal of Social History*, permission to reprint granted by the author. The edited volume received generous and patient support from our editor, Len Husband, and the staff at the University of Toronto Press. Elizabeth Hulse provided, once again, excellent copy editing on what must have been a challenging manuscript incorporating multiple languages, national traditions, and discipline-specific idiosyncracies. Finally, we would like to thank the authors for their excellent contributions.

HISTORIES OF SUICIDE:
INTERNATIONAL PERSPECTIVES ON SELF-DESTRUCTION
IN THE MODERN WORLD

Introduction

DAVID WRIGHT AND JOHN WEAVER

Suicide lies at the crossroads of the religious and the secular, the public and the private, the ancient and the contemporary, the philosophical and the medical. The act itself has been open to various interpretations. For psychiatrists, self-murder is a medical problem, one of the leading causes of 'preventable death' worldwide, with more than one million fatalities each year. For sociologists, suicide is a symptom of societal dysfunction. In many Western countries the rates of suicide in Aboriginal communities have reached epidemic proportions, a pattern that is taken as a sign of the cultural disintegration of specific First Nations communities. By contrast, suicide has often been romanticized in theatre, in music, in novels, and in movies. And assisted suicide remains one of the most widely debated topics in Western bioethics and contemporary politics. It is little surprise, therefore, that scholars of different disciplinary affiliations have fought over the complex and multilayered meaning of this controversial phenomenon.

Despite the fascination with suicide studies amongst social scientists and health researchers, relatively few detailed studies of the *history* of suicide existed before the 1980s, when a series of excellent publications rescued the subject from the periphery of humanistic scholarship. Researchers in the United States, Britain, and France analysed how suicide was secularized and medicalized in Europe and North America during the course of the early modern era, how suicide navigated the voyage from 'sin to insanity' in disparate national contexts. During this period, according to recent scholarship,[1] Western society witnessed the 'birth of modern suicide,' by which is meant a decriminalized, secularized, and mostly medicalized act that increased in frequency. Suicide was no longer the province of the church; it became a social phenomenon that engaged the sociologist and the physician. Religious denunciations of suicide that typified much of the medieval period did not diminish necessarily; they were merely crowded out by more tolerant and sympathetic views from within and without the church. Concurrent with this shift, magistrates and juries by the seventeenth and eighteenth centuries were becoming reluctant to impose centuries-old penalties on self-murderers (and their families) through the traditional means of refusing Christian burials, desecrating bodies, or penalizing estates. This transformation in social values predated the articulation of new treatises by the eighteenth-century *philosophes*; rather than breaking new ground, these Enlightenment intellectuals gave articulate voice to ideas in currency at the popular level. By the late eighteenth century a 'modern' conception and treatment of suicide had come to dominate western Europe.

By the early nineteenth century, there had been a perceptible shift from suicide as a predominantly religious and legal concern to one in which medical men began to play a prominent role. Those specializing in mental diseases, or alienists, as they often styled themselves in the nineteenth century, pressed for institutional treatment and control by asserting that suicide was overwhelmingly a consequence of insanity. They alleged that self-murder could be avoided if action was taken at an early enough stage of the (mental) illness. They boldly suggested that suicide was preventable, given appropriate medical oversight and scientific investigation. Suicidality became a pathological symptom of ill individuals, something to be identified, classified, institutionalized, and prevented.[2] Such optimistic and interventionist assumptions were enshrined in nineteenth-century lunacy legislation that gave medical men and magistrates the legal right to involuntarily detain individuals who were a 'danger to themselves,' a precedent that continues to this day in most Western jurisdictions.

By the middle of the nineteenth century, Western nations had begun civil registration of vital statistics, compiling, amongst other things, cause-of-death data. One of the many consequences of this surveillance of life-course events was to generate regional and national data on self-destruction. Prominent intellectuals, from the Belgian Louis Adolphe Quételet to the Czech Tomáš Masaryk to the Italian Enrico Morselli, analysed these new suicide statistics.[3] They compared rates for men and women, for cities and countryside, and for religious groups. Amidst fears of racial deterioration, these intellectuals could not help but infer from these statistics the state of their respective nations. From an early nineteenth-century medical emphasis that favoured individual case-based studies, research momentum between 1850 and 1890 thus swung over to treatises that reviewed aggregate data for fairly large areas. Suicide was no longer solely about the individual body or mind; it was now about the corporate whole.[4]

The most notable individual to arise from this systematic analysis of suicide statistics was the Frenchman Émile Durkheim, whose Le suicide (1897) remains the single most influential treatise on self-murder. He famously postulated that suicide could be traced to the degree of social integration within a particular society. According to Durkheim, social forces unique to each country or region compelled a suicidogenic impulse or 'current' that shaped distinctive rates. Social forces, conducive to low or high social integration, produced distinctive types of suicide that he arranged in pairs: anomic and egoistic; altruistic and fatalistic. The pairs straddled a hypothetical balance between social cohesion and individuality. Individuals dissociated from their groups were prone to egoistic suicides. Communities with inadequate beliefs to meet social realities were susceptible to anomic suicide. The difference between anomic and egoistic suicide was that the social force lacking in the former was deficient collective activity, and the force missing in the latter was society's restraining influence on individual passions. Too much cohesion weakened individuality and led to altruistic suicide.[5]

By introducing a tendency that impelled people to suicide, Durkheim evaded individual situations and specific historical events; he assumed, rather than proved, his generalizations about social integration; he made it theoretically impossible to eliminate suicide but feasible to moderate the rates. For the post–Second World War era,[6] Durkheim's postulates would loom over the literature on the social causes of suicide, guiding methodological inquiries into a predominantly quantitative framework.[7] Social scientists subsequently published scores of papers comparing historical suicide rates to every conceivable measurable aspect of the human condition: to socio-demographic variables (such as sex, age, and marital status); to temporal variables (time of day, seasonality); to geographical variables (urban verses rural, latitude of country); to economic variables (occupation, unemployment, class, income, economic cycles); to the impact of migration (new immigrants versus native-born) and of war (on civilian populations, or the home front). Many of these papers were 'historical' inasmuch as they utilized time series data dating back to the nineteenth century.

By the 1980s, however, academic historians began to question many of Durkheim's connections between modernization and suicide rates. In a landmark paper in *Past & Present*, Olive Anderson, for example, challenged any symmetrical relationship between industrialization in England and suicide rates. She concluded that there was no statistical basis for Durkheim to assert that suicides were higher in 'industrial' areas than in 'rural' areas.[8] As quantitative and qualitative research accumulated in the 1980s and 1990s, many historians became sceptical of the utility of Durkheim's late nineteenth-century framework. Demographers such as L.H. Day overturned Durkheim's axiom that suicide rates were higher amongst Protestants than Catholics.[9] Victor Bailey concluded that the Frenchman's basic dictums need to be 'substantially modified' in any future empirical study of suicide.[10]

Historians of early modern Europe also contributed to new perspectives on the emerging academic debate over the history of suicide. Michael MacDonald and Terence Murphy chose to reorient the historical study of suicide from one preoccupied (in a Durkheimian sense) with suicide rates and industrialization (or modernization) to one grounded more in social and cultural history. They suggested that any apparent rise or decline in the reported rate of suicides in the eighteenth century might well represent a statistical artefact, a reflection, amongst other things, of the greater willingness of some authorities to report suicides accurately.[11] For them, suicide had become steadily secularized (and medicalized) in the seventeenth and eighteenth centuries, a result of a shift in popular sentiments towards the act of self-murder. MacDonald's thesis of a 'ground-up' secularization of and growing tolerance towards self-murder has been extremely influential in early modern studies on the subject, such as Jeffrey Watt's examination of early modern Geneva.[12] As Georges Minois has suggested, the analysis of suicide for pre-modern historians has been less about uncovering the statistical 'truth' of suicide rates as about detecting the way in which the discussion, reception and punishment of 'voluntary death' reflected the core values of different societies.[13]

The historical study of suicide has also occasioned a certain degree of interdisciplinarity – a sensitivity to the biological, a grounding in the social, an eye to the cultural, and an ear to the verbal.[14] An important aspect of all four has been the growing recognition of the importance of aging and the different crises faced by men and women, as Anderson perceptively recognized.[15] Simon Cooke, writing about suicide in the Australian state of Victoria, documented the importance of the interaction of the social and biological; aging brought dependence, and differences between the life courses of men and women were embodied in the distinct methods of suicide.[16] Bailey chose to use life cycle as the prism through which he analysed suicide in nineteenth-century Hull, England.[17]

Despite the new interdisciplinary approaches, historians of suicide have mined a fairly common set of primary sources: religious and medical treatises, coroners' and medical examiners' reports, police and jail records, hospital and asylum admission books, and newspapers and popular magazines. Each set of sources poses challenges for historical interpretation, not least of which is that many were the (re-)constructions of witnesses and juridical authorities collected or imagined after the event. Only extant suicide notes can be said to incorporate the 'voice' of the suicide, but even those are subject to multiple posthumous interpretations. Like the history of madness, contemporary accounts of the causes of self-murder tell us as much about the attitudes and cultural frameworks of witnesses as they do about the act itself.

Trends in psychiatric and historical research have also reoriented recent academic research into the history of self-murder. As Western-based academics reflect more and more on the Eurocentricity of much scholarly teaching and research, there has been a desire to expand the scope of inquiry, to look more 'globally' and transnationally at different historical phenomena. Parallel to this trend, one can identify the important, if challenging, implications of transcultural psychiatry, a field that explores the multi-faceted nature of the experience,[18] understanding, and treatment of mental disorders beyond the implicit universalism of the modern DSM (Diagnostic and Statistical Manual of Mental Disorders) and ICD (International Statistical Classification of Disease). Both trends have prompted scholarly collections on the history of mental health to engage more actively with transnational and cross-cultural themes that look beyond the traditional focus on Europe and North America.

The contributions to this edited volume build on recent scholarship in the history of suicide by widening the geographical remit of the countries under inquiry and by bridging edited collections on the history of suicide in early modern Europe with more contemporary debates. The chapters examine some twelve different national contexts, from South Africa to Japan, from Australia to Scotland, from Soviet Russia to Peru. They are written from a variety of academic perspectives – historical, to be sure, but also criminological, anthropological, and sociological. Despite these differences in disciplinary approach, the arguments emerging from these chapters intersect and complement one another. The authors grapple with many of the defining themes of the history of suicide. To what extent did the professionalization of medicine involve a reconceptualization of self-murder? How do we account for popular attitudes to voluntary death that appeared to be softening over the course of the nineteenth and twentieth centuries? Can one reconstruct, with any degree of confidence, demographic trends in national, regional, and sex-specific suicide rates over the modern era? And if so, what do these look like? How did self-destruction become conflated with the dominant debates over 'modernity' and the expression of nineteenth- and twentieth-century anxieties over urbanization, secularization, and racial diversity? Why has suicide, as a field of study, become the domain of so many different professional communities?

There has certainly been a recurrent perception amongst the elite members of Western industrializing countries that suicide was (and is) on the rise. Indeed, the laments of 'suicide epidemics' that wax and wane in the modern era first became prominent in eighteenth-century Europe. As Jeffrey Merrick demonstrates, the frightening rise of suicide as a subject of popular fascination and elite discussion in late eighteenth-century Paris fuelled a debate over the cause of this perceived decline in personal morality. Religious authorities, of course, blamed contemporary epidemics of suicide on the creeping secularization of society, encouraged by the liberal ideas of the Enlightenment. Others mused about the debilitating and demoralizing effects of rural depopulation and urban living. Cities were fingered as both the locus and the engine of prostitution, crime, and licentiousness, which, mixed together, provided an iniquitous environment ripe for such egregious behaviour as self-murder. In this way the metropolis became inextricably linked to professional discourses on the relentless rise of suicide. Whether Paris, Lima, St Petersburg,[19] London, or Tokyo, national elites, ironically themselves the product of the same modernizing forces and most often living in urban environments, blamed cities for moral and physical degeneration.

The city as a *physical* location that distorted and weakened the emotional and psychological sensibilities of its inhabitants was only one aspect of the pernicious effects contemporary social commentators identified in the process of modernization. As the city gained in size and influence, the countryside became increasingly romanticized as a fading emblem of community, kinship, health, and moral behaviour. Thus the twinning of suicide and the city was also a lament for a bygone era of a harmonious, quieter life that, regardless of its historical 'accuracy,' resonated with many nineteenth-century urban commentators. As Howard Kushner clearly articulates in his chapter, nineteenth-century thinkers in western Europe and North America took it as axiomatic that cities *must* have higher (real) rates of suicide and dismissed counter-arguments that such data were merely statistical artefacts of more organized urban civil bureaucracies or of rural under-reporting. The dominant discourse was not about *whether* the urban environments had higher rates of suicide but *why* and *to what extent.*

As the nineteenth century evolved, the emerging tendency to biologize social problems affected this professional preoccupation. The 'slums' became a synecdoche for the city and code for the physically degenerate, as well as racially marginalized, populations. As theories of (urban) degeneration took hold in many industrializing societies in the last quarter of the nineteenth century, self-murder became one of the subjects of eugenic-inspired public inquiries and medical treatises. Thus, as Paulo Drinot observes, Lima intellectuals wrote about suicide not only as an *urban* phenomenon or strictly as a *medical* problem but also as a sign of national decline, of the insidious effects of Asian immigration to the Peruvian capital and the dangers of interracial marriage.[20] Similarly, Julie Parle illustrates how (East) Indians in South Africa were targeted as degenerate (and therefore dangerous) social elements as a result of their very high rates of suicide. The Western medicalized discourse about suicide at the turn of the twentieth century thus became integral to the emerging justification for racial differentiation and civil disenfranchisement that characterized the twentieth-century history of many Western countries.

Professional discourses about suicide and race could manifest themselves in a multitude of often contradictory ways. Parle explains how the lower rates of suicide amongst black South Africans were also used to signify evolutionary backwardness. According to the then predominant medical discourse, South African blacks were considered to be 'immune' to suicide because of their 'undeveloped natures.' Paradoxically, both the higher rates amongst Indians and the lower rates amongst blacks were used to justify racial segregation. Such self-serving medical treatises are strikingly similar to the early twentieth-century United States, where, as Andrew Fearnley argues, it was widely held that African Americans had *lower* rates of suicide than 'white' Americans. When postwar suicidology emerged as an organized scholarly discipline in the United States and its practitioners discovered that blacks had equal or higher rates of suicide, black suicides became framed in a particular manner, emphasizing youth and masculinity. Just as a lower rate of black suicide had justified racial segregation in the pre-war United States, a higher rate of black suicide in the volatile 1960s was identified as a possible danger of racial integration and radical politics. Whites engaged in 'passive,' 'introspective,' and 'non-threatening' suicide; black suicide was characterized as 'dangerous,' 'aggressive,' and 'violent.' Suicide rates, and the way suicide was framed, could be used to reinforce power relations in a multitude of ways.[21]

Social and political imperatives thus informed the professional investigation of suicide in the twentieth century. Such contextual factors influencing the 'scientific' examination of 'objective' data can be seen most starkly in Junko Kitanaka's examination of Japan. The long-standing cultural legitimization of what was known as the 'suicide of resolve' (rational suicide) in Japan led to a crisis amongst Japanese psychiatrists, who were caught between Westernizing influences of Kraepelinian classification and centuries-old cultural validation (and aestheticization) of honourable death. As a consequence, psychiatrists in Japan had limited impact on the (re-)conceptualization of suicide in their own country. A similar crisis emerged in Soviet Russia. Since suicide was considered a bourgeois act of self-indulgence, Bolshevik commentators in the 1920s were faced with explaining the persistence of suicide concurrent with the construction of a socialist utopia. Using Bolshevik party records, Kenneth Pinnow illustrates how party apparatchiki were forced to perform intellectual gymnastics in their attempt to explain how party members succumbed to such individualist temptations.

Any edited volume on the history of suicide must ultimately grapple with one overarching theme that has dominated the historical literature for the last quarter-century, namely, the impact of the rise of the medical profession in the nineteenth century. The case for the medicalization of suicide is strong, particularly when one examines the changing language used to describe the (mental) state of the individual suicide. The eighteenth-century Western world inherited significant legal penalties that were inflicted upon the suicide's family if a sudden death was labelled an intentional suicide, rather than 'accidental' or arising from a state of mental disorder. Individuals who committed suicide were culpable of a *felo de se* (a felony against oneself), resulting in the seizure or forfeiture of property as well as non-Christian burial. As a result, families (and sympathetic witnesses and coroners) might have constructed posthumous accounts of the death that would obviate this determination as a possibility, either through narratives that implied that the person in question could never have committed suicide (and thus the death had to be an accident) or through anecdotal reconstructions suggesting the person was *non compos mentis*. Thus in turn-of-the-nineteenth-century London, Paris, and Edinburgh, the rise of verdicts of lunacy might well have represented a softening of public attitudes towards suicide and a desire not to further punish families already suffering the pain and torment of the death of someone close to them. A *non compos mentis* verdict served several social and emotional ends.

Although medicalized language in nineteenth-century witnessed depositions became more and more common, several of our contributors question whether increasing references to mental illness should be interpreted as the *medicalization* of the suicide act. For Rab Houston, no such medicalization occurred in England and Scotland before the mid-nineteenth century. In the jurisdictions under study, he found that the 'involvement of medical practitioners in uncovering or certifying suicide was limited to the forensic side and to physical signs, rather than psychological symptoms.' The understandings of suicide for lay people, Houston concludes, became medicalized only in a growing expectation that medical men would be involved in the physical care of attempted suicides and in the identification of suicidal death as different from accidental, natural, or homicidal. Houston's findings are part of a broader re-evaluation of medicalization in the history of madness,[22] one that sees it as less comprehensive – and indeed, occurring much later – than a previous historiography of the all-powerful medical profession would suggest. If one can generalize from the variety of chapters and conclusions that fill this book, it is that the process of medicalization was patchy and uneven and the widespread *psychiatrization* of suicide was more often than not a contested twentieth-century phenomenon. Indeed, Junko Kitanaka argues that the 'broad-scale' medicalization of suicide in Japan is only now under way.

Other contributions to this volume have reworked and nuanced the concept of medicalization. For Kevin Siena, the medicalization of language surrounding a suicide that was evident from the eighteenth century onwards was intimately connected to suicide in ways distinct from emerging narratives of insanity. He makes a strong case for rational suicide as an 'illness strategy' in late eighteenth-century England. Doctors' treatises, Siena affirms, were 'rife with discussions of patients expressing a preference for death to continued suffering.' Rarely were these sufferers labelled insane by understanding practitioners, who knew all too well the reality of mercurial treatment for syphilis or the terrifying ordeal of surgery before anaesthesia. Such choices prefigure the current debate over 'euthanasia' and doctor-assisted suicide.[23] And yet medicalized (or psychiatrized) language did slowly sink into professional parlance and popular patois. Lunacy verdicts clearly increased in prominence in the eighteenth and nineteenth centuries. And by the early twentieth century, one sees the ubiquitous (if vague) transnational diagnosis of 'neurasthenia.' Long discussed by academic historians in the context of 'shell shock' and 'trauma,' neurasthenia became a convenient and less stigmatizing label to help explain away suicides, particularly amongst former soldiers in the interwar period. It appears as an aetiological catch-all in Lima, Tokyo, rural Queensland, and Paris, a sign of the internationalization of many psychiatric ideas by the dawn of the twentieth century.

The competition of discourses – religious and lay, medical and popular, cultural and 'scientific' – remains an important aspect of the history of suicide. Indeed, one could argue that, taken to its logical extreme, the history of suicide is all about discourses – the impromptu narratives of witnesses, the formal construction of medical treatises, the traumatized accounts of family members, the insidious formulation of theories of degeneration, the bureaucratic validation of Soviet collectivism. To focus exclusively on these discourses, however, risks de-emphasizing some of the humanistic aspects of self-murder. We must remember that suicide was a violent act that horrified witnesses, destabilized communities, and threw distraught families into the worst sort of financial and emotional maelstrom. Many chapters illustrate the horror of the days leading to the suicidal act and the heart-wrenching circumstances of the end of life through their sensitive use of coroners' reports, the depositions of witnesses and relatives, and indeed, the voices of the deceased themselves (in suicide notes). Whether these were young women who had been 'interfered with,' demoralized but proud men who could not find work in Depression-era Australia, French soldiers returning from the trenches of the First

World War, or culturally displaced indentured Indians in South Africa, the qualitative sources highlighted in these chapters bring us as close as we may ever come to a real empathy with tragic consequences of intense suffering in the past.

It may well be that some individuals made entirely rational decisions to end their own lives – what appears to be a rational catalogue of reasons for 'choosing death.' Kevin Siena's contribution to the current volume marshalls evidence from a variety of sources, including some coroners' inquests, to show that physical illness and injury in eighteenth-century England made suicide 'an option at least worthy of consideration.' The extraordinary suicide notes of Richards and Weaver's Queensland study are remarkable for their lucid accounts of life's travails. As one world-weary individual concluded pithily before killing himself: 'No wife, no home, no work & no money.' Other suicides appeared to be labouring under various delusions or to be melancholic. The 'great despondency' was identified in so many of the depositions, and some suicides had recently been discharged from lunatic asylums. Other desperate and deranged states of mind were aggravated by drink. Indeed, 'the bottle' appears as a remarkably ubiquitous contributing factor to male suicides in these chapters.

In his examination of Geneva, Jeffrey Watt identifies a widening gap between female and male suicides, in the manner in which they murdered themselves: men more violently (such as by gunshot); women by drowning or poisoning. In addition, women attempted suicide more often; men completed suicide at a rate of three to four times that of women. Some explanation for these differences may simply be the result of availability: women had access to household poisons and appliances; many men worked or travelled with guns, shears, and long knives. As Howard Kushner points out, suppositions about the trials and woes that plagued men conditioned gendered explanations (from Durkheim onwards) for women's lower suicide rates – 'the immunity that women enjoy'[24] – and an avoidance of evidence as to the considerable numbers of women who attempted suicide.[25] But the chapters in this edited volume testify to the persistence of this gender difference in rates and methods across national, cultural, and temporal boundaries, suggesting that individual and social contexts cannot alone explain these differences.[26] Indeed, the differences in methods exhibited by men and women, as Rosemary Gartner and Bill McCarthy recount, are sharply delineated in the special instance of murder-suicide.

The ubiquity of guns in nineteenth- and twentieth-century society made it one of the weapons of choice for men. This was no more true than for the self-murder of (male) soldiers.[27] As Janet Padiak and Patricia Prestwich demonstrate, in their analysis of British soldiers in Gibraltar and French soldiers during and after the First World War, the rate of soldier suicide was one that deeply troubled politicians, families, and communities on the home front. Soldiers had long been the emblem of masculinity, pride, and self-confidence. To commit suicide was not only to engage in a terrible act of self-destruction; it also challenged important national and cultural stereotypes of the courageous male war hero. Just as shell shock became a lightning rod for socio-cultural crisis during the First World War, so too did suicide.[28] Unfortunately, the high rates of suicide amongst soldiers continued, and even escalated, when retired soldiers grew older or attempted, often unsuccessfully, to reintegrate into society.

The grisly minutiae of self-murder surely are rendered even more horrific by the act of murder-suicide, when individuals chose not only to take their own lives but to take others along as well. This book includes two excellent large-scale studies of this particular act of self-destruction. Rosemary Gartner and Bill McCarthy illustrate the long-term trends in murder-suicide in four North American cities during the twentieth century. They found that most offenders were males and most victims were females; men's victims were usually their intimate female partners (or the objects of delusional amorous beliefs), whereas women's victims were typically their children. Most homicide-suicides can be classified as 'familicides,' which were almost always committed by males. Gartner and McCarthy remain unconvinced of any straightforward relationship (either positive or inverse) between homicide rates and suicide rates.[29] Their conclusions are rather unnervingly replicated in the work by Richards and Weaver on murder-suicide in Queensland, Australia. While these authors agree with the aggregate findings of Gartner and McCarthy, the coroners' reports upon which they rely reveal the remarkable diversity of individual situations that render generalizations extremely difficult and at times problematic.

The modern understanding and professional examination of suicide emerged in part from the nineteenth-century fascination with numbers – with the power and objectivity of statistics, a cultural preoccupation that continues to this day with the rise of evidence-based medicine in formal clinical practice and medical scholarship. Thus in capitalist, mixed, and socialist countries, the generation of social data was crucial to measuring (and advancing) national progress. As Kenneth Pinnow demonstrates, the Soviet Union established a Department of Moral Statistics, an institution that carried out extensive surveying of suicide in post-revolution Russia. This new bureaucratic entity generated suicide questionnaires which themselves had pre-formulated concepts, classifications, and categories that shaped the outcomes sought by officials.[30] As Fearnley argues in his examination of suicidology in the postwar United States, suicide statistics were thus not solely about divining social scientific laws; they were a larger project of building up professional academic disciplines (such as sociology), legitimating power relations, and justifying the subsidiary role of women, races, and the working classes. Ironically, one of the principal goals of the statistical analysis of suicide – to identify populations 'at risk' and thus institute preventative measures – seems to have had only modest impact on the longer-term historical trends in suicide rates.

This volume has attempted to push the historical examination of suicide beyond its traditional Euro–North American boundaries by including chapters on South America, South Africa, Japan, and Australasia. But despite its wider geographical remit, this book cannot be considered comprehensive in its coverage. We failed to include chapters on countries in South Asia, Northern Africa, Scandinavia, or Southeast Asia. The omission of a country such as Sri Lanka is particularly notable, as this country has witnessed the most dramatic rise of reported suicide in the contemporary world.[31] We hope, however, that the book serves as a useful contribution to transnational themes in the social history of medicine. In a subject area so crowded by social scientists and the helping professions, historians have been too reluctant to contribute to the debate over suicide. We believe that the chapters contained in this book resonate with themes that cut across national boundaries and cultural differences and, by doing so, illuminate cross-cultural perspectives on mental disorder more generally. That many of these chapters are acutely sobering and at times distressing makes them no less important.

NOTES

1 For an excellent edited volume on various early modern European juridisctions, see Jeffrey R. Watt, ed., *From Sin to Insanity: Suicide In Early Modern Europe* (New York: Cornell University Press, 2004).

2 These themes were redolent in the works of the famous French alienists,

but they can be detected across various Western jurisdictions. For a French example, see Jean-Étienne-Dominique Esquirol, *Mental Maladies: A Treatise on Insanity*, translated by Raymond de Saussure (New York: Hafner Publishing Company, 1965; reprint of 1845 edition).

3 *Louis Adolphe Quételet, Sur l'homme sur le développement de ses facultés; ou, Essai de physique sociale* (1835), translated as *A Treatise on Man* (1842); Thomas (Tomáš) Masaryk, *Suicide and the Meaning of Civilization*, translated by William B. Weist and Robert B. Batson with an introduction by Anthony Giddens (Chicago: University of Chicago Press, 1970) first published as *Der Sebstmord als sociale Massenerscheinung der modernen Civilisation* in 1881; Henry (Enrico) Morselli, *Suicide: An Essay on Comparative Moral Statistics* (New York: D. Appleton and Co., 1881).

4 For a discussion of this theme, see Ian Hacking, *The Taming of Chance* (Cambridge: Cambridge University Press, 1991), 105–24.

5 Émile Durkheim, *Le suicide* (Paris: 1897).

6 For most of the interwar period, studies of suicide reflected a strong psychoanalytic approach, as exemplified in the work of Karl Menninger. See Menninger, *Man against Himself* (New York: Harcourt, Brace & Company, 1938). For a discussion of the rise of psychoanalytic interpretations of suicide in American psychiatry, see Howard I. Kushner, 'American Psychiatry and the Cause of Suicide, 1844–1917,' *Bulletin of the History of Medicine* 60 (1986): 36–57. By the early 1960s, as psychoanalysis's power began to decline, Durkheim was 'rediscovered' in the social sciences. For an example of this, see Ronald Maris, 'Suicide in Chicago: An Examination of Emile Durkheim's Theory of Suicide' (Unpublished PhD dissertation, University of Illinois, 1965).

7 Durkheim's work was translated into English in 1951; see Durkheim, *Suicide: A Case Study in Sociology*, trans. John A Spaulding and George Simpson (New York, 1951).

8 Olive Anderson, 'Did Suicide Increase with Industrialization in Victorian England?' *Past & Present*, no. 86 (February 1980): 149–73. See also Olive Anderson, *Suicide in Victorian and Edwardian England* (Oxford, 1987).

9 L.H. Day, 'Durkheim On Religion and Suicide – A Demographic Critique,' *Sociology* (Great Britain) 21 (1987): 449–61. Day explored census data from Prussia, Switzerland, and the Netherlands.

10 Victor Bailey, *This Rash Act: Suicide across the Life Cycle in the Victorian City* (London, 1998).

11 Michael MacDonald and Terence Murphy, *Sleepless Souls: Suicide in Early Modern England* (Oxford, 1990).

12 Jeffrey R. Watt, *Choosing Death: Suicide and Calvinism in Early Modern Geneva* (Kirksville: Truman State University Press, 2001).

13 George Minois, *Histoire du suicide: La société occidentale face à mort volontaire* (Paris: Fayard, 1995); translated by Lydia G. Cochrane as *History of Suicide: Voluntary Death in Western Culture* (Baltimore: Johns Hopkins University Press. 1999).

14 As Howard Kushner concluded in his innovative and interdisciplinary *Self-Destruction in the Promised Land*, historians must 'understand suicide by integrating social, psychological, and biological factors.' See Kushner, *Self-Destruction in the Promised Land: A Psychocultural Biology of American Suicide* (New Brunswick, NJ: Rutgers University Press, 1989), 177.

15 Anderson, *Suicide in Victorian and Edwardian England*, 418–19.

16 Simon Cooke, 'Terminal Old Age: Ageing and Suicide in Victoria, 1841–1921,' *Australian Cultural History* 14: (1995) 76–91; Cooke, 'Secret Sorrows: A Social History of Suicide in Victoria, 1841–1921' (PhD dissertation, University of Melbourne, 1998).

17 Bailey, *'This Rash Act.*

18 As exemplified in the journal of the same name: *Transcultural Psychiatry*.

19 Susan K. Morrissey, 'Suicide and Civilization in Late Imperial Russia,' *Jahrbucher fur Geschichte Osteuropas* 43 (1995): 201–17.

20 Cf. Susan Johnston's original article on how in Canada, British Columbians inscribed their fears of sexual disorder and racial miscegenation on the bodies of the suicides. See Johnston, 'Twice Slain: Female Sex-Trade Workers and Suicide in British Columbia, 1870–1920,' *Journal of the Canadian Historical Association* 5 (1994): 147–66.

21 For an unusual perspective on suicide and race, see the following historical article written in 1969: Sheldon Hackney, 'Southern Violence,' *American Historical Review* 74 (1969): 906–25.

22 See, for example, Akihito Suzuki, *Madness at Home: The Psychiatrist, the Patient, and the Family in England, 1820–1860* (Berkeley: University of California Press, 2006).

23 Ian Dowbiggin, *A Merciful End: The Euthanasia Movement in Modern America* (New York: Oxford University Press, 2003).

24 Jack Porter Gibbs, 'A Sociological Study of Suicide' (PhD thesis, University of Oregon, 1957), 258.

25 See Howard I. Kushner, 'Women and Suicide in Historical Perspective,' *Signs* 10 (1985): 537–52.

26 Within the social sciences, there is a cluster of papers on modernization and sex differences in (completed) suicide. See, for example, Catherine Krull and Frank Trovato, 'The Quiet Revolution and the Sex Differential

in Quebec's Suicide Rates: 1931–1986,' *Social Forces* 72 (1994): 1121–47.

27 See also Norbet Ortmayer, 'Selbstmord in Osterreich 1819–1988 [Suicide in Austria, 1819–1988],' *Zeitgeschichte* (Austria) 17 (1990): 209–25.

28 It is for this reason (and others) that soldier suicide was largely marginalized from discussion by Durkheim and others, as Kushner insightfully argues.

29 In contrast to Lane's controversial 1970s thesis on Philadelphia. See Roger Lane, *Violent Death in the City: Suicide, Accident, and Murder in Nineteenth Century Philadelphia* (Cambridge: Harvard University Press, 1979).

30 For a competing view, see Gabor T. Rittersporn, 'Le message des données introuvables: L'État et les statistiques du suicide en Russie et en URSS' [The Message behind the Missing Data: The State and Suicide Statistics in Russia and the USSR],' *Cahiers du monde russe* (France) 38 (1997): 511–23.

31 See Robert N. Kearney and Barbara D. Miller, 'The Spiral of Suicide and Social Change in Sri Lanka,' *Journal of Asian Studies* 45 (1985): 81–101. See also David C. Purcell, 'Suicide in Micronesia: The 1920s and 1930s,' *Pacific Studies* 14 (1991): 71–86.

1 Suicide, Gender, and the Fear of Modernity

HOWARD I. KUSHNER

In the early nineteenth century, numerous European and North American commentators warned that the growth of cities threatened social cohesion and individual tranquility. The assertion in 1820 by Étienne Esquirol, the leader of the French asylum movement, that 'madness is the disease of civilization' was emblematic of these views.[1] The rise of factories, which led to the downgrading of traditional skills, was portrayed as particularly disruptive. The family was depicted as the primary defence against the forces of social disintegration. Because middle-class ideology emphasized the role of women as mothers and as guardians of the family, theorists assumed that they were better positioned than men to resist the chaos ascribed to modernity.

This analysis was sustained by the new science of social statistics, whose initial findings seemed to provide empirical evidence attesting to the negative impact of urban life. Compilations of rates of disease, insanity, and violence reinforced ancient suspicions about the evils of the city.[2] Self-destructive behaviour became a prima facie example of the corrupting effects of urbanization and the incidence of suicide developed into a barometer for social health.[3] Given the assumptions that had informed the collection of these data, what constituted a suicide would be defined in ways that reinforced assertions about the disruptive consequences of urbanization and modernization. What commentators considered to be self-destructive behaviour was framed by their assumptions of what caused self-destructive behaviour and who (men) would be most susceptible to it. These beliefs were enshrined in Émile Durkheim's definitive Le suicide (1897) and have remained undisputed ever since.[4]

From the very first, hypotheses about the causes of suicide were tied to sentimental visions of the family and to an ambivalence toward social change. Thus warnings of nascent suicide epidemics were coupled with nostalgic portraits of rural life. Since the nineteenth century, experts have concluded that the best safeguards against suicide lay in the restoration of traditional values, especially the patriarchal family.[5] Given the logic of these assumptions, it was a foregone conclusion that women would prove more immune to suicide than men. A gendered analysis, however, not only challenges that assumption but also calls into question the entire statistical enterprise that has informed our understanding of suicide since the early nineteenth century.[6]

The City as Killer

The connection between suicide and urban life has deep roots in Western thought. As early as the seventeenth century, clergymen and moral philosophers portrayed urban dwellers as at much greater risk of suicide than their country cousins. For instance, in 1653 the English Puritan minister Sir William Denny connected what he alleged was an outbreak of suicides to the growth of London as an urban centre.[7] By the eighteenth century the city became a metaphor for those habits – intemperance, idleness, melancholy, decline of religious faith, and licentiousness – which sermons since the seventeenth century had connected with suicide. The reason there were 'fewer suicides in the country than in cities,' wrote Voltaire, was because 'in the fields it is only the body which suffers; in the city it is the mind. The ploughman doesn't have time to be melancholic.'[8] Like Voltaire, Jean Dumas (1773) tied the putative increase in suicide to the decline of the traditional social and moral order brought on by the growth of cities.[9] A decade later the French playwrite Louis Sébastien Mercier claimed that urban conditions had made 'suicide ... more common in Paris today than in all the other cities in the known world.'[10]

The association of suicide, vice, urbanization, and modernity gained intensity in the beginning of the nineteenth century as the generalized anxieties of earlier eras were translated into social 'facts' by swelling urban populations. Informing and exacerbating all of this was a fear of gender chaos: women, it seemed, were becoming more like men, and men more like women. These concerns had surfaced in revolutionary France, but they intensified throughout the nineteenth century.[11] Thus, as experts defined suicide as a male activity, they simultaneously labelled women who killed themselves 'masculine.' Women were warned that if they persisted in acting like men, they endangered not only themselves but also their families. Often this connection was explicit. Sometimes these issues were submerged in a formulaic and generalized set of caveats about the dangers of urban life which portrayed those most subsumed in it as at greatest risk of suicide. In this construction, women rarely appear. This absence, however, both obscures and reveals concrete fears that increasing numbers of working urban women were themselves among the forces of modernity that posed a 'threat' to the moral fabric.[12] So, while anxiety about the changing role of women was no mere abstraction, any more than the fear of class conflict was, it remained subterranean in the highly structured and ritualized jeremiads about the connections between suicide and urban life. It is these later texts and warnings that we examine first, before reconnecting them with the more explicit discussion of women, gender, and suicide.

'Every day,' wrote the Prussian diplomat J.F. Reichardt in 1803, 'one hears talk of murders and suicides among the people and the petty bourgeoisie' of Paris.[13] In the New World, Americans also uncovered an urban suicide epidemic. In *The Guilt, Folly, and Sources of Suicide,* two sermons delivered and published in 1805, Presbyterian minister Samuel Miller of New York proclaimed that suicide was 'a crime which has become alarmingly frequent ... in our city.' The rate of suicide, he insisted, was tied directly to 'the progress of vice in our city.'[14]

These examples, along with those that opened this section, expose two strands of anti-urban thought, one religious and the other secular. Like Denny and Miller, ministers enunciated the Calvinist belief that the temptation to suicide was best held at bay by tight authoritarian communities. When communitarian controls were relaxed and moral choices multiplied, as they tended to in cities, ordinary people would find it difficult to resist temptation. The secular view, as evidenced in Voltaire, Dumas, and Mercier, contrasted the sheer exhaustion and emotional equilibrium of rural life with the putative psychological anxiety of urban existence. At bottom, however, both religious and secular assertions that modernity led to suicide were founded on the shared belief that humans were unable to negotiate the variety and choice that urban life offered. By the early nineteenth century, these two strands became conflated and difficult to disentangle.

This merging of religious and secular fears of modernity found its clearest expression in the medical rhetoric of 'moral treatment.' Its advocates believed in an environmental view of the aetiology of disorder. Health depended upon the combination of diet, atmosphere, climate, work, and lifestyle; disease, even lesions in the brain, resulted from imbalance of these elements. Fed by a belief that, like the environment, individuals were malleable, suppressive modes of control were de-emphasized in favour of more repressive behaviours. Reflecting wider cultural, economic, and political developments, the moral treatment stressed self-discipline as an alternative to external authority.[15]

The assumptions of the moral treatment were especially useful for explaining the aetiology of non-specific psychiatric disorders such as suicide. Even though its proponents had their own agendas, the moral treatment provided a 'scientific' vocabulary, as well as a common ground, for religious and secular assertions that suicide was a function of modern urban life. And more than any other group, alienists (nineteenth-century forerunners of psychiatry) provided the perfect combination of scientific and moral rhetoric to legitimize the popular and religious beliefs that had connected modernity with increased suicides.

In alienists' hands, social descriptions mutated into diagnosis. And given the protean nature of suicide, these diagnoses could only be expressed metaphorically. Thus 'civilization' became a metaphor for modern urban society, while 'education,' 'ennui,' and the breakdown of social distinctions were its signifiers. When the French alienist Jean-Pierre Falret (1822) asserted that 'civilization plays a great role in the production of suicide,' it was quite clear to his readers, particularly to other alienists, that 'civilization' was synonymous with contemporary urban life. For while 'civilization' exposed the brain to increased stresses and excited an excess of passions and desires that could not be satisfied, these pressures, wrote Falret, were 'almost unknown' in rural regions of Europe.[16] An 1836 review of suicide statistics published in *Annales d'hygiène publique* connected increasing European suicide rates with rising social aspirations. 'Suicides,' according to this analysis, were 'more common where education is more widespread' and less frequent where education was restricted. The rate of suicide would be reduced 'if the education of youth was more in conformity to that of their relatives, and to the real needs of the social sphere' into which they were born.[17] 'In all countries of the world,' wrote the French alienist Louis Bertrand in 1857, 'suicides are most common where education is the most diffused.'[18]

Across the Channel, the sentiments were the same. 'There cannot be a doubt,' wrote Forbes Winslow (1840), editor and founder of the British *Journal of Psychological Medicine*, 'but that the general diffusion of knowledge, and the desire to place within the command of the humblest person the advantages of education, have not a little tended to promote the crime of suicide.' For, Winslow argued, 'in proportion as the intellect becomes expanded, knowledge and civilization diffused, the desire to commit self-murder would be engendered.' 'It is an indisputable fact,' he concluded, 'that insanity in all its phases marches side by side with civilization and refinement.'[19]

Modernity (or 'civilization') led to suicide because it subverted traditional forms of deference. 'Man needs an authority to direct his passions and govern his actions,' wrote Esquirol. Because lines of authority were clearer in the countryside than in the cities, one could be certain, he added, that 'in comparing the number of suicides in cities ... with the number of suicides in the countryside,' the cities would always produce more suicides.[20]

The opinions of French, British, and American alienists about modernity and suicide were reinforced by republication and translation of one anothers' writings in psychiatric journals such as the *Annales d'hygiène publique*, the *Annales médico-psychologiques*, the *Asylum Journal of Mental Science*, the *Journal of Psychological Medicine*, and the *American Journal of Insanity*.[21] For instance, in an 1855 article entitled 'De l'influence de la civilisation sur le suicide,' Alexandre Brierre de Boismont, editor of the *Annales médico-psychologiques*, cited the work of his New and Old World colleagues to support his contention that modernity underlay an increase in the number of suicides: 'The time in which we live is not only wrought by *ennui*, this sickness of advanced civilizations,' but also by 'a universal confusion of ideas, a general weariness, the complete disillusionment with everything we have praised and adored.'[22] An 1858 article in the London *Journal of Psychological Medicine* drew on French sources that 'proved that among the inhabitants of large cities suicides are more frequent than in rural districts.'[23]

The assertion by the Belgian statistician Adolphe Quételet that suicide rates followed a statistical 'law' which could be 'confirmed year after year' provided additional authenticity for assertions that increases in suicide were a function of the complexity of urban life.[24]

Extending Quételet's law, the editors of nineteenth-century psychiatric journals regularly published suicide rates as evidence of the relationship between the city and the rising incidence of suicide. Even though these statistics often were ambiguous or questionable, the underlying assumption of the connection between modernity and suicide was sufficient to ensure that the data would be interpreted as an indictment of urban life.[25] The French asylum (Liancourt) director Jean-Baptiste Cazauvieilh collected rates of suicide for rural France and found that, in many cases, rural suicide rates exceeded those in cities. Lack of 'restraint' combined with ambition (for more land), greed, and alcoholism were, according to Cazauvieilh, the reasons for the high rate of suicide in the countryside.[26] Nevertheless, subsequent studies, including Brierre de Boismont's influential *Du suicide et de la folie suicide* (1856), cited Cazauvieilh's *Du suicide* (1840) as evidence for the urban nature of suicide.[27]

In the United States, Dr Amariah Brigham, the superintendent of the New York State Lunatic Asylum in Utica and editor of the *American Journal of Insanity*, used incomplete and questionable data for his assertions in 1845 that suicide had reached epidemic proportions in American cities.[28] Brigham's conclusions were based on statistics supplied by Dr E.K. Hunt of Hartford, Connecticut. To this data, Hunt had appended the caveat that he was 'far from claiming that an accurate estimate can be made from the data before us, as to the number of suicides committed throughout the country, or in any particular portion of it.' Suicides, he explained, were much more likely to be reported in large cities than in rural areas.[29] Although he faithfully published Dr Hunt's warnings about the defects of suicide statistics, Brigham nevertheless used the data as if their veracity had been established. He was not trying to deceive anyone (he did, after all, publish Hunt's caveat); rather, Brigham and his readers shared a set of beliefs that established the rules for determining which data were valid and which were not.[30] Therefore Brigham's *Journal* continued to rely on similar sources that seemed to confirm a growing disparity between urban and rural suicide.[31]

Statistics demonstrated, according to Dr Petit, the director of the asylum at Rennes (France), that 'the most industrial areas, are also those which count the most suicides.'[32] 'The conclusion to draw from these facts is evident,' wrote Brierre de Boismont. 'The rate of suicide increases progressively with the increase of the population of cities, and decreases progressively with the increase in the population of the countryside; the rise or fall of the rate of suicide in all districts thus corresponds directly to the relative strength of the urban or rural component.'[33] Dr Brierre de Boismont had proved, 'by authentic and exact statistics,' wrote a reviewer in the *American Journal of Insanity*, 'that the number of suicides is in direct proportion with the advance of civilization.'[34] Carrying this conviction to its logical conclusion, American and British asylum superintendents had constructed their asylums in rural locations. Indeed, bound up with the 'moral treatment' was the belief, shared by French, British, and American alienists, that removal of the insane from urban to rural settings provided powerful therapeutic benefits.

Nineteenth-century psychiatry not only lent credibility to popular beliefs about the nexus between modernity and suicide but also provided a 'scientific' vocabulary for others who wished to medicalize the causes of suicide.[35] This medical language and diagnosis also infected the discussion of suicide in the British, French, and American popular press. Thus in August 1859 the *New York Times* attributed 'A New Epidemic' of suicides to the conditions fostered by urban life.[36] Building on these clinical views, the periodical press emphasized the affinity between urban vice and suicide. 'History shows,' explained a writer in *Harper's New Monthly Magazine* (1859), that suicide increases 'among nations sunk in enervating luxuries and vices' as a consequence of the 'extraordinary degeneracy of public and private morals in those countries.'[37] Suicide was 'never less than five times higher [in cities] than in villages,' according to an 1880 article in *Blackwood's Magazine* (Edinburgh and London), because in cities there was 'more misery and more despondency, with less encouragement of restraint.'[38] And repeating sentiments first expressed by Esquirol three-quarters of a century earlier, a writer in the British *Pearson's Magazine* insisted that 'careful study of statistics for the last half century proves that [the increase in] suicide ... can only be attributed to that complex influence we call civilization.'[39] These views were summed up by the British commentator Reginald Skelton, who, writing in the last year of the nineteenth century, asserted that 'the increase and extension of education has contributed in no small degree to the general *malaise*. The enlightened masses have become dissatisfied with their social condition,' and 'it is a marked characteristic of the present epoch that a considerable increase in worldly ambition ... has pervaded every class of society.' This 'social capillarity' Skelton diagnosed as a 'social disease,' of which he 'unhesitatingly affirm[ed] the increase of suicide to be a symptom.'[40]

In the final decades of the nineteenth century, two influential and sophisticated (in terms of methodology) statistical studies of suicide appeared which confirmed the link between modernity and the alleged increasing incidence of suicide: Enrico Morselli's *Il Suicidio* (*Suicide: An Essay on Comparative Moral Statistics*; 1879) and Tomáš Masaryk's *Der Selbstmord als sociale Massenerscheinung der modernen Civilisation* (*Suicide and the Meaning of Civilization*; 1881). For Morselli, professor of psychological medicine at the Royal University of Turin, these statistics demonstrated that 'in the aggregate of the civilized States of Europe and America, the frequency of suicide shows a growing and uniform increase ... since the beginning of the century' that multiplied 'more rapidly than the geometrical augmentation of the population and of general mortality.' These factors convinced Morselli that suicide was the 'fatal disease of civilized peoples.' 'Suicide,' he insisted, was 'an effect of the struggle for existence and of human selection, which works according to the laws of evolution among civilized people.' Urban (modern) societies had more suicides than rural (traditional) ones because in the city the struggle for existence was more intense. Although Morselli admittedly was influenced by the language of Spencer, Darwin, and Wallace, his conclusions reflected the assumptions that had informed the investigations of his psychiatric colleagues throughout the nineteenth century.[41]

Like Morselli, Tomáš Masaryk argued that suicide rates were directly proportional to social complexity. According to the Austrian-trained academic and future liberal democratic founder of Czechoslovakia, 'primitive people showed no suicide tendency at all,' but 'civilized peoples, on the other hand, show a very intensive one.' Masaryk argued that the decline of religious faith, which resulted from the overthrow of the traditional social order, was the fundamental cause of a modern suicide epidemic. Suicide, according to Masaryk, was 'the fruit of progress, of education, of civilization.'[42]

Both Morselli's and Masaryk's views were echoed by the British psychiatrist and barrister S.A.K. Strahan in his *Suicide and Insanity: A Philosophical and Sociological Study* (1893). Like Morselli, Strahan relied on Spencer's sociology for 'scientific' authority: 'Where civilisation is highest the struggle for life is fiercest, and there we meet the greatest number of breakdowns ... It is a sad fact that suicide, all the world over, occurs in inverse ratio to ignorance. To the untutored savage it is almost unknown, and it increases regularly as we rise step by step through the various grades of civilisation.'[43]

This review of nineteenth-century experts' belief that suicide increased with the growth of 'civilization' confirms the assertion of historian Olive Anderson that 'Victorian ideas about the incidence of suicide were illustrated by statistics rather than founded upon them.'[44] In fact, given the seemingly overwhelming 'common sense' that informed the connection between modernity and self-destruction, it is difficult to imagine how Europeans or Americans could have read suicide statistics in any way other than one which reinforced their pre-conceptions.[45] In any case, the connection between modernity and suicide was so firmly established by the end of the nineteenth century that experts would see their task as uncovering precisely *why* rather than *whether* this was so.[46]

The Immunity of Women

Modern urban life was identified as the cause of suicide, and traditional familial values were presented as the best protection against self-destruction.[47] The replication of an ideal 'family' was often the aim of the 'moral treatment' in British, French, and American asylums, even among those who, like Philippe Pinel, advocated removing patients from particular familial situations that they saw as contributing to a disorder.[48] As Brierre de Boismont argued in 1856, the 'treatment that renders the greatest service' to the suicidal is 'family life,' which itself can remove 'the moral suffering in the vast majority' of cases.[49] Reviewing European and American suicide statistics, Albert Rhodes, an American author who lived in Paris and whose articles on 'social issues' appeared regularly in American, French, and British periodicals, concluded in 1876 that 'these figures are eloquent pleaders in favor of family ties as conservators for life.'[50] As one British writer explained in 1883, 'domestic ties, religious training in youth, and a sense of the duties that each of us owes to society, are the best safeguards against the growing evil' of suicide.[51]

It became axiomatic that, if traditional family life protected its members from suicide, those most subsumed in traditional roles – women – ought to demonstrate the greatest resistance to suicide. Not surprisingly, this was exactly what the earliest statistics showed – that approximately three out of every four completed suicides in both Europe and North America were men.[52] 'Although women were more exposed to mental illness than men,' wrote Esquirol in 1821, 'suicide is less frequent among them. Observers from all nations are in agreement on that issue.'[53] Esquirol attributed this outcome to women's 'overexcitement of their sensibilities, their flights of imagination, their exaggerated tenderness, their religious attachments,' all of which 'produce in them illnesses opposed to suicide, in addition to which their mild character and natural timidity distances them' from suicidal thoughts.[54] The reason that suicide was 'less frequent among women,' wrote Falret in 1822, was to be found 'in the weakness of their physical constitution, in the sweetness of their temperament, in their natural timidity, which saves them from these murderous excesses.'[55]

Esquirol's and Falret's explanations for women's resistance to suicide reflected widely held assumptions that were repeated reflexively throughout the century. While 'civilization' was attached to male behaviour, 'mother,' 'wife,' and 'woman' served as representations of a set of socially constructed behaviours attached to females that translated vaguely into an assortment of attributes which included passivity, frailty, modesty, patience, loyalty, acceptance, and self-renunciation. In this scheme 'civilization' and 'women' were opponents if not opposites. Social constructions (gender), as opposed to biological distinctions (sex), became the operative metaphors used to explain the alleged immunity of women to suicide. This circumstance, of course, did not preclude the conflation of gender and sex; rather, it ensured it.

Thus rudimentary and incomplete statistics were proof enough for the editors of the *Annales d'hygiène publique* in 1829 'that women are able to bear the vicissitudes of life better than men.'[56] 'There are more suicides among men than women,' according to Forbes Winslow, writing in 1840, which 'will not surprise those who know the energy, courage, and patience of women under misfortune; men more readily give way to despair, and to the vices consequent upon it.'[57] Women proved more resistant to suicide, wrote Brierre de Boismont in 1856, because suicide required 'a degree of energy, of courage, of despair, which is not in conformity with the weak and delicate constitution of women.' Moreover, women's heightened attachment to 'family affections' and 'religious principles' were, according to Brierre de Boismont, 'obstacles that struggle victoriously against the idea of self-destruction.'[58] Bertrand in 1857 tied the 'difference in frequency of suicide between the two sexes' to the fact that women were more sedentary, followed more regular practices, and were more religious, more resigned to life, and better able to bear the incessant pain of life than men.[59]

Indeed, the same reasoning continued to be presented throughout the century with such regularity, that hardly anyone doubted the assertion, in a widely republished 1881 British article entitled 'Suicidal Mania,' that 'religious restraints' and the possession of 'a larger measure of that hope which springs eternal in the human breast,' accounted for the fact that women 'were less prone to commit suicide ... than men.'[60] From a more secular point of view, a writer in London's *Contemporary Review* (1883) explained 'that three-fourths of the cases [of suicide] are males, which shows that if the female intellect be less powerful than man's, it is at the same time better balanced, or at least more capable of standing against reverses of fortune, and facing the battle of life.'[61]

Even when Darwinian metaphors replaced earlier nostalgic portrayals of family life, the conclusions were familiar. 'It is easy to understand the great male preponderance [of suicide],' wrote Morselli in 1879. 'The difficulties of existence, those at least which proceed from the struggle for life, bear more heavily on man. Woman,' he insisted, 'only shares in these through the affections, and although she has a more impressionable nervous temperment, yet possesses the faculty of resigning herself more easily to circumstances.'[62] 'The comparative immunity of the female sex from self-destruction,' according to Strahan in 1893, 'depends in part upon the relatively less harassing part she takes in the struggle for existence; in part upon the less indulgent and vicious life she leads; and in part upon her lack of courage and natural repugnance to personal violence and disfigurement.'[63]

No matter what the statistics showed, the fact remained that *some* women committed suicide. Commentators explained this phenomenon in two ways. First, they insisted that the motives for male and female suicides were very different. Suicide among women was portrayed as an individual emotional act, and thus inconsequential, while male suicide was seen as a barometer of national economic and social well-being. Second and building on the first assumption, because male suicide was a consequence of the stresses inherent in men's roles and responsibilities (i.e., the price of 'civilization'), female suicide occurred when women *deviated* from their less conflicted (traditional) roles.

The contrast between men's and women's motives reflected what Barbara Welter has described as the 'Cult of True Womanhood,' in which failure by a woman to adhere to the virtues of 'piety, purity, submissiveness, and domesticity ... brought on madness or death.'[64] Although Welter was describing American attitudes, she could have as easily turned to France for confirmation of her argument.[65] Again, Esquirol's explanations were emblematic. 'Women kill themselves more rarely than men,' he wrote in 1821, and when they do, 'more often it is [amorous] passion that impels them to this aberration.'[66] Back in the United States, an anonymous 'Southern Physician' wrote in the *Whig Review* in 1847 that 'in men, real or fancied impotence is very apt to induce self-destruction; – and among women, we cannot help always suspecting the dread of the consequences of secret loss of honor.'[67] Three decades later Rhodes explained that women committed suicide for very different motives from those of men: 'Women appear to be more subject to moral influences, such as disappointed love, betrayal, desertion, jealousy, domestic trouble, and sentimental exaltation of every description.' Men, on the other hand, 'are rather affected by trials of a material order, such as misery, business embarrassments, losses, ungratified ambition.'[68] Morselli found that men's suicides were caused by 'financial embarrassments,' 'weariness of life,' and other 'egoistical motives, whilst among women, after mental diseases, there predominate passions, domestic troubles, shame and remorse.'[69]

Popular nineteenth-century fiction reinforced these characterizations in works such as Nathaniel Hawthorne's *The Blithedale Romance* (1852), Gustave Flaubert's *Madame Bovary* (1857), Leo Tolstoy's *Anna Karenina* (1875), and Edith Wharton's *The House of Mirth* (1905). In all of these an illicit love affair led the despairing woman to suicide. This was, of course, a literary convention, but one that gained credence from its similarity to nineteenth-century French, British, and American newspaper accounts, which invariably connected women's suicide to real and imagined loss of purity.[70]

If women's suicide could not be attributed to dishonour, it invariably was tied to their adopting roles that nature and society had assigned to men. When women left the security of their families, explained Brierre de Boismont in 1856, they substantially increased their risk of suicide.[71] The higher suicide rates of women who 'take an active part in the business of life,' according to an 1883 English essay entitled 'Insanity, Suicide, and Civilization,' 'serve as a caution to prevent them from taking part in politics, or matters best suited for men.'[72] 'It has been observed,' wrote the American Richard N. Reeves in 1897, 'that as woman approaches man in her mode of life she also becomes more familiar with those abnormal conditions which have previously been peculiar to man.' This experience leads to an increase in suicide among women because 'the comparative immunity of women from self-destruction in the past has depended greatly upon the relatively less harassing part she has taken in the struggle for life.' As women moved 'deeper into ... vocations' such as 'art, literature, finance, and even politics,' they 'must expect to suffer the consequences.' 'Already,' Reeves warned, 'it is noticeable that feminine suicide is not entirely due to the sentimental causes of disappointed love, desertion, and jealousy, but to those trials of a more material order such as have led men to the act of self-destruction.'[73]

Joining the chorus of his French and American cousins, Reginald Skelton in 1900 summed up the view that had become commonplace: a woman was 'exempt from many of the factors most favourable to suicide' because 'her affection for home and children is greater, and the religious sentiment has diminished less in woman than in man; her intellectual faculties are usually less developed, and hence also her sensibility to mental pain; inured to continual petty troubles, her patience is fortified to resist greater ones.' However, warned Skelton, in cities 'these factors tending to the exemption of women from suicide largely disappear.'[74]

Durkheim and Women

Nineteenth-century assumptions about women and suicide were codified in Durkheim's *Le suicide* (1897). Although Durkheim was not a physician, his work nevertheless serves as one of the best expressions of nineteenth-century medical thinking about suicide.[75] As Durkheim explained in *Règles de la methode sociologique* (*The Rules of the Sociological Method*; 1895), he hoped that his sociology would transform the statesman into 'the physician [who] ... prevents the outbreak of illnesses by good hygiene, and [who] ... seeks to cure them when they have appeared.'[76]

Along with his medical and moral predecessors, Durkheim assumed that 'mental illnesses go hand in hand with civilization' and that insanity was more common 'in towns than the countryside, and in large rather than small towns.' He connected suicide with modernity. What appeared to be suicide among primitive people, he characterized as not 'an act of despair but of abnegation ... On the contrary, true suicide, the suicide of sadness, is an endemic state among civilized persons.' Its incidence is a function of 'the level of civilization,' with the greatest numbers of suicides occurring among the most developed societies. 'Everywhere,' wrote Durkheim, 'suicide is more prevalent in towns than in the country-side. Civilization is concentrated in large towns, as is suicide.'[77]

Given these views, it was not surprising that Durkheim reached the same conclusions that his predecessors had about the protective influence of the traditional family against suicide. In an 1888 essay entitled 'Suicide et natalité: Étude de statistique morale,' he linked low birth rates in France to increases in the rate of suicide. 'If suicide progresses when the birthrate declines,' he wrote, 'it is that these two phenomena are equally due in part to a decline of domestic sentiments.'[78] 'All facts,' he insisted, 'demonstrate that where the family exists, it protects against suicide and that it has even more of this protective force when it is ... dense enough.' Durkheim claimed that areas with the lowest birth rates experienced the highest rates of suicide. A 'good' birth rate was 'only possible where ... domestic solidarity' was chosen over a life of 'material ease.'[79] Thus, the more children a family produced, the safer its members were from self-destruction: 'the individual becomes part of the solid mass with which he is unified and which multiples his strengths: his power of resistance is thus increased.' But, Durkheim warned, 'where on the contrary families are sparse, poor, or meagre, individuals, less closely joined to one another, allow spaces between them where the cold wind of egoism blows, freezing their hearts and weakening their courage.'[80] Because the health of society depended upon the density of families, women were expected to be mothers of many children. And by extension, women were healthiest and least prone to suicide themselves to the extent that they were subsumed in traditional roles. 'Woman is less concerned than man in the civilizing process,' Durkheim asserted in 1893, 'she participates less in it and draws less benefit from it. She more recalls certain characteristics to be found in primitive natures.'[81] His assertion in Le suicide that 'in all the countries of the world, women commit suicide less than men,' was based, then, not only on the statistical data of his predecessors but also on their gendered assumptions.[82] Thus Durkheim attributed what he called the relative immunity of women to suicide to the fact that they were 'fundamentally traditionalist by nature, they govern their conduct by fixed beliefs and have no great intellectual needs.'[83] Although he insisted that his explanation for the incidence of suicide rested on social factors, throughout his study he also ascribed the low incidence of women's suicide to organic influences.[84] For instance, in explaining the immunity of women to suicide, he concluded that 'being a more instinctive creature than man, woman has only to follow her instincts to find calmness and peace.'[85]

Indeed, whenever it came to issues of gender, Durkheim's sociology was displaced by biologisms.[86] In *De la division du travail social* (*The Division of Labor in Society*; 1893), drawing upon Lamarck's 'law of use and disuse' and Gustave Le Bon's neo-Lamarckian writings, Durkheim argued that as the division of labour increasingly separated men from women in modern societies, it had the effect of enlarging men's brains (and intelligence) while diminishing women's: 'Woman had long withdrawn from warfare and public affairs, and had centered her existence entirely around the family. Since then her role has become even more specialized. Nowadays, among civilized peoples the woman leads an existence entirely different from the man's. It might be said that the two great functions of psychological life had become as if dissociated from each other, one sex having overcome the affective, the other the intellectual function.' These sexual divisions in labour, Durkheim asserted, were 'made perceptible physically by the morphological differences they have brought about.' As a result, 'not only are the size, weight and general shape very dissimilar as between a man and a woman, but ... with the advance of civilization the brain of the two sexes has increasingly developed differently.'[87]

At least when it came to issues of gender, Durkheim's view of suicide was less a novel contribution than a restatement of a widely accepted convention.[88] His conventional views on women's intelligence and social roles may seem somewhat perplexing to those familiar with his sometimes otherwise unconventional views that traditional moral values could no longer effectively regulate modern, industrial society. Unlike many of his more nostalgic contemporaries, Durkheim sought adoption of a moral system more attuned to the social realities of modern life.[89] To a great extent, a similar project underlay and informed much of his *Suicide*. Nevertheless, a number of scholars have found Durkheim's assumptions to be more conservative than his rhetoric.[90] Nowhere does that conservatism display itself more clearly than in his discussion of gender. His conventionality resulted, in part, from his failure to extend the logic of his social critique of morality to the issue of women's suicide. But this was no mere oversight, for Durkheim's entire project rested on assumptions about the (natural) immunity of women to suicide. If he had challenged this notion, the foundation of the rest of his enterprise would have been considerably undermined. What was new, then, in Durkheim's *Suicide* was not his presentation of the aetiological role of social disintegration or the immunity of women to suicide, but a definition and a classificatory system (typology) that allowed him to use the incidence of suicide as a yardstick for social pathology.[91]

Durkheim's definition of suicide as 'death resulting directly or indirectly from a positive or negative act of the victim himself, which he knows will produce this result' was, on the one hand, irrelevant to the statistics he used, while, on the other, it ensured that suicidal behaviour by women could not be considered suicide.[92] It was irrelevant because all of Durkheim's conclusions about the incidence of suicide were drawn from official statistics which defined suicide in ways that were incompatible with his definition. For instance, those who sacrificed their lives for others ('un acte positif') were never listed as suicides in official statistics. And those whose deaths resulted only 'indirectly' from their acts generally did not appear in the statistics either.[93] Indeed, Durkheim must have known that those officials charged with the determination of whether an act was a suicide almost always labelled antisocial (socially disintegrative) acts as suicide, while they almost never called a socially sanctioned (integrative) behaviour (heroism) suicide. The unquestioned assumption that suicide was an antisocial act was, after all, why Durkheim had chosen it as an indicator of social pathology in the first place. Apparently he never considered the possibility that the belief – shared by official statistics collectors and interpreters of suicide – that suicide was antisocial behaviour had, a priori, distorted suicide statistics.

In addition, Durkheim's definition guaranteed that attempted suicide, the most commonly acknowledged women's suicidal behaviour,[94] would be excluded from consideration. For, although he admitted that attempted suicide fitted his definition of suicide *as a behaviour*, he excluded it from his typology because it fell 'short of actual death.'[95] By confining his categories to completed suicides, Durkheim excluded most suicidal behaviour by women from subsequent investigations of suicide.[96] If he had included attempted suicides, women rather than men would have emerged as the group at greatest risk of self-destructive behaviour.[97]

Moreover, data just as good (or just as bad) as those on completed suicides were available had Durkheim's preconceptions not prevented him from considering them. For instance, beginning in 1826 (and until 1961) the French Administration de la justice criminelle, under the direction of the minister of health, published suicide statistics that made no distinction between attempted and successful suicides ('suicides tentés ou effectués'). In the nineteenth century these were published in the *Annales d'hygiène publique*, which recorded the incidence of suicide (including but not separating out attempted suicides) by age and by sex. Although these statistics suffered from the same weaknesses as data on completed suicides, there was no 'objective' reason why they could not have been considered.[98] The decision to exclude attempted suicide from consideration was odd because the entire enterprise of the sociological study of suicide was aimed at describing social behaviour. Certainly, attempting to kill oneself must be considered suicidal behaviour. Yet suicidologists since Durkheim have relied on statistics which, by defining only completed suicide as suicide, have effectively eliminated most suicidal behaviour from their analysis of such behaviour.

The data on attempted suicide could have been used to demonstrate that women were less content with their social roles than men were. Curiously, no suicide study has ever come to that conclusion. Thus, while suicidologists continue to refine their statistical methods, they have rarely questioned the assumption that only completed or successful suicides should constitute the database for suicidal behaviour.[99]

If Durkheim's definition of suicide ensured that women's suicidal behaviour would be trivialized, his typology guaranteed that even those women who completed suicide would be excluded from the suicide equation. That is, in creating a 'scientific' sociology, Durkheim enshrined the unquestioned assumptions about both the effects of modernity and the immunity of women to suicide. Thus his classificatory system contributed to and sustained the under-reporting of women's completed suicides.[100]

Durkheim described four types of suicide – altruistic, egoistic, anomic, and fatalistic. He elaborated only the first three and assigned the fourth, fatalistic, to a footnote. Because he wanted to demonstrate that the rate of suicide provided a way to measure social pathology, his typology was created to uncover the 'regular and specific factor[s] in suicide in our modern societies.' As Durkheim defined them, both anomie and egoism resulted from the collapse of traditional restraints, and thus their incidence could be used as an index for social pathology. The rate of anomic suicide measured alienation, while the rate of egoistic measured the decline of self-restraint. Altruistic suicide, on the other hand, reflected socially sanctioned self-sacrifice. Although the construct of altruistic suicide makes theoretical sense, such acts (heroism) were never reported as suicides.[101] Fatalistic suicide, however, as Durkheim explained in his footnote, 'derives from excessive regulation, that of persons with futures pitilessly blocked and passions violently choked by oppressive discipline.' He declined to look in detail at this type of suicide because he claimed that 'it has so little contemporary importance and examples are so hard to find ... that it seems useless to dwell upon it.'[102] Given the way social statistics were collected, the reported number of anomic and egoistic suicides would always be significantly greater than altruistic and fatalistic suicides. This, of course, served Durkheim's larger project of measuring the breakdown of social integration (which he attributed to anomic and egoistic behaviour).

Like others before him, Durkheim assumed that suicide was exacerbated by social disintegration. Accepting the belief that traditional family life offered the best safeguard against suicidal behaviour, he never questioned the supposition that those most subsumed in the family (women and children) would be most immune to suicide.[103] Given this paradigm, suicide and integrative (women's) behaviour – what Durkheim labelled 'fatalism' – were opposites. Because social integration was alleged to be the cure for suicidal ideation, there was no way for him to suppose that suicide could be a female behaviour. Thus classifying women's suicide as fatalistic guaranteed that they would be defined a priori as immune to suicide.

However, Durkheim's data could be read as evidence that those who were most subsumed in social institutions were at greater risk of suicide than those who were less socially integrated. Even if one were to accept the equivocal data that women completed suicide less frequently than men, the high rate of attempted suicide by women indicates that suicidal behaviour was more common among women than men. Given the social place of most nineteenth-century women, it is fair to assume that submersion in the family provided no special protection for them from suicidal behaviour.[104] Although his evidence was no more 'value-free' than Durkheim's, Steinmetz in 1894 found that women living in the most socially integrated societies had a greater incidence of suicide than men.[105] Kathryn Johnson has suggested that women most submerged in the family display the greatest female suicidal behaviour.[106] Her views have been affirmed by recent reports that the highest rates of suicide in the world are found among rural Chinese women.[107] This phenomenon reinforces the suggestion of historian Roger Lane, who found that, contrary to Durkheim's assumptions, increases in suicide rates were linked to social integration. He discovered that as nineteenth-century Philadelphia urbanized, its suicide rate grew proportionally greater than its homicide rate. Lane reasoned that the increasing incidence of suicide in late-nineteenth-century cities served as a barometer of social integration because suicide, unlike homicide, indicated internalization of social anger.[108] S. Kunitz's study on the effect of overintegration in the family among Navajos in the southwestern United States supports the views of Johnson and Lane. Social relations within extended Navajo families, Kunitz found, often resulted in negative health outcomes, including significantly higher rates of depression and self-destructive behaviours.[109]

The greatest challenge to the belief that social integration provided protection from suicide, however, came from Durkheim's own data. Official statistics consistently reported that the highest rates of suicide were in the military. 'It is a general fact in all European countries,' wrote Durkheim, 'that the suicidal aptitude of soldiers is much higher than that of the civilian population of the same age.'[110] His definition of fatalistic suicide as resulting 'from excessive regulation,' whose 'passions [were] violently choked by oppressive discipline,' seemed to describe nineteenth-century military life perfectly. Durkheim's understanding of official statistics and his own typological definitions could have led him to classify military suicide as fatalistic. Given the reported incidence of military suicide, he could have concluded that fatalism was the most important type of suicide.[111]

Durkheim, however, overcame the obvious inconsistency that military suicide exposed for his typology by arbitrarily classifying it as 'altruistic,' even though the greatest number of reported military suicides could hardly be attributed to self-sacrifice.[112] Given his familiarity with suicide statistics, he must have known that those who sacrificed their lives for their military comrades in battle were never categorized as a suicide in any official statistics. Indeed, to be reported as a suicide, a military death would have to have occurred *outside* a combat situation.

Durkheim was not the only commentator who was forced to perform logical and classificatory gymnastics to account for the extraordinary rate of military suicide. Skelton, whose explanations for the immunity of women to suicide mirrored Durkheim's, tied what he found to be the 'truly appalling' rates of military suicides to 'training' that 'is essentially destructive of individualism.' Laying out a pattern of socialization that could have as easily described women as it did soldiers, Skelton attributed military suicide to the fact that a soldier 'learns to consider himself a mere unit in a huge aggregate of individuals ... The soldier's very trade consists in placing at the disposal of others that of all possessions most valued by man – his life. Is it, then, surprising that he should have less hesitation than other men in removing it?'[113]

Given their assumptions about the 'nature of women' and the prophylactic impact of family life, neither Skelton nor Durkheim could acknowledge the parallels that they had drawn between soldiers' and women's social situations. The point, of course, is *not* that women's and soldiers' socialization was the same. Rather, Durkheim's description and discussions of military suicide fit into his category of fatalism more clearly than it fit into altruism. The reason that he could not acknowledge this discrepancy was that he was tied to a set of rules which assumed that high rates of suicide were attached to the anomy and egoism brought on by modern urban life. If military suicide were categorized as fatalistic, Durkheim would have had to question his basic assumptions. This he could not do because it seemed self-evident to him that low rates of suicide were associated with social integration. Since fatalism was attached to social integration, women's low rates of suicide could be categorized as fatalistic – so infrequent a cause as to be hardly worthy of notice. Because the high rate of military suicide (at least Durkheim and most others *believed* it to be high)[114] could not be attributed to modernity, it was placed in a special category, altruism, which effectively eliminated it from consideration.[115] Altruism became the baseline of suicide that all societies could condone – sacrifice for others.

This is not to suggest that Durkheim (or for that matter, Morselli, Masaryk, or Skelton) consciously set out to distort evidence. Rather, he was bound to a set of assumptions that framed his conclusions before he began his research. Given these assumptions, it would have been surprising if Durkheim had reached different conclusions. Thus his typology sanctioned the anti-modernity and nostalgia that had 'discovered' the suicide 'problem' in the first place. His sociology provided (and continues to provide) 'scientific' justification for traditional assumptions about women's behaviour.[116] Had it been otherwise, Durkheim's *Suicide* might never have achieved the overwhelming influence that it has.

Conclusion

No conspiracy existed to exclude women's suicides from consideration. Rather, we must return to the rules that shaped Western considerations of suicide in the first place. That is, the fear of modernity was based upon a set of nostalgic beliefs that identified the growth of urban society as a challenge to traditional (patriarchal) authority. In this context, the motivation for the collection and analysis of suicide rates was to illustrate that modernity caused self-destructive behaviour. Given these preconceptions, it was assumed that women were insulated from suicide to the extent that they were subsumed within the bounds of traditional family life. In other words, given the set of rules for defining and classifying suicide, there was no way in which it could have been seen as a female behaviour. By refusing to re-examine these assumptions about women's roles and behaviour, Durkheimian sociology was doomed to endorse the underlying values that Durkheim had hoped to challenge. As a result, neither he nor his followers could construct a classificatory system or adopt a methodology that would expose traditional life to the same scrutiny as they had insisted upon when it came to modernity. This conclusion serves to reenforce Joan Scott's wider caveat that statistics 'are neither totally neutral collections of fact nor simply ideological impositions. Rather they are ways of establishing the authority of certain visions of social order, or organizing perceptions of "experience."'[117]

NOTES

This chapter was revised and updated by the author from his article 'Suicide, Gender, and the Fear of Modernity in Nineteenth-Century Medical and Social Thought,' which was published in the *Journal of Social History*, 26 (Spring 1993), 461–90. The author thanks Elizabeth Colwill, Lisa Lieberman, Carol R. Kushner, Fred Matthews, and David L. Ransel for their critical comments. All translations from French are the author's, unless otherwise noted.

1 Jean-Étienne Esquirol, 'De la lypémanie ou mélancolie,' reprinted in *Des maladies mentales*, 2 vols. (Paris: J.-B. Baillière, 1838), 1:400–1. By mid-century this view had become commonplace. For instance, the American alienist Edward Jarvis attributed insanity to 'the price we pay for civilization. The causes of the one increase with the developments and results of the other.' See Jarvis, 'On the Supposed Increase of Insanity,' *American Journal of Insanity*, 8 (April 1852), 333–64, esp. 364.

2 For more, see Theodore M. Porter, *The Rise of Statistical Thinking, 1820–1900* (Princeton: Princeton University Press, 1986), 18–70, esp.

28–31, 36–9. Statistics were collected in ways that reinforced assumptions that rural life produced healthy and hardy people. See Marie-Noëlle Bourguet, *Déchiffrer la France: La statistique départementale à l'époque napoléonienne* (Paris: Éditions des Archives contemporaines, 1989), esp. 218–24, 274–9.

3   'Suicide,' writes Barbara T. Gates, 'took on the status of trope quite readily.' It 'became an indicator of social illness, a measure of what was wrong with late Victorian Britain and her institutions.' See Gates, *Victorian Suicide: Mad Crimes and Sad Histories* (Princeton: Princeton University Press, 1988), 155. See also Ian Hacking, The Taming of Chance (Cambridge: Cambridge University Press, 1990), 64–72.

4   Émile Durkheim, *Suicide: A Study in Sociology* (1897), translated by John A. Spaulding and George Simpson (Glencoe, Ill.: The Free Press, 1951), 166. Also see Christian Baudelot and Roger Establet, *Durkheim et le suicide* (Paris: Presses universitaires de France, 1984), 9, and Howard I. Kushner and Claire E. Sterk. 'The Limits of Social Capital: Durkheim, Suicide, and Social Cohesion,' *American Journal of Public Health*, 95 (July 2005), 1139–43.

5   For instance, in their critical reexamination and reformulation of Durkheim's *Suicide* (1897), Baudelot and Establet concluded that the deeper an individual was subsumed in the family, the greater her/his protection from suicide. See Baudelot and Establet, *Durkheim et le suicide*, 99–104, esp. 101. For more on how this view continues to inform experts' thinking about suicide, see Howard I. Kushner, *Self-Destruction in the Promised Land: A Psychocultural Biology of American Suicide* (New Brunswick: Rutgers University Press, 1989; republished as *American Suicide: A Psychocultural Exploration* [Rutgers, 1991]), 100–1.

6   I draw on Joan W. Scott's notion that gender is the grammatical way of describing the properties associated with the distinctions of sex. See Scott, 'Gender: A Useful Category of Historical Analysis,' *American Historical Review*, 91 (December 1986), 1053–75, esp. 1067, 1070. See also Joan Wallach Scott, *Gender and the Politics of History* (New York: Columbia University Press, 1988), esp. 2–8; and Linda Alcoff, 'Cultural Feminism versus Post-Structuralism: The Identity Crisis in Feminist Theory,' *Signs: Journal of Women in Culture and Society*, 13 (1988), 404–36.

7   William Denny, *Pelecanicidium; or, The Christian Adviser against Self-Murder* (London, 1653), book I: 1.

8   François-Marie Arouet de Voltaire, 'De caton et du suicide,' *Dictionnaire philosophique*, vol. 2, in *Les oeuvres complètes de Voltaire* (Paris: Société Littéraire-typographique, 1774), 38: 394.

9 Jean Dumas, *Traité du suicide, ou du meurte volontaire de soi-même* (Amsterdam: D.J. Changuion, 1773), 2.

10 Louis Sébastien Mercier, *Tableau de Paris*, nouv. éd. (Amsterdam, 1783), 3: 188.

11 Elizabeth Colwill, 'Transforming "Women's Empire": Representations of Women in French Political Culture, 1770–1807' (Ph.D dissertation, State University of New York at Binghamton, 1991).

12 Judith DeGroat, 'The Work and Lives of Women in Parisian Manufacturing Trades, 1830– 1848' (Ph.D. dissertation, University of Rochester, 1991). Also see Christine Stansell, *City of Women: Sex and Class in New York, 1789–1860* (New York: Knopf, 1986).

13 J.L. Reichardt, *Un hiver à Paris, 1802–1803: Sous le Consulat* (Paris: E. Plon, Nourrit, 1896), 438–9.

14 Samuel Miller, *The Guilt, Folly, and Sources of Suicide: Two Discourses* (New York, 1805), 13, 54–7. Also see Joseph Lathrop, *Two Sermons on the Atrocity of Suicide, and the Causes Which Lead to It* (Springfield, Mass., 1805), 17–36.

15 For a discussion of the origins and development of the moral treatment in France, see Jan Goldstein, *Console and Classify: The French Psychiatric Profession in the Nineteenth Century* (New York: Cambridge University Press, 1987), 65–6, 80–119. For Britain, see Andrew Scull, *Museums of Madness: The Social Organization of Insanity in Nineteenth-Century England* (New York: St. Martin's Press, 1979), and Scull, 'Moral Treatment Reconsidered: Some Sociological Comments on an Episode in the History of British Psychiatry,' *Madhouses, Mad-Doctors, and Madmen: The Social History of Psychiatry in the Victorian Era*, ed. Scull (Philadelphia: University of Pennsylvania Press, 1981) 107–18. For the United States, see Constance M. McGovern, *Masters of Madness: Social Origins of the American Psychiatric Profession* (Hanover, NH: University Press of New England, 1985), 62–85; Charles E. Rosenberg, 'The Therapeutic Revolution: Medicine, Meaning, and Social Change in Nineteenth-Century America,' in *The Therapeutic Revolution: Essays in the Social History of Medicine*, ed. Morris J. Vogel and Charles E. Rosenberg (Philadelphia, 1979), 5–6; and Kushner, *Self-Destruction in the Promised Land*, 37–51.

16 Jean-Pierre Falret, *De l'hypochondrie et du suicide* (Paris: Croullebois, 1822), 76–7, 93–4, 104–11.

17 M. Brouc, 'Considérations sur les suicides de notre époque,' *Annales d'hygiène publique et de médecine légale*, 16 (1836), 252, 261.

18 Louis Bertrand, *Traité du suicide: considéré dans ses rapports avec la philosophie, la théologie, la médecine, et la jurisprudence* (Paris: J.B. Baillière, 1857), 93.

19   Forbes Winslow, *The Anatomy of Suicide* (London: H. Renshaw, 1840; reprint, Boston: Longwood Press, 1978), 338.

20   Jean-Étienne Esquirol, 'Du suicide' (1821), reprinted and revised in *Des maladies mentales*, 1: 588–90.

21   For instance, the *American Journal of Insanity* printed both reviews and extensive excerpts of European works on suicide. See reviews of Gustave-François Étoc-Demazy, *Recherches statistiques sur le suicide, appliques à l'hygiene publique et à la médecine legale* (Paris: Germer-Bailliere, 1844), reviewed in 1 (April 1845), 383; Alexandre Brierre de Boismont, *Du suicide et de la folie suicide*, reviewed in 12 (April 1856), 351–3; and Louis Bertrand, *Traité du suicide*, reviewed in 14 (October 1857), 207–14. Reprints included the work of British epidemiologist John Netten Radcliffe, 'The Aesthetics of Suicide,' ibid. 16 (April 1860): 385–409, originally published in *Journal of Psychological Medicine*, 12 (October 1859), 582–602. On the French side, Brierre de Boismont drew on Brigham's American statistics for evidence of the role of urban forces in the increase of suicides. See Brierre de Boismont, 'De l'influence de la civilisation sur la suicide,' *Annales d'hygiène*, 2nd series, 2 (1855): 164–5; and *Du suicide et de la folie suicide, considérés dans leurs rapports avec la statistique, la médecine, et la philosophie* (Paris: J.-B. Baillière, 1856), 370–1.

22   Brière de Boismont, 'De l'influence de la civilisation sur la suicide,' 179–80; for citation of Brigham, see 164–5. Brierre de Boismont republished this essay in *Du suicide et de la folie suicide*, in chapter 5: 'De l'influence de la civilisation sur le développement du suicide,' 352–89; text quoted, 386–7; Brigham, 370–1.

23   'On Suicide,' *Journal of Psychological Medicine*, 11 (1858), 419–20.

24   Adolphe Quételet, *Du système social et des lois qui le régissent* (Paris: Guillaumin, 1848), 88–9.

25   For a parallel example of how preconceived values framed statistical investigations, see Joan Wallach Scott, 'A Statistical Representation of Work, *La statistique de l'industrie à Paris*,' in Scott, *Gender and the Politics of History*, 113–38.

26   Jean-Baptiste Cazauvieilh, *Du suicide, de l'alienation mentale et des crimes contre les personnes, compares dans leur rapports reciproques* (Paris: J.-B. Baillière, 1840), 2–3, 250. Also see Brierre de Boismont, *Du suicide et la folie suicide*, 359.

27   Brierre de Boismont's claimed that Cazauvieilh had demonstrated that increases in rural suicides resulted from the influence of urban culture on rural life. See Brierre de Boismont, *Du suicide et de la folie suicide*, 359.

Morselli, on the other hand, faithfully reproduced Cazauvieilh's conclusions but disputed his findings. See Henry (Enrico) Morselli, *Suicide: An Essay on Comparative Moral Statistics* (New York: D. Appleton and Co., 1882), 174. See also Anthony Giddens, 'The Suicide Problem in French Sociology,' *British Journal of Sociology*, 16 (March 1965), 4n10.

28 Brigham asserted that 'as many [suicides] have been committed some years in the city of New York alone, as are assigned to the whole State.' See 'Statistics of Suicides in the United States,' *American Journal of Insanity*, 1 (January 1845), 232–4.

29 E.K. Hunt, 'Statistics of Suicides in the United States,' *American Journal of Insanity*, 1 (January 1845), 231–2.

30 Not much has changed in regard to suicide statistics since Brigham's time. Most contemporary studies begin with a caveat about the unreliability of suicide statistics and then ignore their own warnings. For example, O'Carroll admits that 'there is an enormous body of literature that questions the validity and reliability, and thus the usefulness of suicide mortality statistics.' Nevertheless, he insists that 'there are, of course, a number of compelling reasons to use suicide mortality data' (1). See Patrick W. O'Carroll, 'A Consideration of the Validity and Reliability of Suicide Mortality Data,' *Suicide & Life-Threatening Behavior*, 19, no. 1 (Spring 1989), 1–16. 'Although there are persistent doubts about the validity of suicide data,' write Stafford and Weisheit, they conclude that 'there is no practical alternative to using them.' See Mark C. Stafford and Ralph A. Weisheit, 'Changing Age Patterns of U.S. Male and Female Suicide Rates, 1934–1983,' *Suicide & Life-Threatening Behavior*, 18, no. 3 (Summer 1988), 149–63.

31 Discovering that 'the occurrence of suicide has been more than four times as frequent in the city of New York, as in all other parts of the State,' Brigham suggested a mathematical formula for the calculation of urban suicide: '*in great cities* when compared with the country, all human passions are exercised with more than fourfold constancy and intensity, and that reverse of fortune and disappointments of desire are more frequent by fourfold, and are accompanied by a shock of the intellect or affections, more than four times as severe, and by more than four times the liability to that temporary or continued overthrow of reason, which induces self-destruction.' See Brigham, 'Statistics of Suicides,' *American Journal of Insanity*, 4 (January 1848), 247–9 (italics in original).

32 Petit, 'Recherches statistiques de l'étiologie du suicide: Tableaux synoptiques' (Thèse., Paris, 1850), in Brierre de Boismont, *Du suicide et de la folie suicide*, 84. Similar views are found in Gustave-François Étoc-Demazy,

Recherches statistiques sur le suicide, appliques à l'hygiene publique et à la médecine legale (Paris: Germer-Bailliere, 1844).

33 Brierre de Boismont, *Du suicide et de la folie suicide*, 358. Brierre de Boismont cited both Brigham's and Petit's studies in *Du suicide et de la folie suicide* (84, 370–1) and in his essay 'De l'influence de la civilisation sur la suicide,' 151–2, 164–5. For more on Brierre de Boismont, see Ian Dowbiggin, 'French Psychiatry and the Search for a Professional Identity: The Société Médico-Psychologique, 1840–1870,' *Bulletin of the History of Medicine*, 63 (Fall 1989), 348.

34 H.T. 'Suicide and Suicidal Insanity,' *American Journal of Insanity*, 12 (April 1856), 352.

35 See Marc Saint-Marc Girardin, *Cours de littérature dramatique, ou de l'usage des passions dans le drame*, 5 vols. (Paris: Charpentier, 1843), 1: 90.

36 In the rural United States, the *Times* explained, men and women were so wrapped up in their daily chores that they had no 'time for any mischievous thoughts of ropes, razors and morphine.' Transfer these same people to cities, warned the editorial, and a combination of rising aspirations, leisure time, and temptations to vice would form 'the train of causes that lead to self-destruction.' See 'A Chapter of Suicides,' *New York Times*, 3 August 1859, 8: 2; 'The Alarming Increase of Suicides,' ibid., 4: 4.

37 C. Nordoff, 'A Matter of Life and Death,' *Harper's New Monthly Magazine*, 18 (March 1859), 516–20, esp. 516, 519.

38 'The preponderance of suicides' in cities, this author asserted, 'is not exclusively a product of the greater suffering they contain in comparison with the country, but also, and quite as much, of the lesser disposition to support that suffering.' See 'Suicide,' *Littel's Living Age*, 146 (10 July 1880), 71–2, reprinted from Frederick Marshall, 'Suicide,' *Blackwood's Magazine*, June 1880, 719–35.

39 J. Brand, 'Is Suicide a Sign of Civilization?' *Pearson's Magazine* 2 (July–December 1896): 666–7.

40 Reginald A. Skelton, 'Statistics of Suicide,' *The Nineteenth Century*, 48 (September 1900), 466–7. Also see Gates, *Victorian Suicide: Mad Crimes and Sad Histories*, 152–7.

41 'The whole cure is ... preventive, and is contained,' wrote Morselli, 'in this one precept: To develop in man the power of well-ordering sentiments and ideas by which to reach a certain aim in life; in short, to give force and energy to the moral character.' Like his predecessors, Morselli found that 'the proportion of suicides in all Europe is greater amongst the condensed population of urban centres than amongst the more scattered inhabitants of the country.' See Morselli, *Suicide: An Essay on Com-*

parative Moral Statistics, 29, 13, 169, 354, 373–4 (italics in original).
Morselli's book was quickly translated into English and found a wide
readership in both Britain and the United States. The first British edition
was published by Kegan Paul in 1881. For a discussion of Morselli's
influence on British thinking about suicide, see Barbara T. Gates, 'Suicide
and the Victorian Physicians,' *Journal of the History of the Behavioral Sciences*, 16 (1980), 169–70, and Gates, *Victorian Suicide*, 18–19.

42 Tomáš G. Masaryk, *Suicide and the Meaning of Civilization* (*Der Selbstmord
als sociale Massenerscheinung der modernen Civilisation*, 1881), translated by
William B. Weist and Robert G. Batson (Chicago: University of Chicago
Press, 1970), 140–70, 3–4, 112.

43 S.A.K. Strahan, *Suicide and Insanity: A Philosophical and Sociological Study*
(London: Swan Sonnenschein & Co., 1893), 174.

44 Olive Anderson, 'Did Suicide Increase with Industrialization in Victorian
England?' *Past & Present*, 86 (February 1980), 167.

45 A good example of this is found in the careful statistical studies of the
English epidemiologist John Netten Radcliffe, who cited studies which
demonstrated that 'the most probable cause of great differences observed
in the annual average of the mortality from suicide in the different countries, is the greater or less degree of imperfection of their statistics.' Radcliffe nevertheless ignored the implications of this observation when
reaching his conclusions about the distribution of suicide. See Radcliffe,
'The Method and Statistics of Suicide,' *Journal of Psychological Medicine*, 12
(1859), 209–23, esp. 218–19.

46 Shared assumptions about the connections between modernity and
suicide made it extremely difficult for medical and social experts to
understand suicide in any way other than they did. Not until 1980 did a
serious challenge to the urban/rural contrast emerge in Olive Anderson's
analysis of suicide in nineteenth-century England and Wales. Anderson
found that young men and women living in rural towns and villages
were more likely to kill themselves than their cohorts in industrial cities.
This finding, she argued, 'casts doubt both on the traditional sociological
theory that the spread of modern industrial society was accompanied by
high general levels of anomie and egoism, and upon the rather newer
school of sociology which associates it [suicide] with local social disor-
ganization and ecological problems.' See Anderson, 'Did Suicide Increase
with Industrialization in Victorian England?' 149–73, esp. 165–6. Also see
Anderson, *Suicide in Victorian and Edwardian England* (Oxford: Oxford
University Press, 1987), 54, 83–91, 101–3. For a nuanced view of the connection between urban life and suicide based on an examination of life

cycles, see Victor Bailey, *This Rash Act: Suicide across the Life Cycle in the Victorian City* (Stanford: Stanford University Press, 1998), esp. 253–66.

47 Looking at the assumptions of nineteenth-century French statistical investigations of work Joan W. Scott found that the family was portrayed as 'the natural environment that fostered those qualities of individual discipline and orderliness necessary for the health and prosperity of society.' See Scott, 'A Statistical Representation of Work,' 115, 129.

48 For more on this, see Robert Castel, *The Regulation of Madness: The Origins of Incarceration in France*, translated by W.D. Halls (Berkeley and Los Angeles: University of California Press, 1988), 201–5.

49 Brierre de Boismont, *Du suicide et de la folie suicide*, 633.

50 Albert Rhodes, 'Suicide,' *The Galaxy*, 21 (February 1876), 195.

51 M.G. Mulhall, 'Insanity, Suicide, and Civilization,' *The Contemporary Review*, 63 (January–June 1883), 908.

52 Falret, *De l'hypochondrie et du suicide*, 17–18; Adolphe Quételet, *Sur l'homme et le développement de ses facultés*, 2 vols. (Paris: Bachelier, 1835); Quételet, *Du système social et des lois qui le régissent* (Paris: Guillaumin et Cie, 1848); A.-M. Guerry, *Essai sur la statistique morale de la France* (Paris, 1833); Winslow, *The Anatomy of Suicide*, 276; Étoc-Demazy, *Recherches statistiques sur le suicide*, 212; E.K. Hunt, 'Statistics of Suicide in the U. S. [for 1843],' 225, 229–32; George P. Cook, 'Statistics of Suicide, Which Have Occurred in the State of New York from Dec. 1st 1847 to Dec. 1, 1848,' *American Journal of Insanity*, 5 (April 1849), 308–9.

53 Esquirol, 'Du suicide' (1821); republished in *Des maladies mentales*, 1: 584.

54 Ibid., 1: 584–5.

55 Falret, *De l'hypochondrie et du suicide*, 17–18.

56 Quoted in Louis Chevalier, *Labouring Classes and Dangerous Classes in Paris During the First Half of the Nineteenth Century*, translated by Frank Jellinek (London: Routledge & Kegan Paul, 1973), 285.

57 Winslow, *The Anatomy of Suicide*, 276.

58 Brierre de Boismont, *Du suicide et de la folie suicide*, 63, 65–6.

59 Bertrand, *Traité du suicide*, 75. Almost exactly the same words could be found in the popular press; see 'Suicides in New York City in 1860,' *New York Times*, 17 January 1861, 2: 1.

60 William Knighton, 'Suicidal Mania,' *Littel's Living Age*, 148 (5 February 1881), 376.

61 Mulhall, 'Insanity, Suicide, and Civilization,' 907. That women should have been viewed as less suicidal than men is particularly puzzling, given the long-held connection between suicide and insanity. See Elaine Showalter, 'Victorian Women and Insanity,' in *Madhouse, Mad-Doctors, and*

Madmen, ed. Scull, 313–31; esp. 315–16. See also Showalter, *The Female Malady: Women, Madness, and English Culture, 1830–1980* (New York: Random House, 1985), esp. 51–73.

62 Morselli, *Suicide*, 195, 197.

63 Strahan, *Suicide and Insanity*, 178. As I have demonstrated elsewhere, even within the set of rules used by statistics gatherers, both nineteenth- and twentieth-century official suicide statistics can be characterized as having under-reported the number of completed suicides by women. See Howard I. Kushner, 'Suicide, Gender and the Fear of Modernity in Nine- teenth-Century Medical and Social Thought,' *Journal of Social History*, 26 (Spring 1993), 461–90. Although official statistics continue to report that men are three to four times more likely to commit suicide than women, as Jack D. Douglas demonstrated, these statistics are fatally flawed. See Douglas, *The Social Meanings of Suicide* (Princeton: Princeton University Press, 1967), 163–231, esp. 215.

64 Barbara Welter, 'The Cult of True Womanhood: 1820–1860,' *American Quarterly*, 18 (Summer 1966), 151–5. Gates (*Victorian Suicide: Mad Crimes and Sad Histories*, 125) argues, somewhat inexplicably, that 'despite all evi- dence to the contrary, most Victorians ... wanted and expected suicide, like madness, to be a "female malady."' Her sources for this conclusion are Showalter (*The Female Malady*) and an 1857 essay by George Henry Lewes ('Suicide in Life and Literature,' *Westminster Review*, July 1857, 52–78). But contrary to Gates's assertion, neither supports her claim. Although Showalter (see note 61) does discuss the predominance of women among mental patients, she does not discuss the incidence of suicide among women. Lewes (71), on the other hand, not only pointed out that women had a lower incidence of suicide than men, but also, like his contemporaries, he attached this 'fact' to women's 'greater timidity' and to 'their greater power of passive endurance, both of bodily and mental pain.'

65 For a discussion of suicide as a literary convention in nineteenth-century France, see Lisa J. Lieberman, 'Romanticism and the Culture of Suicide in Nineteenth-Century France,' *Comparative Studies in Society and History*, 33 (July 1991), 73–85, and Lieberman, *Leaving You: The Cultural Meanings of Suicide* (Chicago: Ivan Dee: 2003), esp. 70–7.

66 Esquirol, 'Du suicide,' 585.

67 'A Southern Physician,' 'Suicide,' *American Whig Review*, 6 (August 1847), 142. This essay was widely circulated and reprinted in several journals, including the *Democratic Review* in 1854 and *Harper's New Monthly Maga- zine* in 1859. See the *Democratic Review*, 34 (November 1854), 405–17; C.

Nordhoff, 'A Matter of Life and Death,' *Harper's New Monthly Magazine*, 18 (March 1859), 516–20.

68 Rhodes, 'Suicide,' 192, 194.

69 Morselli, *Suicide*, 305.

70 Gates, *Victorian Suicide*, 125–50; Silvia S. Canetto, 'She Died for Love and He for Glory: Gender Myths and Suicidal Behavior.' *Omega*, 26. (1992–93), 1–17. Also see Margaret Higonnet, 'Suicide: Representations of the Feminine in the Nineteenth Century,' *Poetics Today*, 6: 1–2 (1985), 103–18, esp. 113–18.

71 Brierre de Boismont, *Du suicide et de la folie suicide*, 66.

72 Mulhall, 'Insanity, Suicide, and Civilization,' 908.

73 Robert N. Reeves, 'Suicide and the Environment,' *Popular Science Monthly*, 51 (June 1897), 189–90.

74 Reginald A. Skelton, 'Statistics of Suicide,' *Nineteenth Century*, 48 (September 1900), 471.

75 Dominick LaCapra, *Émile Durkheim: Sociologist and Philosopher* (Ithaca: Cornell University Press, 1972), 7; Robert A. Nye, 'Heredity, Pathology, and Psychoneurosis in Durkheim's Early Work,' *Knowledge and Society: Studies in the Sociology of Culture Past and Present*, 4 (1982), 103–42, esp. 130–2. Also see Kushner, *Self-Destruction in the Promised Land*, 58–9.

76 Émile Durkheim, *The Rules of the Sociological Method*, 8th ed. (1895), translated by Sarah A. Solovay and John H. Mueller (New York: The Free Press, 1938), 75.

77 Émile Durkheim, *The Division of Labor in Society* (1893), translated by W.D. Halls, with an introduction by Lewis Coser (London: Macmillan, 1984), 215, 191–2. This is a more up-to-date and better translation than the standard Simpson 1933 American translation. I have, however, changed the spelling to correspond more closely with North American usage. See also Émile Durkheim, *De la division du travail social*, 7th ed. (Paris: Presses Universitaires de France), 1960. For more on Durkheim's connection of suicide with the 'intensity' of modern urban civilization, see Nye, 'Heredity, Pathology, and Psychoneurosis in Durkheim's Early Work,' 132–3, and Bailey, *This Rash Act*, 15–33.

78 Émile Durkheim, 'Suicide et natalité: Étude de statistique morale,' *Revue philosophique de la France et de l'étranger*, 26 (1888), 446–63, quotation from 462.

79 Ibid., 462.

80 Ibid., 663.

81 Durkheim, *The Division of Labor in Society* (Halls translation), 192.

82 G.E. Berrios and M. Mohanna argue that Durkheim drew selectively from the writings of nineteenth-century psychiatrists, exaggerating alienists' linking of suicide with psychopathology. Nevertheless, there was a congruence of Durkheim and nineteenth-century psychiatrists on the characterization of the aetiology of women's suicide. See Berrios and Mohanna, 'Durkheim and French Psychiatric Views on Suicide during the 19th Century: A Conceptual History,' *British Journal of Psychiatry*, 156 (1990), 1–9.

83 Durkheim, *Suicide*, 385, 166.

84 For a discussion of this contradiction in Durkheim's *Suicide*, see Philippe Besnard, 'Durkheim et les femmes, ou le suicide inachevé,' *Revue française de sociologie*, 14, no. 1 (1973), 27–61, esp. 29–33.

85 Durkheim, *Suicide*, 272.

86 For a discussion of Durkheim's debt to the degeneration model, see Nye, 'Heredity, Pathology and Psychoneurosis in Durkheim's Early Work,' and Robert A. Nye, *Crime, Madness, & Politics in Modern France: The Medical Concept of National Decline* (Princeton: Princeton University Press, 1984), 144–154. Also see Ian Dowbiggin, 'Degeneration and Hereditarianism in French Mental Science 1840–90: Psychiatric Theory as Ideological Adaption,' in *The Anatomy of Madness: Essays in the History of Psychiatry*, vol. 1, ed. W.F. Bynum, Roy Porter, and Michael Shepherd (London and New York: Tavistock Publications, 1985), 188–232. For a comprehensive discussion of degeneration, see Daniel Pick, *Faces of Degeneration: A European Disorder, c. 1848–c. 1918* (Cambridge: Cambridge University Press, 1989), esp. 7–17.

87 Durkheim, *The Division of Labor in Society* (Halls translation), 20–1. Also see Stephen Jay Gould, 'Measuring Heads: Paul Broca the Heyday of Craniology,' in *The Mismeasure of Man* (New York: W.W. Norton, 1981), 73–112.

88 Silvia Sara Canetto, 'Gender and Suicidal Behavior: Theories and Evidence,' in *Review of Sociology, 1997*, ed. Ronald W. Maris, Morton M. Silverman, and Silvia Sarah Canetto (New York: The Gilford Press, 1997), 138–67.

89 Durkheim, *The Division of Labor in Society* (Halls translation), 329–41.

90 For a discussion of this see LaCapra, *Emile Durkheim: Sociologist and Philosopher*, 1–26.

91 Ibid., 144.

92 Durkheim, *Suicide*, 44 (italics in original). See Durkheim, *Le suicide. Étude de sociologie*, nouv. éd., 10e tirage (Paris: Presses Universitaires de France, 1986), 5.

93   For a discussion of the failure of official statistics to report those (particularly women) who die indirectly from their suicidal acts, see Howard I. Kushner, 'Women and Suicidal Behavior: Epidemiology, Gender, and Lethality in Historical Perspective,' in *Women and Suicidal Behaviour*, ed. Silvia Sara Canetto and David Lester (New York: Springer Publishing Co., 1995), 11–34, and Kushner, *Self-Destruction in the Promised Land*, 103–4.

94   Silvia S. Canetto, 'Epidemiology of Women's Suicidal Behavior,' in *Women and Suicidal Behavior*, ed. Silvia S, Canetto and David Lester (New York: Springer Publishing Co., 1995), 35–57.

95   Durkheim, *Suicide*, 44.

96   For a discussion of gender and attempted suicide, see Silvia S. Canetto and David Lester, 'Gender, Culture, and Suicidal Behavior,' *Transcultural Psychiatry*, 35 (June 1998), 163–90.

97   Estimates since the early nineteenth century have indicated that for every completed suicide there have been six to eight attempts. These same statistics have concluded that women attempt suicide at a rate approximately 2.3 times greater than men. See Edwin S. Shneidman and Norman L. Farberow, 'Statistical Comparisons between Attempted and Committed Suicides,' in *The Cry for Help*, ed. Farberow and Shneidman (New York: McGraw-Hill, 1961), 24–37; Ronald Maris, *Pathways to Suicide: A Survey of Self-Destructive Behavior* (Baltimore: Johns Hopkins University Press, 1981), 243, 268; Louis Israel Dublin, *Suicide: A Sociological and Statistical Study* (New York: Ronald Press, 1963), 3; Herbert Hendin, in *Suicide in America* (New York: Norton, 1982), 49, sees the ratio as 10:1.

98   See Baudelot and Establet, *Durkheim et le suicide*, 66–7; Chevalier, *Labouring Classes and Dangerous Classes*, 470–3.

99   Although suicidologists have offered various *ex post facto* explanations justifying the exclusion of attempted suicides from measures of suicidal behaviour, none of these can be sustained on close examination. This decision has no logical basis other than one of convenience – that is, completed suicides are readily available to researchers as part of national vital statistics on death rates. It seems bizarre that suicide attempts should have been excluded from all considerations of the incidence of suicide just at the moment when sophisticated statistical methodologies were developed that could have been used to include attempted suicide – that is, unless, of course, the reason for excluding attempted suicide from the equation rested ultimately upon a set of beliefs that only could conceive of suicide as a male behaviour.

100 Although twentieth-century psychiatrists tended to emphasize intra-
psychic conflict at the expense of social causes, they nevertheless continued to view women's suicide in the framework laid out by Durkheim.
See Kushner, *Self-Destruction in the Promised Land*, 100–2.

101 Durkheim, *Suicide*, 241–58, esp. 246, 252, 258.

102 Ibid., 276. Most subsequent studies, even those that claim to re-evaluate
Durkheim's *Suicide*, have ignored fatalistic suicide.

103 Durkheim, 'Suicide et natalité,' 450.

104 For more on this point, see Kushner, *Self-Destruction in the Promised Land*,
109–11.

105 S.R. Steinmetz, 'Suicide among Primitive Peoples,' *American Anthropologist*, 7 (January 1894), 55–60.

106 Kathryn K. Johnson, 'Durkheim Revisted: Why Do Women Kill Themselves?' *Suicide and Life-Threatening Behavior*, 11 (Summer 1981), 143–5.

107 E. Rosenthal 'Suicides Reveal Bitter Roots of China's Rural Life,' *New
York Times*, 24 January 1999, 1: 1; A. Bezlova, 'Women Suicides Reflect
Drudgery of Rural Life,' *IPS*, 21 September 1998; URL:
http://www.hartford-hwp.com/archives/55/353.html; accessed on 1
November 2006.

108 Roger Lane, *Violent Death in the City: Suicide, Accident, and Murder in
Nineteenth Century Philadelphia* (Cambridge: Harvard University Press,
1979), 33–4, 115–34.

109 S. Kunitz, 'Social Capital and Health,' *British Medical Bulletin*, 69 (2004),
61–73.

110 Durkheim, *Suicide*, 228. Also see Morselli, *Suicide*, 256–61; Skelton, 'Statistics of Suicide,' 473–5.

111 As early as 1821, Esquirol had attributed the high incidence of military
suicide to factors that seem consistent with Durkheim's fatalistic category; see Esquirol, 'Du suicide,' 590.

112 Durkheim, *Suicide*, 228–39. As Besnard points out, 'Après tout, le seul
exemple "moderne" qui soit donné [par Durkheim] du suicide altruiste
est le suicide militaire qui pourrait d'ailleurs tout aussi bien être inter-
prété en termes de régulation excessive (Durkheim évoque la discipline
rigide, "compressive de l'individu") qu'en invoquant la trop forte inté-
gration en l'en-groupe.' See Besnard, 'Durkheim et les femmes,' 42.

113 Skelton, 'Statistics of Suicide,' 473, 475.

114 Masaryk's explanation for the high suicide rate in the military was especially convoluted given his algebra of the more 'civilized' a society, the
greater its suicide rate. 'The philosophy of life, which at present is mani-

fested by the military services,' he wrote in 1881, 'is wanting throughout in either true moral or religious content, and suicide therefore appears more frequently among soldiers than among civilians.' See Masaryk, *Civilization and the Meaning of Civilization*, 171. For Morselli's discussion of military suicide, see Morselli, *Suicide*, 256–7.

115 If Durkheim contradicted his own logic by portraying military suicide as altruistic, he ignored entirely the fact that official statistics regularly reported extremely high rates of suicide among prisoners. 'Prison life,' according to Masaryk, 'disposes very strongly to suicide, as the relatively high frequency of among prison inmates indicates.' Given his typology, Durkheim would have had to categorize the majority of prisoner suicides as fatalistic. See Masaryk, *Suicide and the Meaning of Civilization*, 39. Recent studies continue to report high rates of prisoner suicides: 'In most countries,' according to Kerkhof and Bernasco, suicide 'in correctional institutions is higher than in the population at large.' See J.F.M. Kerkhof and Wim Bernasco, 'Suicidal Behavior in Jails and Prisons in the Netherlands: Incidence, Characteristics, and Prevention,' *Suicide and Life-Threatening Behavior*, 20 (Summer 1990), 123–37. See also Jean-Claude Bernheim, *Les suicides en prison* (Montréal: Edition du Méridien, 1987), 315–17.

116 See Kushner and Sterk, 'The Limits of Social Capital,' 1139–40.

117 Scott, 'A Statistical Representation of Work,' 115.

2 Suicide as an Illness Strategy in the Long Eighteenth Century

KEVIN SIENA

Illness was omnipresent in eighteenth-century discussions of suicide. Initially, this observation may not seem very revealing. After all, the dominant paradigm to explore suicide in the Enlightenment has been medicalization; suicide came to be understood through the prism of medical science, most especially described in terms of mental illness.[1] The intimate connection between mind and body in Enlightenment thought meant that the presumed diseased mind of the suicide was frequently linked to his or her diseased body. Thus historians of Enlightenment suicide have had much to say about medical issues. Rather than putting illness on suicide's historiographical map, this chapter seeks to offer a slightly different and, it is hoped, complementary way of interpreting the connection between sickness and suicide. The evidence for the medicalization of suicide in the Enlightenment is ample. However, we miss an opportunity to appreciate what the sources have to teach us if we allow the paradigm of medicalization to alone explain the mountain of evidence connecting illness and suicide in the eighteenth century.

The difference in approach may be as simple as where to place the suicide in our teleology of analysis. Explorations of medicalization have tended to explore suicide records from the perspective of those interpreting the phenomenon after it has happened. In other words, the event of a suicide acts as a catalyst initiating survivors' reconstructions, which scholars then analyse.[2] Medicalization is in some ways, then, a kind of intellectual history after the fact: how did survivors explain suicides after they had happened?[3] This approach is natural considering that the bulk of records pertaining to suicide in the period, such as coroners' records, were created after the fact. Nevertheless, suicide seems odd as a starting point. It is more commonly configured as a conclusion. It may therefore be fruitful to explore the material on illness within a different set of narratives – narratives that end with suicide rather than ones that begin with it. What role did illness and injury play in motivating people to consider and commit suicide in the eighteenth century? This seems a worthwhile, if basic, question since the most focused study of motivations for suicide, Michael MacDonald's chapter on the subject in *Sleepless Souls*, omits discussions of illness. In his analysis, illness is confined to describing how contemporaries understood suicides, but it is not considered as a factor in why people actually killed themselves. For motivations, MacDonald instead points to shame and poverty as the two most important influences on suicide in the period.[4] Reinterpreting coroners' inquests in light of documents such as medical treatises and trial records suggests that illness needs to be added to, and perhaps even placed atop, this list. For the eighteenth-century ill, the battle against disease was arduous and fought on multiple fronts with a wide range of resources. For some, the choice to end suffering was merely the last card played in a very long game, finally admitting defeat with a kind of self-euthanasia.[5] We therefore need to conceptualize suicide as an illness strategy. Indeed, we pay respect to our historical actors by considering the possibility that frequently such decisions represented rational choices and not merely the products of the 'diseased minds' that their survivors were so certain they possessed.

Of course, the material needs to be handled carefully. While suicides were frequently described as being sick during the period leading up to their decision to kill themselves, the prominence of sickness in suicide records may simply mark the pervasive nature of medicalization in the period. Enlightenment science offered medicalized explanations for many phenomena, and suicide was no different; in this case doctors increasingly presented it as a form of mental illness. In 1793 physician William Rowley argued that even contemplating suicide was, by definition, evidence of madness. 'It is certainly clear, that when a man mediates [on self-murder] ... he is no longer *compos mentis*; the commission, therefore, of suicide, must, necessarily, be always an act of insanity.'[6] The rising force of medical science in the period meant that by the late eighteenth century many confronting suicide were predisposed to highlight medical issues.

Moreover, we also know that families of suicides actively sought to entice coroners' juries to return verdicts of *non compos mentis* to free loved ones from the felony charge of *felo de se*, which could result in the state confiscating the felon's possessions and prohibiting his or her burial in a Christian cemetery. Highlighting mental illness was the best way to do this. Commenting on the paucity of suicides recorded in the *Bills of Mortality*, physician William Black lamented in 1789 that coroners were frequently bribed for this very reason.[7] MacDonald has made a strong case that a culture of leniency towards suicide grew in the Enlightenment, so that coroners' juries indeed became more sympathetic to insanity defences.[8] If James Parkinson's 1800 text for surgical students is to be believed, so too did doctors. Look long and hard, Parkinson told them, to find evidence of a disordered mind. He went so far as to present it as an act of mercy to conjure up such evidence. Even in cases where the deceased was cogent right up to the end, he asked, 'can you pretend to say that the act was not committed during a [sudden] fit of frenzy [?] ... Surely there can be no risque in imputing so dreadful an action to the sudden deprivation of reason' out of kindness for the family.[9] Readiest at hand for surgeons or coroners wishing to declare a suicide *non compos mentis* was fever. Through the matrix of the nerves that linked mind and body, bodily illnesses such as fevers were commonly said to disrupt the mind and cause delirium.[10] It is thus quite possible that many of the coroners' inquests for suicides that emphasize bodily illness represent either eighteenth-century folk steeped in a medicalized view of suicide looking to somatic causes or else the fabrication of evidence in the name of steering the verdict.

Some cases read this way. Elizabeth Horrell hanged herself in 1765 and was declared a 'lunatick' by the Westminster coroner. That verdict surely arose from the testimony of her husband, who emphasized the fever under which Elizabeth had suffered for the two weeks leading to her death. She was declared out of her senses. However, the husband's testimony also reveals that Elizabeth Horrell had tried to kill herself many times during the previous decade and spoke of suicide frequently. Nevertheless, despite evidence of at least ten years of suicidal tendencies, her widower emphasized her very recent fever as the main culprit, disrupting her mind and momentarily sapping her of reason. In such a case, testimony about bodily illness can hardly be taken at face value. And yet we also have a glimpse of Horrell's words. She was reported to complain about her physical pain during the week before her death, stating of her illness that 'if she could not get some ease she would make away with herself, for her punishment was more than she could bare.'[11] What do we have here, then – a family colluding to emphasize sickness in order to obtain an insanity verdict or a sick woman choosing to endure her physical suffering no longer?

It may well have been the former. However, if it was the latter, there is a lot of evidence that Horrell would have been very far from unique. For example, doctors' published treatises are rife with discussions of patients expressing a preference for death to continued suffering. Here again the material needs to be handled carefully. Doctors sometimes tossed around the rhetoric of suicide liberally, even comically. For example, writers on regimen often accused those who lived an unhealthy lifestyle of choosing behaviour that hastened death and thus of committing slow suicide.[12] By this rationale, drinkers committed 'suicide,'[13] as did sexual libertines,[14] masturbators,[15] those who patronized quacks,[16] and those who tried the controversial practice of inoculation.[17] Patients occasionally employed the rhetoric of suicide as liberally as their doctors. Women with reproductive complaints reluctant to be examined by male doctors frequently reported that they would 'rather die' than suffer the indignation of a physical exam.[18] And it was certainly an exaggeration when gout patients advised to give up rich foods and wines exclaimed that 'they would rather choose to die than continue to live, thus excluded from all the social comforts of life.'[19] Some medical rhetoric on suicide was clearly hyperbole.

But other instances are much harder to dismiss. Time and again doctors reported patients at the height of suffering invoking suicide or otherwise alluding to chosen death.[20] This was especially common when patients confronted surgery or other forms of rough eighteenth-century treatment. In 1714 surgeon Daniel Turner said of his patients that 'many of them rather choose to die than suffer the knife.'[21] We have examples of patients undergoing abdominal surgery said to be 'afflicted with such cruel pains that [they] desired Death every moment.'[22] Thomas Fuller recorded that a smallpox patient bled so copiously that he exclaimed 'he should much rather die quietly than endure such Pangs to save his life.'[23] Surgeons reported patients using similar terms when undergoing or facing the prospects of amputation or being cut for the stone, in some cases refusing surgery altogether. A case recorded by the Society of Physicians in London in 1776 reveals that a thirty-year-old man facing lithotomy 'would not consent, protesting obstinately that he would rather die,'[24] while surgeon Richard Wiseman failed to convince a Scottish soldier shot in the arm at the battle of Worcester to submit to amputation. 'Give me Drink, and I will die,' responded the soldier to the suggestion of the operation; he died the following day.[25]

Without modern anaesthesia, such operations were dreadfully painful; without antiseptics, they were highly risky. No surgery was minor in this period, and all surgical patients knew that they might not survive. Surprisingly, some patients actually embraced the possibility of death on the surgical table. In contrast to the patients above who choose death over the travails of surgery, other patients expressed their preference for death to continued suffering in a different way, seeing the possibility of surgical death as a relief from anguish. Wiseman relates the case of a cancer patient told that his survival rested on a painful and highly risky operation. 'God's will be done,' the patient replied, 'for I had rather die than live thus.'[26] When consulting with surgeon James Latta on whether to undergo lithotomy, another patient asked if the operation might alleviate his pain if he survived it. When Latta replied that it would, the patient replied, 'I have made up my mind upon it: You are to cut me immediately at my own desire; death being to me more desirable than a life of such pain.'[27]

Such discourse needs to be read within the context of the early modern doctor-patient relationship, a fluid negotiation based heavily on the rhetorical give-and-take between doctor and patient.[28] In some instances, patients seem to have invoked a preference to die as part of a narrative aimed at conveying to their doctors the gravity of their situation and ensuring that they be taken seriously. At times, patients even employed such language to convince surgeons to undertake operations about which they were reluctant. A patient only known as Mr B—— suffered a lengthy bout with the respiratory wasting condition known as phthisis. His physician, William Withering, recorded that the man was confined to his room and that 'his breathing became so extremely difficult and distressing, that he wished rather to die than live, and urged me warmly to devise some mode to relieve him.' Note here how the invocation of preferred death is followed immediately by the request for treatment, hinting at a discursive strategy at work. Although little acquainted with the disease, Withering offered a speculative operation that he could only theorize might work. Despite the doctor's quite limited confidence, the patient submitted eagerly.[29] Barthélemy Saviard relates a similar case involving a women suffering from an anal fistula. After examining her, he decided that an operation was in order. However, he judged the patient too weak to endure it. Regarding the operation as 'both uncertain and dangerous,' he advised her to wait until she had gained strength enough to proceed. Not satisfied with his diagnosis, the woman consulted several other practitioners. She must have been in quite poor health because all of them concurred that patience was the best course of action. Determined to undergo the operation, the woman now invoked preferred death. 'But her Impatience, added to the Pains she endured induced her in a short Time to a Re-consultation upon her Distemper, telling those she consulted that she had rather die than suffer any longer. *Upon this resolve they determined to perform the Operation.'* Again, the surgeons acquiesced upon the hint of hastened death. In the event, the operation was 'long, laborious, and attended with a considerable Loss of Blood,' and she died within two days.[30]

Still other forms of eighteenth-century medical treatment frequently drove patients to invoke preferred death. Mercurial salivation for syphilis is especially notable in this regard. In an excruciating procedure involving what we would now call heavy metal poisoning, patients consumed significant quantities of mercury, and doctors monitored them as they salivated more than a pint per day. Patients described the treatment, typically lasting more than a month, as excruciating.[31] John Martin, Walter Harris, Jean Astruc, Gerard van Swieten, Henry Eyre, and Nicholas Robinson all reported patients who resisted salivation or refused it outright by claiming that they would rather die than endure it.[32] Again, individual instances might easily seem like inflated turns of phrase. However, some reports came from patients who had already endured the procedure. In 1709 John Sintelaer related the case of a patient who told him 'that he had gone thro' no less than five most violent Salivations, but instead of being better, found himself worse now than ever before, and that therefore ... he would rather die than submit to so much Misery once more.'[33]

Powerful evidence of a different kind suggests that this was not hyperbole, and here we see the value of reading multiple kinds of sources in tandem. The Westminster coroner's inquests for the 1770s and 1780s record four separate suicides linked directly to mercurial salivation for syphilis. Domestic servant William Pearson contracted the so-called foul disease in the summer of 1772 and underwent salivation under the direction of a Dr Henry. Fellow servant Willis Richards deposed that Pearson 'spit very much for about six weeks' and 'was in great agonies and pain' on his last morning alive. When asked if there was anything Richards could do to help, Pearson replied, 'Nothing,' and departed, claiming that he was going to the doctor. In fact, Pearson sneaked into his master's stable and hanged himself in the hayloft.[34] A parallel case involves Mary Elson, who was similarly right in the midst of mercurial salivation when she leaped to her death from the window of a London workhouse infirmary on 25 April 1780.[35] Soldier John Jackson survived his salivation in a Westminster military hospital in May of 1773, but barely. He had already endured the operation several times without success, and his multiple trials of mercury clearly took a toll because a fellow soldier testified that Jackson looked 'worse than he used to' when he emerged from the hospital. Described by acquaintances as 'weak' and 'low spirited,' Jackson shot himself just days later.[36] Finally, a man named Richard Miller arranged for a bed in London's Lock Hospital to receive mercury treatment in March 1770. However, friends described him as 'melancholy and uneasy about his distemper' in the days leading up to his admission. If he feared the travails of salivation, it was with good reason; they were widely known and even the stuff of rough comedy.[37] Whatever the case, he was not optimistic, for he hanged himself in a barn the night before he was scheduled to enter the hospital.[38] The records of such desperate actions demand that we take seriously patients' words recorded in doctors' published treatises. Surely, doctors' stories about patients' wishes for hastened death must be understood to fall along a wide spectrum. Some expressions clearly reflect patients' narrative strategies or doctors' inflated rhetoric. However, many of the reports of patients invoking preferred death point to a simpler truth: that the eighteenth-century ill not infrequently considered suicide.

Moreover, closer inspection of medical treatises reveals evidence beyond vague exclamations of suffering and, like coroners' inquests, uncovers reports of actual suicides. In 1796 Erasmus Darwin recorded the case of a fifty-year-old man suffering from a poorly treated head wound: 'during the time he took in healing, he was indignant about it, and endured life, but soon afterwards shot himself.'[39] In 1780 John Hunter reprinted a most telling first-person account by a patient who had survived a bout with a contagious fever that gripped his ship. The man's journal describes day-by-day suffering marked by agony that drove him to 'a strong desire to put an end to his existence.' Moreover, he was not alone; many of his fellow sufferers 'roar[ed] hideously under the violence of the pain' and shared his 'strong desire for self-destruction.' It was not long before one of his shipmates took the next tragic step. 'We had a fatal instance of it in our party. Mr. Brown, the second day of his fever, being left alone, got to his pistols, and, throwing in four or five balls, discharged it into his breast, and was found dead a few minutes afterwards.' It was not the only instance. Days later, a second sufferer 'opened a vein in his arm and bled to death, most probably intentionally.'[40]

It is notable that in these accounts the link between physical illness and madness is frequently absent. Commentators did not always attribute patients' suicidal thoughts to their disordered minds. This last case of fever patients is particularly revealing, because delirium was so commonly associated with high fevers. Yet the surviving diarist did not excuse his suicidal shipmates through the convenience of fever-induced madness, which was ready at hand. Quite the opposite: he sympathized with them, exclaiming, 'I believe every one of us at times would have done the same, had we been possessed of the means of accomplishing it.' Moreover, he underscored their rationality to the end. 'Mr. Robson died the third day of his fever in great agonies, but perfectly sensible.'[41]

This absence of links to madness is especially notable in case studies involving women. Enlightenment medicine held that women's physiology, especially their reproductive organs and weaker nerves, powerfully predisposed them to mental illness, notably hysteria.[42] And yet we find no dearth of case studies involving women – even those suffering from reproductive disorders – wishing for death, in which the expected jump from bodily disorder to mental illness is absent. In terms that readers will by now find familiar, female patients with severe uterine complaints told doctors such as Frederick Ruysch, Charles Jenty, and John White that they would rather die than continue suffering. Ruysch's patient suffering from an ulcerated uterus can stand in for the others: 'The intolerable pains which she felt in those parts made her often wish for death.'[43] These doctors would have been forgiven had they ascribed their patients' wishes for hastened death to the madness-inducing effects of their diseased uteruses, the organs that give us the very word 'hysteria.' That they do not is telling. Like those of the patients described a moment ago, their exclamations were instead couched in terms of physical suffering, the fear of its continuance, and the quite rational decision that death might be an option at least worthy of consideration under the circumstances. In short, while medical treatises provide much evidence to support the medicalization thesis and the link to mental illness, they also supply no shortage of instances connecting sickness and suicide in different terms.

So pain, whether the pain of illness or the pain of eighteenth-century medicine, could lead to thoughts and acts of suicide. However, it was not just immediate pain but patients' long-term prospects for suffering that also had this effect. Here it is worth pointing out how limited medicine's powers were believed to be. Despite the optimism of Enlightenment science, nobody fooled themselves; eighteenth-century folk well understood that many sick people could not be cured. It was for this reason that the term 'incurable' still had enormous currency in the eighteenth century.[44] Indeed, the term referred to an entire category of patients whom, it was well known, hospitals refused because their ailments were considered beyond help. A woman known only as Jane died in the street on a cold night in January 1765 soon after she had been discharged from St George's Hospital, 'turned out from thence as incurable.'[45] The eighteenth-century sick knew all too well that medicine might fail, that recovery was far from certain, and that lingering sickness and slow death could well lie ahead. So it was that we find individuals such as John Clifton, a man of seventy long suffering from gout, violent headaches, and pain in his limbs, reporting to his doctor that he 'despaired of ever getting better in this world.'[46] Further eighteenth-century case studies are similarly rife with patients who 'despaired of ever being cured' or 'despaired of ever getting better.'[47]

Noting the despair about future prospects begins to point to the utility of painting illness in its broadest terms and setting it within patients' wider life experiences. As it does today, illness in the eighteenth century brought much more than merely physical suffering. It generated and was forever accompanied by other cultural, economic, and psychological dilemmas. For example, in addition to pain, illness brought reduced physical abilities. For a huge portion of the population, livelihood depended on the body's ability to labour. Disability, then, could be economically tragic.[48] In 1790 John Beck suffered from a severely damaged leg and was reduced to reliance on the workhouse, an institution known to have been a hated last resort for eighteenth-century Londoners.[49] Fellow inmates in the sick ward testified that Beck, no longer able to support himself, complained of his pain and reduced abilities frequently, citing these as the likeliest reasons that he hanged himself.[50] Records relating to the attempted suicide of a miller's apprentice similarly point to the impact that illness had on the young man's capacity to labour. Though he had partially recovered from his bout with an ague, his ability to work was diminished, bringing upon him the wrath of his master, who beat him viciously, worsening the man's physical abilities and, according to reports, leading to his attempt to hang himself in 1745.[51]

The economic impact of illness and injury means, therefore, that we must connect illness and poverty. MacDonald was absolutely correct to point to poverty as a major motivation of suicide in the eighteenth century.[52] But rather than merely adding illness *alongside* poverty on the list of motivations for suicide in the period, we must recognize the dynamic interplay between the two. Consider William Cole. A sixty-year-old carpenter treated as an outpatient in Middlesex Hospital, he expressed death wishes during his arduous battle with a range of awful symptoms. No longer able to control his bowels, he was incontinent six to seven times a day. Complaining of violent internal pains, he was frequently dizzy, unable to remain standing, and finally unable to work. 'By these complaints his life was so miserable that he wished for death,' reported his doctor, John Brisbane. However, Brisbane emphasized that it was his anxiety about unemployment and his dramatically reduced station that Cole feared the most. 'But he was unable to work, and was afraid, after a healthy and laborious life, to be obliged to go upon the parish, though he had reared a numerous family by his own labour only.'[53] It was a point of pride for working-class Londoners to avoid the workhouse and to support themselves through honest labour, a point about which Cole had been clearly proud but which his physical reduction now threatened. His despair therefore needs to be understood through a complex interplay between illness, poverty, impotence, and masculinity.

The travails brought on by a combination of illness and poverty in the long eighteenth century are also well captured in criminal court records. A twenty-six-year-old man named William Trapp suffered a paralytic stroke seven years prior to his trial for assault at London's Old Bailey courthouse. Testimony by family members relates a narrative of decline – physical, emotional, and economic – from the point of his stroke forward. Forced to rely on crutches, Trapp suffered subsequent pain and reduced physical abilities that continally frustrated his attempts to work. He bounced from job to job. For a time he worked as an usher for a school, but his health prevented him from performing the duties required. He subsequently tried his hand at shoemaking, but he was not able to hold this job either once another injury forced him to seek care at the London Infirmary. This was just one occasion on which Trapp's decline necessitated his reliance on others. Indeed, despite his best efforts to work, by the time of the trial his poor health rendered him almost completely dependent. Though an adult, Trapp was still supported by his parents; he was frequently hospitalized, and for a time he was even reduced to the workhouse. All of his relatives who testified related long-standing anxiety that Trapp might kill himself, and all of them pointed to the reciprocal tandem of poor health and economic dependency that fostered his growing depression and inclination towards 'self-destruction.'[54]

As Cole's and Trapp's cases suggest, when sickness, unemployment, and poverty conjoined, eighteenth-century patients were often forced to confront the quite imperfect social welfare network of hospitals, workhouses, and poor relief, bringing new challenges that had the power to intensify suicidal despair. The system, if it can be called that, was difficult to navigate. For example, getting a bed at most English hospitals required networking in order to obtain a nomination from a hospital governor, and many people failed in this endeavour. Robert Munro was one such man. Suffering from syphilis for several years and having once previously been in the Lock Hospital, he sought read-mission in 1762. However, admission to the Lock, as with most hospitals, hinged on securing the nomination of a governor. Somehow, the poor were expected to network to bring their case before one of the rich men who donated money to the hospital. If they could even put themselves in contact with such a man, they then had to hope that their case was made in just the right way to elicit mercy and secure the letter needed to get a bed.[55] (Indeed, some applicants for charitable help invoked suicide in ways that may have been strategies to convince benefactors to pity them.)[56] When testifying to the coroner about why they thought Munro slit his own throat, acquaintances reported that he feared he would never recover his health once he learned that he would not be admitted to the hospital. A gentleman was reportedly working on his behalf to obtain the nomination letter, but shortly before killing himself, Munro learned that his agent had come up empty. One witness put it this way: 'The best account that can be given at present for his doing this act is that he despaired of being cured of his disease (for which he had been in the Lock Hospital before he came here) and have been in expectation of a place, which it is said to have been promised to be given to him, he was acquainted, that he must lay aside all thoughts of it, for it could not be procured for him; and this it is thought was what determined him to put a speedy end to his life.'[57] It is noteworthy that, despite the rich evidence of the impact of disease on this common man's life contained in this inquest, the coroner went on to declare that Munro's illness rendered him delirious and hence insane. This kind of case, then, both supports the medicalization thesis that coroners increasingly described suicide in terms of madness and simultaneously offers considerable evidence for the wider socio-cultural impact of illness in the period.[58]

Just as illness related dynamically to poverty, so too did it link up with MacDonald's other main motivation for suicide, shame.[59] Here the example of syphilis is extremely telling. The effects on reputation from the debilitating, disfiguring, and heavily stigmatized disease were powerful and well known, and public exposure of infection seriously damaged reputations.[60] Patients sought desperately to attain care privately to guard against public exposure, but this was harder to do the poorer one was. For the working poor, reputations damaged by infection could quickly circle back to economics, as in cases when discovery of their illness by an employer cost them their jobs.[61] Infection could also prevent one from ever attaining gainful employment in the first place. Frances Gardner learned this tough lesson while sitting in the venereal ward of the parish workhouse of St George, Hanover Square, in 1796. She was hopeful about her prospects when she was pronounced 'perfectly cured' and awaited dismissal. Her optimism sprang from the promise given her by a gentlewoman to recommend her for a new job, likely in domestic service. Her hopes were dashed when her patron discovered that she had been treated for the pox. She called on Gardner at the workhouse and, according to witnesses, 'told her that she could not recommend her any more, as she has lost her character by having that disorder.' Shortly after the meeting, Gardner hanged herself.[62] Considering the cases of Frances Gardner and Robert Munro alongside those of syphilitics John Jackson, Mary Elson, William Pearson, and Richard Miller, related earlier, gives considerable reason to pause. However, when we reflect on the wider socio-cultural implications of illness in the period, we should not be surprised to find syphilitics so numerous in surviving examples of Enlightenment suicides. Patients were struck by a gruesome disease that was extremely painful. Its main treatment was horrible and frequently failed. Sufferers were visibly disfigured, laden with stigma, and often ground down to poverty and unemployment, if not by their physical debilitation, then by their reduced social standing. In syphilis, pain, poverty, and shame frequently fused in a kind of suicidal perfect storm that all too often led to despair.

Indeed, the evidence even warrants momentary comparison with the present, something that historians of long ago are extremely hesitant to do. However, that eighteenth-century syphilitics appear to have considered and committed suicide so frequently cannot but evoke an obvious comparison with HIV/AIDS patients, who, studies have long established, constitute one of the highest risk groups for suicide today.[63] Like today, the seriously or terminally ill in the eighteenth century frequently saw their prospects for renewed health as bleak enough that suicide became an option worth considering. And like today, those within that group who suffered from a slow, lethal, sexually transmitted disease with limited treatment options faced added social, cultural, and psychological challenges that put them at an even higher risk.

In conclusion, historians would do well to conceptualize suicide as an illness strategy and set it within the longer narratives of patients' struggles. Yet it is currently accepted as such a commonplace that poor health links causatively with suicide that it may seem surprising to some that detailing the link for pervious periods even need be done. That it does powerfully spotlights the influence of the medicalization thesis on the historiography of suicide, steering historians away from exploring the phenomenon in these terms. The omnipresence of sickness in eighteenth-century suicide records certainly has a lot to do the rise of medical science at the dawn of modernity. Moreover, there can be no denying the increased tendency to account for suicide by way of mental illness in the period. By the late eighteenth century, medico-scientific discourse was employed to explain almost everything, and suicide was no exception. The medicalization thesis holds. However, not all discussions of sickness in suicide records lead to mental illness, the linchpin in medicalization arguments, and some even ring hollow, providing telling evidence of just how devastating illness and injury could be in the long eighteenth century. If we allow the large body of evidence connecting suicide and sickness to be explained by way of medicalization alone, we run the risk that some readers may conclude that the evidence is essentially fictional; looking to secure an insanity verdict, survivors invented or exaggerated stories of physical sickness as a way to facilitate arguments about madness. Such a reading would be unfortunate. It is even conceivable to turn the thing on its head. It is possible that discussions of madness were made possible by the fact that sickness in its many forms was already present in so many stories of eighteenth-century suicide. Perhaps those who so frequently connected the evidence of bodily illness to mental illness needed to take only a small step.

Moreover, taking the time to consider illness as a motivation for suicide allows opportunity for reflection on the powerful drive to cast

suicide as evidence of madness in the eighteenth century. Smart arguments have suggested that the phenomenon represents the Enlightenment at work, embodying its core components of humanitariansim,
secularism, and science. Yet in a different way the flight to madness
may have functioned to *protect* the Enlightenment world view from
frightening truths that seriously threatened to undercut it. For all the
philanthropic energy that went into building hospitals, the welfare
network had massive cracks that too many people fell through. And
for all the faith in science, medicine was still weak. Safer to dismiss the
sick who killed themselves as deranged than to confront the implications if they were not.

NOTES

Thank you to Donna Andrew, Steve King, Alannah Tomkins, and Michael
Stolberg for reading drafts of this chapter.

1   Medicalization has sat at the centre of a range of related debates about
    the rise of secular and lenient attitudes towards suicide in the Enlighten-
    ment and the movement away from religious interpretations of the act as
    a mortal sin, usually inspired by the Devil. See especially Michael Mac-
    Donald and Terence R. Murphy, *Sleepless Souls: Suicide in Early Modern
    England* (Oxford: Oxford University Press, 1990); MacDonald, 'The Secu-
    larization of Suicide in England,1660–1800,' *Past and Present*, 1988, 111,
    50–100; and MacDonald, 'The Medicalization of Suicide in England:
    Laymen, Physicians, and Cultural Change, 1500–1870,' in *Framing Disease:
    Studies in Cultural History*, ed. Charles Rosenberg and Janet Golden, 2nd
    ed. (New Brunswick: Rutgers University Press, 1997), 85–113. Most
    recently see several of the contributions to the aptly titled *From Sin to
    Insanity: Suicide in Early Modern Europe*, ed. Jeffery Watt (Ithaca: Cornell
    University Press, 2004), esp. Paul Seaver, 'Suicide and the Vicar General
    in London: A Mystery Solved?' 25–47, and Vera Lind, 'The Suicidal Mind
    and Body: Examples from Northern Germany,' 64–80. These contribu-
    tions should be read alongside the debate between MacDonald and
    Donna T. Andrew in 'The Secularization of Suicide in England 1660–1800'
    and 'Reply,' *Past and Present*, 1988, 119, 158–70.
2   This is especially true of scholars exploring sources such as coroners'
    records; indeed MacDonald places the coroner's jury, rather than the
    physician, at the centre of the story of medicalization. See, e.g., 'The Med-
    icalization of Suicide in England.'

3 Vera Lind's study is a notable departure, taking the issue of medicalization in a smart direction. Hardly 'after the fact,' she argues that those
   contemplating suicide appropriated the character of the melancholic,
   replete with the prevailing physical and mental symptoms. But here
   again the evidence related to sickness in the records is marshalled as a
   kind of means to an end, rather than as itself a motivating cause. Here
   those contemplating suicide role-played that they were sick. While this
   may have been the case for some, it has the effect (as do presentations of
   survivors emphasizing sickness in pursuit of insanity verdicts, discussed
   below) of rendering evidence of sickness almost fictional, an element of a
   character played by the prospective suicide or a set piece in a tale spun
   by the survivors. See Lind, 'The Suicidal Mind and Body,' 67–74.

4 MacDonald and Murphy, *Sleepless Souls*, 259–300. That bodily sickness
   might have been a causative factor, not linked to mental illness, has been
   occasionally noticed but seldom analysed. See,for example, Jeffery
   Merrick, 'Suicide in Paris, 1775,' in *From Sin to Insanity*, 162–3.

5 On the question of euthanasia in the period, see Michael Stolberg's most
   recent article suggesting that a learned debate churned around the question of euthanasia in the late seventeenth and eighteenth centuries, that
   popular practices to help hasten death for those suffering were well
   known, and that some early modern doctors were sympathetic to the terminally ill who sought help ending their lives. See Stolberg, 'Active
   Euthanasia in Pre-Modern Society, 1500–1800: Learned Debates and
   Popular Practices,' *Soc. Hist. Med.*, 2007, 19, 205–21.

6 William Rowley, *The Rational Practice of Physic*, 4 vols. (London: E. Newberry and J. Hand, 1793), 2: 122.

7 William Black, *An Arithmetical and Medical Analysis of the Diseases and
   Mortality of the Human Species* (London: John Crowder, 1789): 'It is generally believed, that the total amount [of suicides] is concealed in the
   London registers, whereby a considerable emolument is derived by ...
   coroners ... from the relations of the deceased, in order to their procure-
   ment of a different report; such as found dead, suddenly, drowned,
   lunatick' (243).

8 MacDonald, *Sleepless Souls*, 109–43.

9 James Parkinson, The Hospital Pupil (London: H. D. Symonds, 1800),
   156–9.

10 On the centrality of the nerves in Enlightenment physiology (and wider
   Enlightenment thought), see the essays of G.S. Rousseau compiled in
   Nervous Acts: Essays on Literature, Culture and Sensibility (Basingstoke: Pal-
   grave, 2004).

11 Westminster Abbey Library and Muniments Room (hereafter WA), West-

minster Coroner's Inquests, 1760–99, Elizabeth Horrell, 27 November 1765.

12 George Cheyne, *Essay on Long Life*, 4th ed. (London: George Strahan, 1725), 4–5; James Makittrick, *An Essay on Regimen* (London: J. and P. Wilson, 1799), 21.

13 Thomas Hale, *Compleat Body of Husbandry*, 4 vols. (Dublin: P. Wilson and J. Exshaw, 1757), 4: 161; James Nelson, *An Essay on the Government of Children* (London: R. and J. Dodsley, 1753), 287–8.

14 Thomas Beddoes, *A Lecture Introductory to a Course on Popular Instruction on the Constitution and Management of the Human Body* (Bristol: N. Briggs, 1797), 31–2.

15 S.A.D. Tissot, *Three Essays: The First on the Disorders of People of Fashion; Second, on Diseases Incidental to Literary and Sedentary Persons ... Third, on Onanism* (Dublin: James Williams, 1772), 22. On the anti-masturbation campaign, see especially Thomas Laqueur, *Solitary Sex: A Cultural History of Masturbation* (New York: Zone Books, 2003), and Michael Stolberg, 'An Unmanly Vice: Self-Pollution, Anxiety, and the Body in the Eighteenth Century,' *Soc. Hist. Med.*, 2000, 13, 1–22.

16 References to suicide in discussions of quackery clearly need to be understood within the context of the medical marketplace. Some doctors presented the choice of an unlicensed practitioner as a form of suicide (using that term) on the grounds that it was a choice that could lead to one's own death. See Joseph Cam, *A Practical Treatise; or Second Thoughts on the Consequences of the Venereal Disease* (London: G. Strahan, W. Meers, C. King, and E. Midwinter, 1729), 150–1; J.H. Smyth, *A Practical Essay on the Venereal Disease* (London: n.p., 1798), 38; John King, *An Essay on Hot and Cold Bathing* (London: J. Bettenham, 1737), 65; John Leake, *A Dissertation on the Efficacy of the Lisbon Diet Drink* (London: R. Baldwin, 1767), 122. Others told frightening cautionary tales of patients treated by quacks who were so badly off after their inferior care that they were 'pushed ... to acts of suicide, in order to get rid of a life, the continuance of which appears to them more dreadful than death itself.' See Daniel Smith, *An Apology to the Public for Commencing the Practice of Physic* (London: Carnan and Newberry, 1775), 30–1.

17 William Smith, *A New and General System of Physic* (London: W. Owen, 1769), 238.

18 Edmund Chapman, *A Treatise on the Improvement of Midwifery* (London: J. Brindley, J. Clarke, and C. Corbett, 1735), 179; W.S. [William Salmon], *Aristotle's Compleat and Experience'd Midwife* (London: n.p., 1760), iv. On this dynamic, see Roy Porter, 'A Touch of Danger: The Man-Midwife and

Sexual Predator,' in *Sexual Underworlds of the Enlightenment*, ed. G.S. Rousseau and Roy Porter (Manchester: Manchester University Press, 1987), 206–32; and Kevin Siena, 'The "Foul" Disease and Privacy: the Effects of Venereal Disease and Patient Demand on the Medical Marketplace in Early Modern London,' *Bull. Hist. Med.*, 2001, 75, 214–22.

19 Nicholas Robinson, *An Essay on the Gout* (London: Edward Robinson, 1755), 152.

20 For just two examples, consider Thomas Sydenham's description of rheumatism patients suffering for lengthy periods with symptoms that he described as 'dispiriting'; he remarks that they were 'so very unpleasing to the Patient, as to make him almost desire Death to relieve and give him ease.' See Sydenham, *Praxis Medica* (London: J. Knapton and W. Innys, 1716), 53. Naval surgeon John Clark reported a case involving an officer suffering from advanced hepatitis who was 'reduced to a mere skeleton, and all his hopes were an ardent wish for death to put a period to his complicated distress.' See Clark, *Observations on the Diseases in Long Voyages to Hot Climates* (London: D. Wilson and G. Nicol, 1773), 278.

21 Daniel Turner, *De Morbus Cutaneis* (London: R. Bonwicke et al., 1714), 228.

22 Pierre Dionis, *A Course of Chirurgical Operations* (London: Jacob Tonson, 1710), 66–7.

23 Thomas Fuller, *Pharmacopoeia Extemporanea* (London: William Innys, 1714), 258. John Woodward relates a similar case of a smallpox patient, not bled but overly medicated with astringents and purgatives. He writes: 'I found her so extremely shattered, weak and sunk, that she could hardly speak. The most I could perceive was, to beg that she might take no more Physick ... to be short, she desired rather to die, than to take any more of what thus teized, molested, endangered and hurt her.' See Woodward, *Select Cases and Consultations in Physick* (London: L. Davis and C. Reymers, 1757), 326; original emphasis.

24 Society of Physicians in London, *Medical Observations and Inquiries* (London: T. Cadell and E. Johnston, 1776), 82.

25 Richard Wiseman, *Eight Chirurgical Treatises* (London: Benjamin Tooke and John Meredith, 1705), 356.

26 Ibid., 112.

27 James Latta, *A Practical System of Surgery*, 3 vols. (Edinburgh: G. Mudie and Son, A. Guthrie, and J. Fairbairn, 1793), 1: 484.

28 For an introduction, see Dorothy Porter and Roy Porter, *Patient's Progress: Doctors and Doctoring in Eighteenth-Century England* (Oxford: Polity Press, 1989), 70–95.

29 William Withering, *An Account of Foxglove, and Some of Its Medical Uses: with Practical Remarks on Dropsy and other Diseases* (Birmingham: M. Swinney, 1785), 206.

30 Barthélemy Saviard, *Observations in Surgery: Being a Collection of One Hundred and Twenty Eight Different Cases* (London: J. Hodges, 1740), 117–18; emphasis added.

31 For a description of the process, see Kevin Siena, *Venereal Disease, Hospitals and the Urban Poor: London's 'Foul Wards,' 1600–1800* (Rochester: University of Rochester Press, 2004), 22–4.

32 John Marten, *A Treatise of All the Degrees and Symptoms of the Venereal Disease* (London: S. Crouch et al., 1708), 321; Henry Eyre, *A Brief Account of the Holt Waters* (London: J. Roberts, 1731), 105; Walter Harris, *A Treatise of the Acute Diseases of Infants; to Which Are Added, Medical Observations on Several Grievous Diseases* (London: Thomas Astley, 1742), 218; Jean Astruc, *Treatise on the Venereal Disease*, 2 vols. (London, W. Innys, 1754), 2: 159; Gerard van Swieten, *The Commentaries upon the Aphorisms of Dr. Herman Boerhaave*, 18 vols. (London: Robert Horsfield and Thomas Longman, 1773), 17: 360–1; Society of Physicians in London, *Medical Observations*, 402.

33 John Sintelaer, *The Scourge of Venus and Mercury* (London: G. Harris et al., 1709), 154.

34 WA, Westminster Coroner's Inquests, 1760–99, William Pearson, 14 September 1772.

35 Ibid., Mary Elson, 25 April 1780.

36 Ibid., John Jackson, 31 March, 1771.

37 Siena, *Venereal Disease*, 33.

38 WA, Westminster Coroner's Inquests, 1760–99, Richard Miller, 16 March 1770.

39 Erasmus Darwin, *Zoonomia; or the Laws of Organic Life*, 2 vols. (London: J. Johnson, 1796), 2: 373.

40 Society for the Improvement of Medical and Chirurgical Knowledge, *Transactions of a Society for the Improvement of Medical and Chirurgical Knowledge*, 3 vols. (London: J. Johnson, 1793), 3: 53–90, especially 86 and 90.

41 Ibid., 86.

42 For an introduction, see Evelyne Berriot-Salvadore, 'The Discourse of Medicine and Science,' in *A History of Women*, vol. 3, *Renaissance and Enlightenment Paradoxes*, ed. N.Z. Davis and Arlette Farge (Cambridge, Mass.: Belknap, 1993), 360–4.

43 Frederick Ruysch, *The Celebrated Dr. Frederic Ruysch's Practical Observa-*

tions in Surgery and Midwifry (London: T. Osborne, 1751), 37–39; Charles Jenty, *A Course of Anatomico-physiological Lectures on the Human Structure and Animal Oeconomy*, 3 vols. (London: James Rivington and James Fletcher, 1757), 2: 285; Andrew Duncan, ed., *Medical Commentaries for the Year MDCCXCV*, 10 vols. (Edinburgh: G. Mudie and Son, G.G. and J. Robinson, 1795), 10: 258–9.

44 Peter Shaw captured well the tension of 'incurable' patients in an age of enlightened optimism: 'the Cure of Incurables does not only involve a Paradox in the Expression, but in an Age so productive of new Discoveries, and so fertile in Improvements as the present, it generally passes for a desperate Problem; and is apt to be rank'd in the same Class with the Quadrature of the Circle, the Perpetual Motion, and the Philosopher's Stone.' See Shaw, *A Treatise of Incurable Diseases* (London: J. Roberts, 1723), 2.

45 WA, Westminster Coroner's Inquests, 1760–99, Jane [no surname], 16 January 1765.

46 Count Belchilgen, *An Essay on the Virtues and Properties of the Ginseng Tea* (London: n. p., 1786), 25.

47 Henry Boësnier de la Touche, *Some Observations of the Power and Efficacy of a Medicine against Loosenesses, Bloody Fluxes* (London: n. p., 1757), 53–4; and Benjamin Bell, *A System of Surgery*, 7 vols. (Edinburgh: Bell and Bradfute, G.G. and J. Robinson, and Murray and Highley, 1796), 1: 275.

48 On disability in the period, see Anne Borsay, *Disability and Social Policy in Britain since 1750: A History of Exclusion* (Basingstoke: Palgrave, 2005).

49 Tim Hitchcock, *Down and Out in Eighteenth-Century London* (London: Hambledon and London, 2004), 125–49.

50 WA, Westminster Coroner's Inquests, 1760–99, John Beck, 30 October 1790.

51 Simon Mason, *The Nature of an Intermitting Fever and Ague Consider'd* (London: J. Hodges, 1745), 190–1.

52 MacDonald shows that poverty was especially powerful in motivating suicides when it represented a significant reduction in one's status as in cases of suicides by the wealthy who lost their fortunes. See MacDonald and Murphy, *Sleepless Souls*, 260–74.

53 John Brisbane, *Select Cases in the Practice of Medicine* (London: G. Scott, 1772), 38–40.

54 Old Bailey Sessions Papers (hereafter OBSP), William Trapp, breaking the peace: assault, 9 April 1823.

55 Roy Porter, 'The Gift Relation: Philanthropy and Provincial Hospitals in Eighteenth-Century England,' in *The Hospital in History*, ed. Roy Porter and Lindsay Granshaw (London: Routledge, 1989), 165–6.

56 Soldier Donald McDermott was discharged from the army because of a badly dislocated ankle that rendered him unfit for service and unable to work. He petitioned his former commander, hoping for assistance in securing his 'sea money,' stressing that failure might leave him with no option but to kill himself: 'the Joint waas Imposible to be Set I am uncapable of Labouring for My Living So I must Either Rely upon your LordShips Mercy or otherwise be obliged to End My Days.' See Henry E. Huntington Library, Loudoun Papers, North America, 1682–1780, Donald McDermott, Memorial to Loudoun (1757), LO 5199, box 114. I am very grateful to Peter Way for sharing this case with me.

57 WA, Westminster Coroner's Inquests, 1760–99, Robert Munro, 22 November, 1762.

58 Desperation for hospitalization similarly led to acts of theft either to secure the admission funds demanded at some institutions or to seek medical care privately. When confessing to robbery, George Robertson explained his actions thus: 'I was very ill with the foul disease, so as not to be able to walk, I said I wished I had been dead, because I had no money or friend to put me in the hospital.' See OBSP, George Robertson, theft with violence: highway robbery, 02 May 1753.

59 MacDonald and Murphy, *Sleepless Souls*, 274–98.

60 On shame, including humour, see Siena, *Venereal Disease*, 31–41. The pox figured prominently in the period's biting satire. Though he does not cite syphilis, Simon Dickie notes the frequency that noselessness, a telltale sign of advanced syphilis, appeared in rough eighteenth-century humour. See Dickie, 'Hilarity and Pitilessness in the Mid-Eighteenth Century: English Jestbook Humor,' *Eighteenth-Century Studies*, 2003, 37, 2.

61 OBSP, William Frazier, theft: simple grand larceny, 16 October, 1723.

62 WA, Westminster Coroner's Inquests, 1760–99, Frances Gardner, 21 April 1796.

63 A sample of studies include M. Bellini and C. Bruschi, 'HIV Infection and Suicidality,' *J. Affect. Disord.*, 1996, 38, 153–64; P.M. Marzuk et al., 'Increased Risk of Suicide in Persons with AIDS,' JAMA, 1998, 259, 1333–7, and L.R. Slome et al., 'Physician-Assisted Suicide and Patients with Human Immunodeficiency Virus Disease,' *N. Engl. J. Med.* 1997, 336, 417–21.

3 Death and Life in the Archives: Patterns of and Attitudes to Suicide in Eighteenth-Century Paris

JEFFREY MERRICK

In May 1750, toward the end of performances of Marmontel's *Cleopatra*, the defeated Egyptian queen wandered on stage carrying a vase of asps concealed by flowers and declared, 'What a fortunate gift of heaven, to know how to die.'[1] In September 1770, after shooting his dog because he knew the loyal creature would not have wanted to outlive him, a German baron ran himself through with his sword. He was reportedly infected by the widespread 'disgust' for life that afflicted the French or influenced by the 'philosophy of the day' that authorized or even encouraged such desperate acts.[2] Unlike his dog, the baron survived. He explained that an impudent *petit-maître* had stepped on his foot at the Wauxhall, that he had graciously accepted an apology instead of demanding a duel, and that he had subsequently and abundantly regretted that decision, which, as far as he was concerned, left his honour tarnished. To the best of my knowledge, no Parisians committed suicide in 1750 or 1770 for the same reason and in the same manner as the tragic queen or the comic baron.

We know something about literary characters, classical and contemporary, who took their own lives and about a modest number of cases that attracted public attention in the course of the eighteenth century.[3] We know even more about the debates between defenders of orthodoxy and advocates of enlightenment over the legitimacy of suicide.[4] But what about ordinary Parisians who killed themselves out of poverty, misery, or lunacy?[5] The *lieutenant général de police* Feydeau de Marville noted only fifteen cases over five years in his newsy letters to the royal minister responsible for Paris.[6] The duc de Luynes, the marquis d'Argenson, and the lawyer Barbier, who included so much instructive and colourful material about the court and the capital in their journals, mentioned some suicides in preceding and following years but not one in 1750.[7] The printer and bookseller Hardy reported ten in and around the city in 1770, including the drowning of the curé of Saint-Jacques-de-la-Boucherie, which scandalized the parish and embarrassed the clergy.[8] Hardy recorded invaluable information about sensitive cases like this one that are not documented in official sources, but he, like the others, only wrote about what he heard about.

There is one and only one reliable method of locating representative, if not comprehensive, documentation about ordinary Parisians who took their own lives – by searching through the voluminous reports of the forty-eight district police commissioners in the Y (Châtelet, the royal municipal court) series in the Archives nationales. This article is based on the surviving papers of forty-three commissioners from 1750 and forty-six commissioners from 1770. The papers are organized by district and by year, month, and day, but they are not sorted by subject or indexed in any way. Suicides are usually tagged in the upper left-hand corner, but they are interfiled with innumerable thefts, assaults, and many other types of offences. The research is difficult, but the results are instructive. The papers from 1750 and 1770 tell us all that we are ever likely to know about 'homicide of oneself' in those years: who, when, where, how, and why, at least according to relatives, neighbours, and friends who observed and outlived the victims. They include some unusual material, most notably one pair of explanatory notes and one posthumous prosecution, but they also document conventional assumptions about and attitudes toward suicide in pre-revolutionary France. In the last analysis, the papers reveal as much about the living as they do about the deceased.

As guardians of public tranquility and morality, the district police commissioners were expected to complete reports about sudden and suspect deaths, most of which, of course, were not self-inflicted. In the populous and sometimes dangerous city, people fell off roofs and into wells, had seizures or got trampled in the streets, and died quietly in their beds during the night. In 1770 commissioner Touvenot reported the deaths of two dozen Parisians, including a five-year-old girl who fell out a sixth-floor window, a carpenter killed by a block of stone at a construction site, a woodcutter and a coachman who had strokes on the job, and ten men, two boys, and two women who drowned in the Seine. The boys were playing by the river, and one of the men, a painter, was bathing in the river. His wife recognized the body at once because his left index finger was crooked from holding his palette, and his right testicle, from no apparent cause, was much larger than the left one. She acknowledged that he sometimes drank too much but insisted that there was 'every reason' to believe that he was drowned (passive voice) 'by accident.'[9] In more than a few instances, the commissioners were not sure, and we cannot be sure, if individuals died accidentally or deliberately. They generally accepted what the witnesses told them, for example, about the old clerk with bad eyesight who fell into the courtyard as he hung his hat on the peg next to the window and the young chiseller who drank more wine than usual with dinner, opened the window to relieve himself before going to bed, and likewise ended up in the courtyard.[10]

The deaths in the Seine belong in a special category of their own because they are too numerous to list and so difficult to read. In some cases, witnesses saw the victims working, playing, or bathing and then struggling in the water. In other cases, especially if the bodies had spent any length of time in the river, it was impossible to tell how they got there or even who they were. Relatives recognized some, but many ended up, unknown and unclaimed, in the morgue. Anne Baudrillon identified her husband, who wore a vest, shirt, breeches, and stockings, all in 'bad' shape, but had nothing in his pockets, presumably because he had spent much of the afternoon in a tavern with friends.[11] But no one knew the name of the eighteen-to-twenty-year-old woman dressed in a blue and white striped blouse and a blue and white checked shirt, with a small folding knife, several copper thimbles, and two packages of silver thread in her pockets and a cross (with eight 'fake' stones set in it) around her neck.[12] One could read the physical remains and personal effects of the individuals whose lives ended in the Seine, as Richard Cobb did so impressively, but one should remember that many of them drowned accidentally.[13]

For that reason, most of them must be excluded from this study, which is based on the eighteen (fifteen completed and three attempted) suicides in 1750 and twenty-six (twenty-five completed and one attempted) suicides in 1770 documented in the Y series. The numbers are significant but hardly definitive. The commissioners did not identify every single suicide as such, by mistake or by design, and some of their papers were discarded or have been mislaid. The figures from 1750 and 1770 suggest a dramatic increase in the incidence of suicide around the time when contemporaries expressed concern about an epidemic of self-destruction, but the number dropped to twenty in 1775.[14] To the best of my knowledge, no one has counted the cases in other years throughout the century; so we should not automatically assume that the authors of journals and *nouvelles* comprehended and represented disturbing trends accurately.

When municipal guardsmen or ordinary subjects found bodies floating in the water, lying on the pavement, or hanging in the bedroom, they sent for a commissioner, who sometimes needed to have a locksmith open a door and always needed (sooner or later) to have a doctor inspect the corpse. The commissioner completed a report (*procès-verbal*) on the spot and submitted it to the *lieutenant criminel* of the Châtelet, who usually instructed him to conduct an investigation (*information*).[15] Within days in most instances, the commissioner collected testimony about the victim's mental, physical, and emotional state from witnesses: guardsmen, doctors, landlords, and, most importantly, relatives, neighbours, and friends of the deceased. With this additional information in hand, the *lieutenant criminel* decided what to do with the body and whether to initiate posthumous prosecution. In 1750 he authorized burial in seven cases and consigned five corpses (four of the nine men but only one of the six women) to the morgue. Families wished and tried to avoid that outcome in order to avoid distressing publicity and possible prosecution. One woman sought and gained custody of her husband's body, which would have gone to the morgue otherwise, by emphasizing his mental problems, which suggested diminished responsibility. By 1770 the *lieutenant criminel* was much more likely to let spouses and children bury the dead. In the case of one man who jumped out a window, 'given the accident that had caused his death,' the Châtelet had to order the parish priest to allow the body to be interred in consecrated ground.[16] In some instances, the dossiers include not only the report and/or the investigation but also the inventory compiled by the commissioner before he sealed the premises and the documents about the transference of the worldly possessions to the heirs.[17]

In one and only one case of attempted suicide, the commissioner sent the victim *manqué* to prison.[18] In one and only one case of completed suicide, the Châtelet enforced the statutory punishments. Toward the end of May 1750, the fifty-year-old master cobbler Jean Baptiste Faverge locked himself in his fifth-floor room, along with his two little dogs, and hanged himself with a rope attached to a beam above the bed. The neighbours, who were used to seeing him come and go, noticed his absence as well as the stench emanating from his room. When they knocked, the dogs reacted, but Faverge did not. On

Saturday, 30 May, they asked commissioner François Bourgeois to investigate.[19] After assessing the situation, he sent for a locksmith and some guardsmen. They found the corpse hanging off the bed, with the left little finger 'partly eaten.' Bourgeois wrote down but crossed out (without explanation but perhaps out of deference to medical expertise) the following words: 'We also noticed that there was no vestige of the [private] parts of said cadaver, having appeared to us to have been eaten or cut off.' The doctor who examined the body on the same day reported that the 'natural parts' had been 'entirely removed and done away with,' which seemed 'to be done as much through will as torn off by teeth.'[20] On 31 May the *lieutenant criminel* directed Bourgeois to see what he could 'discover' about 'this affair.'[21] When the commissioner recorded the depositions on the same day, the witnesses differed on just one subject, the mutilation of the body. The two neighbours and four of the guardsmen said nothing about it. Two other guardsmen noted the absence of the 'noble parts,' and one of them stated that two left fingers as well as the left ear were 'partly gnawed.' The locksmith used the same phrase, 'noble parts,' and added, without spelling out the scenario, that Faverge had supplied the dogs with bones and water.

At this point, Bourgeois turned the case over to the *lieutenant criminel*, who decided to prosecute. On 12 June, Louis Etienne Desnoyers, the *curateur* (curator) appointed by the Châtelet to speak for the deceased, played the role of devil's advocate, as he was expected to do. He maintained that 'ill-intentioned persons' had hanged Faverge, locked the door, and shoved the key under the door to make it look as if he was responsible for his own death. On 23 June, when Desnoyers confronted the ten witnesses, he repeated that claim more than once.[22] The cobbler had 'no reason' to kill himself and was not 'capable' of doing so. Surely 'others' – 'evil-minded people,' his 'enemies' – were to blame. The judges were not impressed or at least not convinced. They authorized burial on 20 September but convicted Faverge on 3 October. They sentenced him to be dragged through the streets and hanged by the feet in effigy and ordered his property confiscated. The Parlement of Paris confirmed the sentence on 17 October.[23]

It is not clear why the magistrates made examples of Faverge and some, but only some, other men (no women) who committed suicide in the eighteenth century. According to the incomplete but instructive inventory of criminal cases appealed to the Parlement (in the Salle des inventaires at the Archives nationales), the number of prosecutions decreased after 1750 but increased after 1770, perhaps as a result of Chancellor Maupeou's replacement of the *parlements* with less refractory and more 'conservative' tribunals.[24] At the same time, the inventory indicates that the Parlement confirmed most of the sentences pronounced by the Châtelet and other courts within its jurisdiction (a third of the kingdom) in both decades but reduced more sentences in the 1770s than in the 1750s. The trends in jurisprudence are not transparent, especially since we have no documentation about deliberations in criminal cases. In any event, the numbers do not demonstrate linear progress from severity to leniency under the influence of the Enlightenment.

It seems unlikely that any of the men and women who killed themselves in 1750 and 1770 did so because they had read Montesquieu, Voltaire, or Rousseau. The percentage of men increased (from 61 to 73), and the percentage of women decreased (from 39 to 27) over two decades, and this trend continued in 1775. The percentages of married victims, married men, and married women increased but declined in 1775. The average age (of those with specified ages) decreased (from fifty-four to thirty-six), and so did the number in their teens and twenties (from four to zero), but these trends were reversed in 1775. In 1750 and 1770 the vast majority belonged to the working classes: craftsmen, shopkeepers, skilled and unskilled workers, servants, clerks, soldiers, and only one beggar. By 1775 the number of notables had increased significantly.

In 1750, 39 per cent of the victims jumped out the window, and 28 per cent hanged themselves in their rooms. Women were much more likely (57 > 27 per cent) to jump, and men were much more likely (36 > 14 per cent) to hang. In 1770, 27 per cent drowned, 23 per cent jumped, and 23 per cent hanged, with less difference between the sexes. In 1750 and 1770 combined, four men and one woman slashed or stabbed themselves, and two men but no women shot themselves. In 1775, on the other hand, 35 per cent, including the one woman, used knives, and 25 per cent used guns. It would be imprudent to make generalizations based on evidence from just three years, but changes over time, most obviously in the cast of characters and the methods of suicide, might have had something to do with collective anxieties about an epidemic of self-destruction in the 1770s.

After ignoring 'when' (morning was apparently the most popular time of day, and winter was definitely the least popular time of year for suicide) and addressing 'who' and 'how,' what about 'why'? Now and then, witnesses did not know and could not guess what had caused the 'accident.'[25] But more often than not, they had seen and/or heard enough to offer explanations or at least speculations. In most instances, even if they also specified physical or emotional problems, they mentioned mental ones. A journeyman had 'no reason for sorrow or quarrel with anyone'; so he must have hanged himself only because of his 'indisposition.'[26] More typically, after hours, days, or months of illness, the body 'overheated' or 'enfeebled' the mind. Sickness caused the 'delirium' that made one man to jump out the window and the 'mental weakness' that made one woman do the same.[27] Sadness, sorrow, or 'even despair' made a man 'lose his head' and his life.[28] Seven men and one woman lost or at least may have lost their senses in another way, by drinking too much. If the market woman 'had not drunk so much' with her friends, the 'misfortune' of jumping out the window 'would not have happened to her' (as object rather than subject).[29]

Some of the mental problems were provoked by interpersonal difficulties, and others were expressed in imaginary anxieties.[30] One man was distressed because his brother took money from him for weeks, and another was distraught because his wife pursued a lawsuit (for separation of property) against him for months. A third argued with his wife after accepting an informal separation of persons, authorizing her to live on her own and giving her custody of their children. A girl despaired because her parents accused her of not working as much as her younger sister and showered that sister with gifts, including a gold cross that constituted the last straw. A servant who lost her job also lost her mind, and a servant who thought she might lose her job threatened to jump into the well or the river. A stoneworker imagined that doctors wanted to amputate his leg. One woman feared institutionalization by her relatives, and three others feared incarceration in a hospital.[31]

Four individuals were obsessed with and frightened by the prospect of imprisonment, in one case for no reason and in the others for indebtedness, mendicancy (a week after the promulgation of the royal declaration of 20 October 1750 against beggars), or alleged involvement in 'the recent business of the populace,' meaning the 'kidnapping' riots that disrupted Paris in May 1750.[32] The wheelbarrow man Lard worried that the authorities had mistakenly identified him as one of the 'mutineers' who had instigated the 'uprising' by distributing money. He declared that he had no money to distribute and declined to say anything more. The commissioners' papers contain one other remarkable example of the impact of public affairs on the hearts and minds of ordinary Parisians. The retired domestic Bruant was known in his neighbourhood as a 'convulsionary,' a Jansenist who attended clandestine assemblies that sometimes involved strange displays of religiosity.[33] The pious old man jumped out the window in 1770 after his confessor, following the example of zealous clergymen in the 1750s, refused to absolve him because of his unorthodox views.

Witnesses employed an extensive and slippery vocabulary to discuss the causes, nature, and symptoms of mental problems. They used the words loosely; so translations from eighteenth-century French to twenty-first-century English are at best approximate: aberration, absent-mindedness, agitation, anxiety, confusion, debility, delirium, derangement, desolation, despair, distraction, disturbance, fever, frenzy, fury, impairment, insanity, intemperance, lunacy, madness, melancholy, peculiarity, perturbation, vapours, violence, weakness. A few individuals demonstrated their abnormality by talking nonsense, but more did so by expressing themselves in coherent, if sometimes perplexing, terms. A beggar lamented that he was not 'satisfied with his life,' and a student admitted that his life 'was a burden to him.'[34] The student insisted that his (undistinguished) parents were members of the nobility, and a journeyman that his stomach was full of pins. Some not only complained but also threatened. A scribe declared that he would not survive his sorrow and that he had 'to put an end to his pains.'[35] The cobbler Faverge's neighbours did not notice any 'aberration,' but his relatives assured them that he had vowed several times 'to do away with himself.'[36]

Some announced what they intended to do before they did it, and others acknowledged what they had done after they did it. Those who tried and failed to kill themselves had more time but less cause to confess. A woman arrested for wanting to throw herself into the Seine declared she 'never had the intention of doing so,' and a man who tried to hang himself twice in the same day 'denied that he had wanted to do away with himself.'[37] The unhappy girl rescued from the Seine, on the other hand, admitted that she had decided 'to throw herself in so as to perish there.'[38] Several others accepted responsibility for their acts before they died. When asked who was to blame for the state in which he was found, one man pointed to himself. When asked 'in what frame of mind' he had cut his throat, he made unintelligible signs and sounds.[39] Another man managed to tell commissioner Graillard de Graville his name, age, status, place of birth, and place of residence and why he was found lying in the street. He claimed that he jumped out the window because he had been sick for some time. But a witness who heard him make these remarks maintained that they showed that 'he did not have his head about him' and, presumably, should not be taken seriously.[40]

Five individuals tried to make sure that they had the last word about their own deaths by expressing, explaining, or excusing themselves in writing, but the commissioners did not always transcribe the messages. The student Duny left five letters sealed with black wax on a table. Three were addressed to schoolmates, and another to someone who shared his last name (perhaps his father, a musician) at the court of Parma. The scribe Marchand had a letter (as well as a draft memoir) addressed to the *lieutenant général de police* in his pocket. An unidentified veteran asked a wine vendor's wife to mail the letters in which he informed his father and the governor of the Invalides (military hospital) 'that he was going to drown himself.'[41] Louis Jean Lebret, a conscientious postman, handed the letters that he was supposed to deliver to someone else before he deposited his frock coat, vest, and hat on the parapet and jumped into the river. He left a very short note back home with his buckles and watch: 'I commend my wife to my brother and all my friends.'[42] Marie Geneviève Bouloche, a fruit vendor's wife, left two longer notes for her twenty-year-old daughter in pockets in an armoire:[43]

I take my leave of you, having tears in my eyes, and I beg you, my daughter, to continue the business to support your father, your brother, and your sisters, and try to ask [for help from] some good souls who could do you a service. The Lord will reward them. You will tell my brother M[illegible] that he should urge my brother Bouloche to do you some service. Madeleine, I beg you not to abandon your father.

You will urge my nephew T[illegible], him of the ave maria [a confraternity or some other sort of religious association], to loan you some money on security [that] you will give back to him little by little. The Lord will reward him for it. My nephew, I beg you not to abandon my children because they are very much in trouble. Misfortune wished it that I found myself in debt. It was necessary to escape for fear of seeing myself imprisoned. I have gone away without a cent, without a penny. I have taken away nothing but my body and my wretched rags.

By blaming her debts (her daughter estimated them at 15,000 livres) on misfortune and her death (she used the euphemistic language of departure) on necessity, Bouloche minimized or at least mitigated her own responsibility for the problem that she had created and the solution that she had selected. By declaring that she had taken nothing of value with her, she assured her family that she had not done anything more to worsen its financial situation. Lebret did not explain and Bouloche did, but both seemed more concerned about those they abandoned, at the end, than about themselves.

Most of the men and women isolated themselves to commit suicide, by waiting until they were alone in their rooms or by going to the latrine, on an errand, for a walk. One man sent his daughter and grandson away on the pretext that he wanted to sleep for a while. Another man's wife must have had reservations about leaving him alone. She took two of their children to work with her but left the youngest with him. The husband and father sent the boy out to buy some salt and then hanged himself. Most of the victims were on their own at the end, but all of them were connected to others through multiple networks of familiarity and sociability. The witnesses included spouses, parents, siblings, children, aunts and uncles, cousins, nephews and nieces, people who lived on the same floor, in the same building, or in the same neighbourhood, long-time or recent and intimate or casual acquaintances, co-workers, employers, and customers. Relatives, neighbours, and friends observed, listened, consoled, and took care of, and looked out for individuals who ended up killing themselves. One man shared his room and his bed with his brother. One woman lived with her sickly mother, whose husband had abandoned her, and another lived with her sickly aunt, whose husband had predeceased her. A third could not live with or without her feeble-minded grandson. Neighbours helped the elderly up and down the stairs and in and out of bed. Friends visited individuals who were unwell and tranquilized individuals who were upset.

Parisians had another source of support and comfort throughout life and especially in times of sickness and distress: religion. The cobbler Faverge went to mass almost every day. One man carried a breviary, and another carried a crucifix. A third exclaimed, 'My God, take pity on me.'[44] Before they killed themselves, a meat vendor talked to his confessor because he was troubled, and a wine vendor sent for his confessor because he was ailing. After the event, priests arrived in time to administer the sacraments to four individuals who had jumped out the window. In one telling case, the sacraments not only helped the soul on its way to paradise but also helped the corpse on its way to burial. After the wool-worker Jean Moyen jumped into the river, his wife told commissioner Bricogne that she did not know 'how this misfortune happened,' but she was sure he had drowned accidentally.[45] They had been married for twenty-three years, after all, and she had never known him to have any problems that could cause him sorrow. She knew very well, moreover, that he had confessed and communed at Easter and for the jubilee year (1750), 'which proves that it is an accident that is not deliberate on the part of her husband.' A neighbour of the Jansenist Bruant made the same point about religion and suicide when she admitted that she was surprised he had jumped out the window, because 'he was a pious man.'[46]

That neighbour saw Bruant jump from the sixth floor. In other instances, witnesses saw people 'fall' or sometimes 'let' themselves 'fall' out the window or into the river. In just a few cases, witnesses interacted verbally or physically with victims during their last moments. Duny told a schoolmate to leave the room 'if he did not want to see him die.'[47] After trying to persuade him not to carry out 'the bad plan he seemed to have,' the schoolmate ran for help and heard the shot. After embracing her husband, one woman headed for the window and yelled 'leave me alone' at the neighbour who grabbed her petticoat.[48] Two other women, one in a well and the other in the river, seized ropes thrown to them but ignored exhortations to hold on and perished because they let go. Neighbours cut down the man who tried to hang himself twice in one day, but more often than not, witnesses arrived too late to stop or save victims. They heard the noise of bodies falling out windows and landing in courtyards, the groans or cries for help of men and women who did not die quickly, and the shrieks or cries for help of the individuals who discovered the remains. Other deaths, including some hangings and most drownings, came to light well after the fact. A woman whose husband had left for work at 7 a.m. worried when he did not return from work by 6 p.m., and a man whose wife went for a walk with their dog at 3:30 worried when the dog returned at 7 p.m. without her. In both instances, the spouses learned the truth hours later.

Witnesses who recalled how they felt when they observed the act, encountered the corpse, or received the news invariably reported shock, fright, grief, and/or surprise. One, 'upset' by what she had seen, did not know what she was doing but collected herself enough to send for a priest and a doctor.[49] Another, 'frightened' by the servant's body in the kitchen, shouted, 'My God, what a misfortune!'[50] A third, distraught over his wife's death, could not bear to go to the morgue to identify her remains. The other reaction, surprise, is more striking, at least when the deceased had a history of acting and speaking strangely. The rector feared that the unhappy and deluded student might have an 'accident' or do something 'extreme,' and yet he stated that he was 'extremely surprised' by the suicide.[51] The scribe said goodbye to a neighbour, who worried that he might strike a 'bad blow,' but she stated that she 'never' thought 'that he would go so far as to do away with himself.'[52] Whether or not they intended to, witnesses who made such comments excused themselves for not having intervened more expeditiously or efficaciously.[53] The man who provided the most remarkable example of exculpation declared not only that he did not know the cause of his wife's despair but also that he had 'never' given her any 'grounds for complaint.'[54]

Witnesses, of course, were primarily concerned about exculpating relatives, neighbours, and friends who had killed themselves. As indicated above, they claimed that they could not account for some deaths, that many deaths were accidental, and that most victims were not in their right minds. Witnesses did not know how a man found hanged in a locked room 'was strangled' (passive voice), asserted that a woman fell from the fourth floor by mistake, even though she had carefully placed a footstool next to the window and removed her worn red slippers, and insisted that a man who had cut his throat 'did not have his reason at the time.'[55] More often than not, witnesses remembered the events in the past with the needs of the present in mind. With the wisdom of hindsight, they selected and recounted acts and words, which may or may not have struck them in the same way at the time, that documented physical and/or mental problems and culminated in death. These problems did not lead them to expect suicide, which would have required more of them to excuse themselves for not preventing it, but did explain abnormal behaviour that surprised and frightened them. The papers from 1750 and 1770 – who knows about the first half of the eighteenth century and the second half of the seventeenth century? – contain countless variations on the theme of diminished responsibility but not a single animadversion on the subject of suicide. The people who tried to lead the unhappy girl rescued from the Seine away before the guard arrested her were probably influenced by her sex and age, but even witnesses who acknowledged that some took their own lives of their 'own accord' never blamed them.[56] Parisians knew what they were supposed to think, and they presumably thought that suicide was wrong, but they refused or at least declined to condemn the dead. Their connections with and sympathy for the deceased trumped the letter of the law. In this regard, as in so many others, they disregarded religious and secular prescriptions and demonstrated personal and collective agency.

The study of suicide opens a window into the lives and minds of ordinary men and women, those who killed themselves as well as those who talked about those who did so. The papers of the district police commissioners illustrate the intersections of private tragedies with social networks and public affairs and provide raw material for reflections about changes in mentalities.[57] Whether or not the incidence of self-destruction actually increased in the second half of the eighteenth century, many commentators thought it did. Whether or not Parisians more generally thought likewise, they seem to have found suicide more familiar and more thinkable after mid-century – more familiar or even comprehensible inasmuch as they had a standard, if not standardized, mental explanation that they could and did apply to one case after another; more thinkable or even usable insofar as they included suicide in the repertoire of gestures through which humans expressed themselves and maligned others. When the rope broke while the glazier Ménétra was removing debris from a well, someone spread 'vicious rumours that I wanted to do away with myself and that it was out of despair.'[58]

When wives filed complaints against husbands and vice versa, they sometimes accused each other of wanting to take their own lives. More commonly, wives reported that their husbands had threatened to kill them and then themselves. If the men did so, they expected the actual threats to work by scaring their spouses. After telling his wife that he was going to drown himself, a disgruntled silversmith stormed out and walked, not to the river to end his life, but to a café to have a drink.[59] Even if the men did not do so, the women expected the alleged threats to work by damning their spouses. A clerk's wife and a barrister's wife supplemented accusations about verbal and physical abuse by adding charges about suicide threats when they lodged additional complaints.[60] The 91 complaints in 1750 contain only one example of the use of such threats as an index of marital tensions. The 184 complaints in 1770 contain 11, and the 170 complaints in 1775 contain 7.[61] The direct and indirect evidence from the papers of the district police commissioners suggests some change in attitudes during the course of the eighteenth century. Parisians did not condone suicide, because some philosophes did, but they domesticated it, by making it more understandable and imaginable, well before the Revolution decriminalized it.

NOTES

1 Jean-François Marmontel, *Oeuvres complètes*, 7 vols. (Paris: Verdière, 1819–20), 5: 417.

2 *Mémoires secrets pour servir à l'histoire de la république des lettres en France depuis 1762 jusqu'à nos jours*, 36 vols. (London, 1780–9), 5: 171–2 and 177–8.

3 Some of my other articles and essays explore such cases: 'Suicide, History, and Society: The Case of Bourdeaux and Humain, 25 December 1773,' *Studies on Voltaire and the Eighteenth Century*, 2000, 8, 113–57; 'Rousseau's Suicide Note,' *Rethinking History: The Journal of Theory and Practice*, 2001, 5, 447–50; 'Le suicide de Pidansat de Mairobert,' *XVIIIe siècle*, 2003, 35, 331–40; and 'Suicide and Politics in Pre-Revolutionary France,' *Eighteenth-Century Life*, 2006, 30, 32–47.

4 See Albert Bayet, *Le suicide et la morale* (Paris: F. Alcan, 1922), chap. 3; Robert Favre, *La mort dans la littérature et la pensée française au siècle des lumières* (Lyon: Presses universitaires de Lyon, 1978), chap. 11; John McManners, *Death and the Enlightenment: Changing Attitudes to Death among Christians and Unbelievers in Eighteenth-Century France* (Oxford: Clarendon Press, 1982), chap. 12; and Georges Minois, *History of Suicide: Voluntary Death in Western Culture*, trans. Lydia Cochrane (Baltimore: Johns Hopkins University Press, 1999), chap. 8–11. The forthcoming books by Patrice and Margaret Higonnet on intellectual history and Dominique Godineau on social history will supersede all previous work on eighteenth-century France.

5 For ordinary people in the provinces, see Monique Lemière, 'Morts violentes, morts subites dans le bailliage d'Orbec au XVIIIe siècle,' in Paul Dartiguenave et al., *Marginalité, déviance, pauvreté en France, XIVe–XIXe siècles* (Caen: Centre de recherches d'histoire quantitative en l'Université de Caen, 1981), 82–115; and Alain Joblin, 'Le suicide à l'époque moderne: Un exemple dans la France du Nord-Ouest, à Boulogne-sur-Mer,' *Revue d'histoire moderne et contemporaine*, 1994, 42, 85–120.

6 *Lettres de M. de Marville, lieutenant general de police, au ministre Maurepas*

(1742–1747), ed. Antoine de Boislisle, 3 vols. (Paris: H. Champion, 1896), 1: 4, 11, 21, 79, and 207; and 2: 12, 39, 86–7, 92, 102, 120, and 135. The most remarkable case (2: 86–7) involves a mistreated slave (or at least servant) who shot himself in despair. After the manager of the rooming house summoned a priest, the 'negro' accepted baptism and the last rites, despite the objections of his master from Saint-Domingue. Marville mentioned the address (rue Taranne) and the date (27 May 1745); so it should not be difficult to locate the district police commissioner's report. Years later, another black servant hanged himself because he did not want to return to the Caribbean. See Archives nationales, Y series (hereafter 'Y') 16076, 30 August 1775.

7 Charles Philippe d'Albert de Luynes, *Mémoires sur la cour de Louis XV, 1735–1758*, ed. Louis Etienne Dussieux and Eudoxe Soulié, 17 vols. (Paris: Firmin Didot frères, 1860–5); René Louis de Voyer d'Argenson, *Journal et mémoires*, ed. Edmond Jean Baptiste Rathéry, 9 vols. (Paris: Mme veuve J. Renouard, 1859–67); and Edmond Jean François Barbier, *Chronique de la régence et du règne de Louis XV (1718–63)*, 8 vols. (Paris: Charpentier, 1866).

8 Siméon Prosper Hardy, 'Mes losirs, ou Journal des événements tels qu'ils parviennent à ma connaissance,' Bibliothèque nationale, Fonds français 6680, ff. 103, 106, 108–9, 116, 141, 163, 169, 186–7, 195, and 206. I have analysed the 259 cases recorded by Hardy and addressed a variety of issues about numbers, procedures, and mentalities in 'Patterns and Prosecution of Suicide in Eighteenth-Century Paris,' *Historical Reflections/ Réflexions historiques*, 1989, 16, 1–53.

9 Y 14555, 20 September 1770.

10 Y 13675, 19 April 1770; and Y 15843A, 20 August 1770. For another such case, see Y 13963, 3 July 1770.

11 Y 14542B, 7 July 1750.

12 Y 13375, 27 March 1750.

13 Richard Cobb, *Death in Paris: The Records of the Basse-Geôle de la Seine: October 1795–September 1801, Vendémiaire Year IV–Fructidor Year IX* (Oxford: Oxford University Press, 1978).

14 Jeffrey Merrick, 'Suicide in Paris, 1775,' in *From Sin to Insanity: Suicide in Early Modern Europe*, ed. Jeffrey Watt (Ithaca: Cornell University Press, 2005), 158–74.

15 In a few instances, the commissioner conducted the investigation without waiting for instructions from the *lieutenant criminel*. See, for example, Y 13269, 29 June 1770.

16 Y 13781, 16 October 1770.

17 See, for example, Y 11566, 26 April 1750.

18   Marie Madeleine Potet was confined in the Grand Châtelet on 10 April
      and released on 11 May 1750; see Archives de la Préfecture de police, AB
      202. My thanks to Michael Sibalis for locating this information. Commis-
      sioner Delavergée probably sent the fifteen-year-old girl from the
      suburbs to prison because she might jump into the river again and
      because her parents were not there to take her home. Judging from the
      report (Y 13756, 10 April 1750), they probably left her there for a month
      to teach her a lesson. For another case of imprisonment, this time in 1742,
      see *Lettres de M. de Marville*, 1: 79.

19   Y 11932, 30 May 1750.

20   Y 10136, 30 May 1750. For another case of castration, this time in 1745,
      see *Lettres de M. de Marville*, 2: 135.

21   Y 11932, 31 May 1750.

22   Y 10136, 23 June 1750.

23   For that reason, *procureur général* Joly de Fleury instructed Bourgeois not
      to proceed with the sale of Faverge's few possessions, as his heirs, includ-
      ing his wife and two sisters, had requested. See Y 11932, 27 October 1750.

24   For trends in jurisprudence, see Dominique Muller, 'Magistrats français
      et peine de mort au XVIIIe siècle,' *XVIIIe siècle*, 1972, 4, 79–108; and Jean
      Lecuir, 'Criminalité et moralité: Montyon statisticien du parlement de
      Paris,' *Revue d'histoire moderne et contemporaine*, 1974, 21, 444–93. These
      articles, unfortunately, do not explore the effects of the Maupeou 'revolu-
      tion.' Muller sampled the 1760s and 1780s but not the 1770s, and Lecuir
      analysed 1775 but not 1771–74.

25   For example, Y 13781, 16 October 1750; and Y 13781, 16 October 1770.

26   Y 11695, 6 March 1770.

27   Y 13237A, 12 April 1750; and Y 11566, 27 April 1750.

28   Y 11257A, 30 June 1770.

29   Y 14333, 5 January 1770.

30   The papers from 1750 and 1770 do not contain any examples of thwarted
      or jilted lovers but, for 1770, see Hardy, 'Mes loisirs,' ff. 169 and 206.

31   The first of these cases is the only one of the twenty-six in 1770 men-
      tioned by Hardy. He reported that the elderly woman was seventy-seven
      rather than seventy-five and that she hanged herself with ribbon rather
      than thread. He also noted that she was buried by order of the lieutenant
      criminel. See Hardy, 'Mes loisirs,' f. 163. Unlike the other two women, the
      abbé Olive 'did not want to die in his room' and desperately wanted to
      go to the Hôtel-Dieu. See Y 10860, 31 August 1750.

32   Y 11312B, 30 July 1750. On the riots, see Arlette Farge and Jacques Revel,
      The Vanishing Children of Paris: Rumor and Politics before the French Revolu-

tion, trans. Claudia Miéville (Cambridge: Harvard University Press, 1991).

33 Y 10899B, 27 April 1770. On the origins and legacy of the convulsionaries, see Robert Kreiser, *Miracles, Convulsions, and Ecclesiastical Politics in Early Eighteenth-Century Paris* (Princeton: Princeton University Press, 1978).

34 Y 14310, 30 October 1750; and Y 15054B, 15 October 1750.

35 Y 11489, 28 September 1770.

36 Y 11932, 30 May 1750.

37 Y 11695, 11 March 1770; and Y 15469, 29 October 1770. The woman was released into the custody of her husband, but it is not clear what happened to the man, who had previously looked for a knife in order to kill himself.

38 Y 13756, 10 April 1750.

39 Y 11187, 21 August 1770.

40 Y 10784B, 30 October 1770.

41 Y 15073, 28 August 1770.

42 Y 15842A, 4 March 1770.

43 Y 11257B, 2 October: 'Je vous fait mes adieux ayant les larmes aux yeux et je vous prie ma fille de continuer le commerce pour soutenir votre pere votre frère et vos soeurs et tachés de prier quelques bonnes ames qui puissent vous rendre service le seigneur fera leur récompense vous direz a mon frere M[?] qu'il prie mon frere Bouloche de vous rendre quelque service. Madeleine je vous prie de ne point abandonner votre pere.'

'Vous priez T[?] mon neveu celui de lave maria de vous preter quelquargent sur gages vous lui remettrez petit a petit le seigneur lui en rendra recompense. Mon neveu je vous prie de ne point abandonner mes enfants car ils sont bien dans la peine. Le malheur en a voulu que je me suis trouvée en dette. Il a fallu me sauver de crainte de me voir emprisonnée. Je me suis en allé sans sols sans deniers. Je n'ai rien emporté que mon corps et mes mechantes guenilles.'

44 Y 11257A, 30 June 1770.

45 Y 13103A, 27 June 1750.

46 Y 10899B, 27 April 1770.

47 Y 15054B, 15 October 1750.

48 Y 14333, 5 January 1770. For another such case, see Y 13237A, 12 April 1750.

49 Y 10899B, 27 April 1770.

50 Y 12594, 27 July 1750.

51 Y 15054B, 15 October 1750.

52 Y 11489, 28 September 1775.

53 Unlike the brother and niece of a master cobbler who reported that he had drowned himself out of despair 'because he was in misery' but did not explain why they did not do something to help him. See Y 10900B, 11 December.
54 Y 14310, 30 September 1750.
55 Y 12194, 9 October 1750; and Y 11187, 26 August 1770.
56 Y 10784, 7 March 1770.
57 Suicide is not mentioned in Michel Vovelle, 'Le tournant des mentalités en France, 1750–1789: La sensibilité pré-révolutionnaire,' *Social History*, 1977, 2, 605–29; or Roger Chartier, *The Cultural Origins of the French Revolution*, trans. Lydia Cochrane (Durham: Duke University Press, 1991).
58 Jacques Louis Ménétra, *Journal of My Life*, ed. Daniel Roche, trans. Arthur Goldhammer (New York: Columbia University Press, 1986), 175–6. In the first line of the next paragraph, Ménétra noted that 'it was around the time' of the marriage of the future Louis XVI and Marie-Antoinette, which took place on 16 May 1770.
59 Y 12987B, 7 May 1770.
60 Y 11705, 13 April 1775 (second complaint); and Y 15842B, 20 January 1771 (fourth complaint).
61 Even with adjusted figures (for the difference in the number of commissioners in the two years), the number of examples increased much more dramatically than the number of complaints.

4 The Medicalization of Suicide: Medicine and the Law in Scotland and England, circa 1750–1850

RAB HOUSTON

The results of English coroners' inquests into suicidal deaths have long attracted attention, both in prominent individual cases and in aggregate. An inquest decided on the state of mind (and thus the culpability or otherwise) of a person judged to have died by his or her own hand. People guilty of their own self-murder (*felonia de se*) could be subject to forfeiture of movable estate until 1870 and profane burial – a legal but not statutorily sanctioned punishment – until 1823. Those found *non compos mentis*, lacking wrongful intent, suffered no official penalties. That there had been a major shift in coroners' verdicts on suicide between the mid-seventeenth and the mid-eighteenth century was written about in the nineteenth century, mostly by lawyers.[1] In the sixteenth and early seventeenth centuries nearly all suicides were found *felo de se*; after about 1750 nearly all were *non compos mentis*.

Michael MacDonald sought in 1986 to use that change as an indicator that understandings of suicide became medicalized, secularized, and decriminalized.[2] Yet he is wrong to state that for England at 'some point during the mid-eighteenth century the men of middling rank who served as coroners' jurors adopted the medical interpretation of suicide.'[3] Indeed, as MacDonald himself points out and as will be shown here, medical men almost never supported juries' automatic link between suicide and insanity. It is surprising then that he can claim, 'Medical opinion certainly provided the main rationale for suspending the old penalties for suicide.'[4] Finding someone *non compos mentis* on the basis of the act of suicide alone was no more a respectable medical judgment than it was a tenable legal (or philosophical) one, something that both doctors and lawyers (as well as philosophers) recognized.

In MacDonald's account of changing understandings of suicide (and most others), secularization and medicalization go hand in hand.[5] For George Rosen, the nineteenth century saw suicide 'considered less in moral and theological terms and increasingly as a social and medical problem.'[6] Explicitly or implicitly, medical analysis is a part of the modernization process, science substituting for religion, clinical discourses supplanting religious ones, and doctors replacing clergymen as the interpreters of self-destructive behaviour. Social differentiation, the rise of science, individualism, and pluralism combine to replace the moral absolutes of earlier ages characterized by pervasive religious cultures.[7] Thus for Michel Vovelle, discussing 'the triumph of the cemetery,' 'morality and religion gave way to health.'[8] For Foucault, 'the sacrilege of suicide was annexed to the neutral domain of insanity.'[9]

Some authorities have gone further, seeing a restructuring of power relationships that placed medical professionals in a privileged position over society. Medical priorities came to dominate social ones, and medical interpretations superseded all others. Expressed in Habermasian terms, medicalization is 'the progressive expropriation of health from the public sphere and its relocation in an exclusive professional domain ... [P]reexisting social understandings of and responses to such basic human experiences as pain, illness, and death are seen to be displaced by arrangements that both produce and legitimate a narrower set of expert interventions.'[10] People were either forced or persuaded to accept growing medical involvement in many areas of life, or they decided to do so for their own reasons. However, it is also possible to see a wider context for medicalization as it entered and influenced the broader society. For Paul Weindling, this meant 'the extension of rational, scientific values in medicine to a wide range of social activities.'[11] Social and moral pathologies came to be expressed as signs or symptoms of a disease. More particularly, Roger Smith sees the history of forensic psychiatry as part of the modernization of societies, belonging with other 'attempts to achieve order, regularity, and predictability in modern social organization.'[12] Science was encroaching on all sorts of public discourses in the nineteenth century, and the treatment of 'deviances' such as suicide was only a part of that broader medicalization.[13]

MacDonald's scenario relies in part on a modern intuitive association of suicide with some level of mental dysfunction. Such a biomedical understanding is not without an historical basis. Towards the end of a section on suicide in a 1788 book on female health, the undistinguished surgeon and male midwife William Rowley seemed to express a common view: 'As no rational being will voluntarily give himself pain, or deprive himself of life ... it follows, that every one who commits suicide is indubitably *non compos mentis*, not able to reason justly; but is under the influence of false images of the mind, and therefore suicide should ever be considered an act of insanity.'[14] Rowley's argument was a fashionable philosophical, rather than a medical, one, even if he dressed it up in technical terms. Such a view was certainly current, but contemporaries were more likely to mix different levels of explanation, as did Rowley. Indeed, a 'pure' medical interpretation of suicide was unusual before James Cowles Pritchard's *Treatise on Insanity* in 1835, which introduced the idea of 'moral insanity' leading to 'irresistible impulse,' and Étienne Esquirol's *Des maladies mentales* in 1838, which was influenced by Pritchard.[15] For Esquirol, suicide was always a symptom of mental illness, and thus understanding it was solely an aetiological matter. Suicide, for him, came out of a psychopathology whose causes were biological, not social. Earlier studies such as Jean Pierre Falret's *De l'hypochondrie et du suicide* of 1822 blended 'internal' causes such as hereditary predisposition with external social and other factors (including 'civilization' or urbanization).[16] Indeed, all early modern interpretations of suicidal behaviour potentially had a medical component to them, from the celebrated early seventeenth-century writings of Robert Burton and even earlier in those of the Elizabethan Timothy Bright.[17]

Further, the medical tendency of the early nineteenth century was only one strain of thought. It was contested at the century's end by Émile Durkheim and his followers, who emphasized the impact of *social* processes on the propensity to commit suicide. Writing in 1930, Maurice Halbwachs argued that only a minority of suicides were insane and that most suffered not from medical problems but from social isolation. For Halbwachs, the effect of mental disorder was indirect, separating the individual from his or her environment, including the social supports that might prevent suicide.[18] Beginning in the eighteenth century, debates around the social and moral or the alternative psychological interpretations of suicide pervaded French academia, and Tony Giddens reports, 'In terms of sheer bulk of material, suicide was probably one of the most discussed social problem of the nineteenth century.'[19] It remained subject to social and moral judgments as much as to medical ones until at least the 1960s in Britain.

A full discussion of the alleged secularization of suicide is beyond the scope of this chapter. It focuses more narrowly on the opportunities for understandings of suicide to become medicalized in the investigative systems of two component parts of the United Kingdom. It makes three related arguments: that the involvement of medical practitioners in uncovering or certifying suicide was limited to the forensic side and to physical signs, rather than psychological symptoms; that doctors and lawyers were highly discriminating in their understanding of the relationship between insanity and suicide; and that the understandings of suicide for lay people became medicalized only in a growing expectation that medical men would be involved in the physical care of attempted suicide and in the identification of suicidal death as different from accidental, natural, or homicidal. Scottish suicide was more medicalized than was English, but in rather specific ways that came out of the different professional status of doctors in the contrasting civil societies of the two countries. The treatment here is weighted towards Scotland, as the English procedure is well known and because there are a number of reasons why the Scottish context should have produced greater medical involvement. All were noted by contemporaries, both those who sought to reform the English system and advocates of the Scottish procedures.

Both at the present day and in the historic past, sudden or suspicious death is dealt with differently in Scotland and England. Between 1194 and 1926 suspicious deaths in England were investigated by a coroner working in public with a jury of approximately twelve men on the view of a corpse. Until 1895 suspicious death in Scotland was investigated in private by warrant of sheriffs or their deputies. Scotland had 27 sheriffdoms around 1800, compared with some 330 coroners in England.[20] Scottish magistrates took a 'precognition' designed to uncover the cause of death and therefore to determine if a case needed to be sent to a procurator fiscal (crown prosecutor) for criminal action or (in the case of suicide) could be allowed to lapse because there was no ground for any judicial process.[21] The decision was based on opinion received from Crown counsel (a triad of legal officials). After 1855, when opinion had come from counsel, it was passed to the district registrar to record the death.

The Scottish procedure, more centralized and supervised (and more closely accountable for spending) than that in England, took cognizance of the possible agency, but not the culpability, of the dead person. State of mind, where relevant to survivors, was assessed in a civil court, not as part of the investigation of death, unless it contributed to a presumption of self-murder rather than murder by

another. The penalties for wilful self-murder were forfeiture of mov-
ables (to 1949 but in reality only up to the mid-eighteenth century) and
some sort of popular or judicial desecration of the corpse (without
explicit sanction of law), which was still visited on some suicides up to
the Edwardian era. The aim of the procedure was not (as in France) to
identify a 'suspect' but to determine whether (and in what sense) the
body was a victim.[22] Nor was it the same as in England (or Wales or
Ireland, which both followed English law and practice).

Prior to the eighteenth century, information that triggered an
inquest in either country came primarily from lay people: family,
neighbours, friends, or those who had come casually upon a stranger's
dead body. Only from the end of the eighteenth century were 'police'
(meant as constabulary) routinely involved, though witness depositions suggest that the first reaction of those who found dead bodies
was to publicize the fact to someone in authority; it was also usual to
fetch a physician or surgeon if there was any chance of the person surviving or being resuscitated. On the night of 15 February 1772 John
Moncreiff, a weaver from the village of Broughton outside Edinburgh,
was going home when he was attracted by the sound of 'snoring.' The
noise emanated from the attempts to breathe of Stewart Spence, 'a lad
or young man' whom he found sitting on the road with his throat cut
and vomiting blood; Moncreiff called a surgeon.[23] Officials came to
play more of a role in nineteenth-century Scotland, and writing in the
1890s, the advocate R.W. Renton (himself a sheriff) opined that initial
information normally came from the police and only 'in cases of difficulty or delicacy' did it come directly from members of the medical
profession.[24] Nevertheless, the information that set off the taking of a
precognition came mainly from laity or legal officials.

Once the process had started, an investigating magistrate could
make personal inquiry into any deaths not obviously natural, 'obtain-
ing any medical assistance which he may consider necessary or desirable.'[25] In Scotland it had been both possible and routine since the sixteenth century to summon medical men to testify about cause of death,
physicians and surgeons being called in by Scottish magistrates to
pronounce on wounds or to open cadavers. In the towns this process
was easy because most surgeons and physicians lived there and
because their guild privileges, still active even in the early nineteenth
century and including a range of exemptions from taxation and civic
duties such as jury service and billeting, were 'paid for' by obligations
to the civic body (in all senses of the word).[26] Medical men were part

of the political as well as the social world of the Scottish burgh. Edinburgh surgeons, for example, had an absolute duty to act for the magistrates of the city, 'in so far as concerns the Judgement and Sight of their Craft.'[27] Over time, involvement of medical professionals became routine if there was any doubt that the death was natural. At the end of the eighteenth century Peebles Sheriff Court recorded the following rules for investigating deaths: 'When any dead body is found with the appearance of violence upon it, or where any person dies, and is suspected to have died by violence, the dead body must be opened, and also the head, and a report made of the cause of the death of the person by physicians and surgeons.'[28] Violence here was the illegitimate use of force: the most common synonym for self-murder in early modern Scottish documents is 'laying violent hands in him/herself,' regardless of the method adopted.

At the stage of a precognition, medical participation was confined to pronouncing on physical evidence, as the Peebles extract makes clear. Precognitions that found suicide do not usually survive among documentation because no further process occurred, but in the few that have been located, medical testimony deals solely with the physical causes of death. While opinions from Crown counsel survive in numbers from the 1820s, it is not until the 1840s that a source exists which offers systematic national coverage of suicide. The earliest two surviving registers of sudden or suspicious deaths ('Reports of Deaths') brought to the notice of the Crown Office cover the period 1848–57 and contain notices of approximately 5,000 deaths, of which 224 men and 100 women were suicides.[29] These are brief abstracts, recording bare facts, such as cause and place of death, and the outcome of Crown counsel's deliberations. In just one case was a person's suicide described as happening 'while insane': John Mair at Aberdeen in early May 1850.[30]

That doctors' involvement was principally with physical pathology is evident in the most influential medical lectures in the British Empire during the first half of the nineteenth century. With nine out of every ten British medical graduates around 1800 coming out of Edinburgh, the influence of medical and legal training in that city on English practitioners and academics is clear; through migration, it also had a profound impact on colonial and post-colonial countries throughout the world.[31] The first professor of forensic medicine in England, John Gordon Smith, acknowledged this, as did George Edward Male. Smith wrote in 1821 of medical jurisprudence: 'in Britain it has been suffered to remain in relative obscurity until this day.'[32] 'It has been a just reproach to England that, although she set the example to other nations of bring to its present state of perfection, the system of "trial by jury," she has allowed them to take precedence in the cultivation of medical jurisprudence.'[33]

The flowering of medical education in Georgian Scotland is well known. Professor Andrew Duncan senior began teaching forensic medicine in 1792, as professor of the Institutes of Medicine at Edinburgh University (1790), and published *Heads of Lectures on Medical Jurisprudence* in 1795; in 1801 he began a series of public lectures on medical jurisprudence and medical police and in that year published *Heads of Lectures on Medical Police*. Duncan was influenced by Continental writings and practice, but he produced a version suited to his own political environment, where doctors advised magistrates and advances in public health (such as lunatic asylums) were driven more by private philanthropy than by state intervention. The lack of an absolutist state in Britain, which may partly explain the line Duncan took, did not mean that politics were irrelevant to the symbiotic development of law and medicine in Scotland. Duncan was a Whig, a party popular in Scotland but eclipsed nationally by the Tories in the late eighteenth and early nineteenth century. The Whigs' brief period in power in 1806–7 allowed a number of reforms to be instituted, including a charter for the lunatic asylum at Morningside (to become the Royal Edinburgh Hospital) and the establishment of the chair of Medical Jurisprudence and Medical Police (forensic medicine) at Edinburgh. The chair's title shows the subordination of medicine to law, and the appointment was in the Faculty of Law, which was more Whig-inclined than that of Medicine. Nevertheless, politics continued to play a powerful role in medicine and its development. When seeking to reinforce Robert Christison's claim to the chair of medical jurisprudence in 1821, the principal of Edinburgh University, George Baird, wrote to his patron, Robert Dundas, second Viscount Melville, of 'the soundness of Dr Christison's *political* opinions & principles': 'In an *University* it is of the last [utmost] importance.'[34]

The development of medical jurisprudence and medical police in Scotland was shaped by that country's distinctive political values and in particular the enduring strength throughout the nineteenth century of Whiggism, or Liberalism. Duncan Forbes has called the tendency within that ideology 'scientific Whiggism': a belief in the Enlightenment ideal of progress coupled with a critique of existing socio-political structures and a desire for innovation.[35] The foundation of a second Regius chair of medical jurisprudence (Glasgow, 1839) also occurred during a Whig administration, as did the first lectureship at Aberdeen (made into a chair in 1860).[36] Medical jurisprudence was moved to the Faculty of Medicine at Edinburgh in 1825 and became a part of the medical curriculum in 1833, the year after Christison moved to the chair of materia medica. Making medical jurisprudence compulsory raised both the standing of the subject and the status and remuneration of its teachers.[37] Finally, from 1856 candidates for admission to the Faculty of Advocates had to take a course in medical jurisprudence. Scottish Whigs liked juries. The advocate John Peter Grant wrote condemning the latitude given to judges at the Court of Session, and following this attack, the English system of random selection 'from a jar' was introduced in 1825.[38] Yet juries were never adopted as part of the investigation of suspicious deaths.

Medical men involved with suicide were cautious about psychologizing. The fifth edition of T.R. Beck's *Elements of Medical Jurisprudence* (1836), which ran to over a thousand pages, was dedicated to Robert Christison.[39] Beck was professor of the Institutes of Medicine and lecturer on medical jurisprudence at the College of Physicians and Surgeons of the Western District of New York.[40] Christison was professor of medical jurisprudence at the University of Edinburgh between 1822 and 1832. He posed the problem of identification in his lectures at Edinburgh around 1830: 'it is very rarely possible to distinguish suicide from accident in a satisfactory manner. But this is a matter of little consequence if both can be distinguished from murder.'[41] Christison laid out in great detail how to distinguish between a natural and an unnatural death and how to identify the agent in the latter.[42] There were 'circumstances external to the body': where it was found, marks on surrounding objects (belonging to the deceased or otherwise). Was there a weapon to hand, and if so, did it fit the wound? Was there only one kind of weapon and what kind? Cudgels and axes, for example, more usually indicated murder. If there was no weapon, could the deceased have disposed of it? For the body itself, clothes, attitude, expression, and skin needed to be considered among presumptive proofs.[43] Suicide injuries were rarely on the back and not often on the left side; shooting was usually in the head, stabbing usually in chest rather than the belly or throat; unless delirious, suicides generally only inflicted a single wound on themselves.[44] Clothing was usually disordered with murder victims, whereas 'those who commit suicide take great care of their clothes, and even sometimes fold them neatly on their chair beside them.'[45] 'It is very common for example for girls who drown themselves to leave behind them their shoes, shawl and bonnet.'[46] Did the death take place behind a locked door? Another (inconclusive) indicator was that suicides usually picked secluded spots close to public areas, whereas murderers were opportunist.[47] Beyond these indications, and almost as an afterthought, investigators had to attend to 'the habits and state of mind of the deceased – his liability to insanity, his worldly prospects, his profession and manner of life.'[48] 'If he was subject to mental derangement, chagrined by misfortune, transported by anger, addicted to intoxication or liable to fits of epilepsy or fainting,' then the death may be accident or suicide.[49] A history of mental abnormality *might*, with other evidence, point to suicide, but there was no automatic connection. In short, no cause of death was intrinsically suicidal, but certain forms were more likely to be self-inflicted. For example, asphyxia was usually presumed to be suicide, even if it could sometimes be accidental or murderous – if it was not judicial.[50]

Approving of Continental practice and of Scottish as 'better calculated to secure a full investigation and correct results,'[51] Christison gave short shrift to the quality of investigation conducted by English coroners. He stated that 'the medical facts of cases are collected in a very meagre and imperfect manner, and that the opinions delivered by medical people in their examinations are often hasty, vague and erroneous.'[52] He did not stop there. Despite widespread discussion of suicide in British society, Christison dismissed academic analysis of the topic, instead referring his students to works in German and French: 'There is not any English work of value on the medico-legal relations of the subject.'[53]

It is easy to agree with Christison. Early English texts in forensic medicine were basic and focused on physical symptoms, often failing to discuss suicide at all. When in 1788 Samuel Farr published a much-abridged translation of J.F. Faselius's *Elementa medicinae forensis* (Geneva, 1767), it included no mention of suicide.[54] The omission may have been deliberate. When in 1836 Alfred Swaine Taylor, lecturer on medical jurisprudence and chemistry at Guy's Hospital, wrote *Elements of Medical Jurisprudence*, he could express relief that the question *'Was the drowning the result of accident, of suicide, or of homicide? ...* fortunately does not commonly fall within the province of the medical jurist. It is generally determined by the verdict of the jury from the circumstances proved on the trial.'[55] Indeed, Taylor positively celebrated the lack of specialist input from English medical men in cases of death by drowning. 'It is only from circumstances, sometimes of a moral and sometimes of a physical nature, that we can judge of the fact; and, therefore, the medical jurist is no better provided with the means of deciding, than those who are concerned in the administration of the law.'[56] This pronouncement was flatly against Christison, who roundly condemned the lay (and disapproved of aspects of the legal) emphasis in decision making. 'If what I have said of the vague notions the unprofessional entertain of madness be correct, a jury might just as well assume that they were qualified to decide upon the mortality of wounds, or on evidence of poisoning.'[57] The tradition of combining medical and legal training in Scotland made Scottish-trained doctors more aware of the broader social, legal, and moral implications of their work than was the case for their English counterparts. Directed by Christison (and by their own instinct for preserving their reputations), doctors eschewed all but the most painfully cautious psychological commentary in suicide investigations and in criminal trials.[58]

Christison's commentary is harsh but fair. In England medical witnesses were rarely used, and most decisions were made by coroners and their lay juries on the basis of common-sense standards of proof and on evidence derived from people other than medical professionals.[59] In English inquests and trials, medical and other facts were determined through oral examination and cross-examination of witnesses by coroner, jury, and counsel for parties, without written reports; either side could call medical witnesses.[60] The level of medical independence in England was therefore slight. English doctors were usually the employees of an interested party and, when they spoke before English coroners' inquests, did so to legitimize conventional 'popular' understandings. For example, when Miss Allan's brother took an overdose of laudanum in May 1824, the Durham doctor consulted opined that, during a drinking bout the night before, bad wine had 'caused a stupor or inflammation of the brain' and thus created a temporary insanity.[61] This diagnosis, which resembles part of Robert Burton's early seventeenth-century analysis of the physiology of melancholy, served the needs of the family and that of the coroner's jury.[62] Doctors might be useful for authenticating lay opinions rather than for the critical (academic or professional) purchase that their understandings of insanity and suicide might offer.[63] Their formal involvement was rare. Only 9 medical men are included among 103 witness depositions before inquests in part of Cumberland between 1690 and 1830, appearing in 7 cases of 111, and their testimony was heard in only 1 case out of 28 suicides at Berwick-upon-Tweed in the years 1745–1833.[64]

Most medicalization narratives posit the steady progress of professionalization, but in reality the status of medical practitioners and medical testimony ebbed and flowed. Hal Cook has argued that even in the seventeenth century, physicians' learned interventions were being devalued in favour of remedies for diseases rather than pastoral advice on lifestyle.[65] Paradoxically, the role of medical experts may also have been more independent in the early eighteenth century than in the later. Counsel was not institutionalized at English criminal trials until 1836, but its use became increasingly common from the 1730s. The development of adversarial trials during the eighteenth century involved a subordination of doctors to partisan legal control, something to which Christison was alert, as he had been brought up in a legal system where counsel had been routinely appointed for all defendants since the sixteenth century.[66] He warned his audience more than once to beware of lawyers' attempts to solicit an opinion on the basis of one piece of evidence. 'Lawyers are in the habit of taking your opinion upon such evidence as they can themselves collect, and of relying upon their own ingenuity to discover the validity both of that evidence and of your opinion.'[67]

Until the second quarter of the nineteenth century, the appearance of medical men at coroners' inquests in England was normally at the behest of an interested party. Detailed analyses of toxicology and pathology, of the kind routine in eighteenth- and early nineteenth-century Scottish investigations, rarely surfaced in English inquests, medical men pronouncing primarily on wounds that caused death or the contents of stomachs in the case of suspected poisoning. In contrast, the Roman–canon law system of the Continent lacked juries and required written records of proceedings as well as references to authorities when justifying decisions, all of which helped to create a privileged position for medical evidence – and promoted the development of scholarship on medico-legal proof.[68] On the Continent only the court's official expert could present evidence, usually in writing, and if he did appear personally, only the judge could question him. The differences between the systems highlight varying understandings of judicial, as opposed to scientific, proof; the supremacy of legal over scientific judgments; and the status of legal, compared with medical, practitioners. Where English criminal prosecutions before the nineteenth century depended on private initiative, Scotland had public prosecutors from an early date, and even when professional police were introduced, the Scottish judicial system only became more firmly in the grasp of lawyers. The greater security and social importance of procurators fiscal and sheriffs-substitute pulled medical men along with them.[69] Thus in the Victorian period medical witnesses in Scottish criminal trials became more privileged: they had to be examined separately, but they were allowed to hear the general evidence adduced in court; any testimony they gave had to be on a matter of opinion, not fact.[70]

Criticisms of English coroners are widely known. Writing in 1893, R.W. Renton thought the English system of investigating sudden deaths 'alike cumbrous and expensive.'[71] Contemporaries recognized that Scottish procedure was more sophisticated than English, and some reformers sought to model their proposals on Scotland. In the 1830s important legal and administrative developments occurred, such as a new police force, civil registration, remuneration for medical witnesses, and penalties for non-attendance at inquests. From 1836, for example, English coroners had the power to order and pay for medical examination and testimony, yet only a few authorities such as Manchester ever employed specialist medical investigators; the legislation did not guarantee that the coroner would be reimbursed for them, a major disincentive to hold an autopsy in doubtful cases.[72] The mid-Victorian lobby for better forensic medicine never succeeded in securing the system of investigating suspicious deaths found on the Continent, though it was nearly successful in 1859.[73]

Coroners themselves were elected by the freeholders (as most county ones were) or appointed (in boroughs); in either case, appointments were for life, though coroners were removable for dereliction. The appointment of coroners was usually a routine matter but sometimes spilled over into the political arena.[74] Coroners were generally lawyers, though the only formal qualification was to be an independent freeholder, and generalists rather than experts continued to provide medical examination and testimony.[75] Possibly because of Scottish influence, one coroner for Northumberland for forty-one years was W. Scott, MD, replaced by a surgeon, William F. Pearson, in June 1803.[76] County coroners received fees and expenses for inquests into all types of death only from 1752 (from 1487 they had only been paid for murder and manslaughter investigations) and became salaried officials as late as 1860.[77]

With only its strengths paraded by English reformers, it is worth noting that the Scottish system also had its flaws. For example, Renton ignored the limitations of cost on Scottish procurators fiscal, who had to balance investigation and prosecution against potential accusations of extravagance.[78] Public prosecutors in Scotland were accountable for how money from the public purse was spent. Concern about being labelled profligate may have encouraged procurators to find a death accidental: two doctors were needed for a Scottish autopsy, both requiring fees, and a suicide (or any other death deemed suspicious) would cost more to investigate. Procurators fiscal had to fund a medico-legal inquiry out of a limited supply of rogue money and, in the case of fatal accidents (when fatal accident inquiries began), out of their own funds. Only if the case went up to the Justiciary Court would the procurator's costs be met from central funds. Those suicide pre-cognitions that survive (such as that of Stewart Spence, mentioned above) look like cases that were in the public eye or involved public officials. When means of death can be aggregated, they were more 'violent' than in England (more hangings and use of knives, notably by women), again suggesting that only cases that could not be interpreted otherwise were dealt with by formal investigation. Financial consider-ations may also explain why the rate of post-mortems in nineteenth-century Scotland was lower than England. The comparatively late arrival of death registration (and death certification), not to mention the slow development of policing (constabulary) in Scotland, made it easier to escape the official gaze, especially in remoter areas, and there were numerous complaints from the Registrar General's examiners (inspectors) after registration arrived in 1855 that procurators fiscal were not acting on their information and were failing to investigate suspicious deaths.[79]

Much as it was criticized, the English system had its advocates, especially at the popular level. At the death near Edinburgh of Sir James Standsfield in 1688, an alleged suicide later proven to be murder, expatriate Englishmen called for a public investigation. Standsfield ran a cloth-making enterprise in East Lothian using many English workers. The villain was his son Philip, who was subsequently tried, convicted, and executed for his murder. 'The pannal [accused] did refuse to send for a chyrurgion, and to let his fathers body be sighted, though the minister, and others did expressly demand it; and the *English men* in the *Manufactury*, who were acquainted with the *Crowner-Laws*, they made a mutiny anent the burial, till the corps were sighted, yet the pannal caused bury the corps that same night without shewing them.'[80] Contrary to the claims of the Englishmen, the Scottish system did allow for public 'sighting' of bodies, usually by laying them out in a church for identification and scrutiny. Standsfield's body was exhumed and examined by medical men, accompanied by magistrates (and the son), on the orders of the High Court of Justiciary. It was this examination which made it apparent that Standsfield had been throttled before being dressed and thrown in a river to simulate suicide by drowning. Among other proofs adduced was cruentation, strongly defended by the presiding judge and apparently a powerful influence on the guilty verdict.

The advantages of the English system that Standsfield's expatriate workers clamoured for were its more obligatory investigations and its open and participative quality, both in the election of coroners and in the use of juries. It was thus more socially and politically responsive than the Scottish or Continental model.[81] The campaign to replace the coroner's inquest with something closer to the Scottish or Continental model in the 1850s and 1860s was not driven by the same forces as promoted greater medical involvement in Scotland. Instead, it reflected the desire of English magistrates to reduce the political embarrassments posed by coroners' juries. Prominent among these were findings about death in custody, as suicide remained common in prison in the mid-nineteenth century.[82] Another example is juries' creative use of the medieval device of deodands to punish corporate negligence over accidental deaths during the 1830s and 1840s.[83] Yet coroners' juries remained a necessary part of any English inquest until 1926. Medical expertise had political value too in England in an age when sentencing policy increasingly came under scrutiny. Forensic medicine had political uses for Benthamite reformers by introducing an element of doubt into proceedings and thus preventing what some perceived to be an inhumane outcome.[84]

The distinction between coroners and police, understood as 'polis' or civic government in a Scottish context, may be less than is conventionally assumed.[85] Scottish Police Acts, which covered public health and amenity as well as public order, were administered by police commissioners elected by local property owners and funded by their taxes.[86] There was more accountability than was found on the Continent. Yet aspects of Scottish procedure could also work against medicalization, notably its relative secrecy. Scottish procedure had the further benefit of discretion. Renton proclaimed that 'the privacy, which forms such an essential feature in all Scots criminal procedure, is maintained. The police reports are private, the witnesses are examined privately, and out-with the presence of each other, and the reports by the procurator fiscal and opinions of counsel thereon are also confidential.'[87] The effect on understandings of suicide in society at large was considerable. In the north of England eighteenth- and early nineteenth-century newspapers routinely used the outcomes of coroners' inquests to report suicides. The full spectrum of social classes is therefore included. In Scotland newspapers seldom reported self-killing, and when they did, they tended to be selective of the young, women, the poor, and the criminal, their commentary reinforcing moral messages about the superiority of a middle-aged, male, bourgeois or landed lifestyle. The other mass medium of the early nineteenth century, broadsheets or strips, focused on the suicides of ruined young women.

Where Scottish newspapers did offer more coverage was of *attempted* suicide (and of fatal and non-fatal accidents), something less commonly included in northern English papers prior to the nineteenth century. Inquest results were easy to come by, as they were in the public domain and came from a known source, whereas attempted suicides required more legwork. Here the emphasis *was* medical, but not in the sense of psychological insights. In about a third of Scottish newspaper reports of completed suicide, some reference to mental state is made (such as melancholy, lunatic, low-spirited, or deranged). These references must reflect the influence of English trends in coroners' verdicts, because this finding had no legal value in Scotland, and it was not something the procurator fiscal was charged to do. In comparison, two-thirds of English suicides reported in the *Cumberland Pacquet* (1774–1824) and the *Newcastle Courant* (1711–1823) mention mental state. Importantly, such mentions were uncommon prior to the 1780s in England. Coming two generations after the change in verdicts was more or less complete, this development shows that newspapers lagged far behind the changes they reported and cannot be construed as opinion leaders in this part of the alleged process of medicalization. However, in the case of attempted suicide, where the person lived, two-thirds of reports in both regions mention that medical assistance or 'proper assistance' was sought. The same is true of the reporting of accidents, and it suggests that newspapers helped to reflect and to create the expectation that physicians and surgeons would be employed. As a contribution to medicalization, it was more an addition to what Roy Porter called the 'polyphonous voices of lay medicine' than to professionalization.[88] Added to these factors was, of course, the increased advertisement in newspapers of a growing range of medical services.[89] Such publicity may have continued a trend towards the use of medical practitioners that had begun in the sixteenth century.[90]

English newspapers did sometimes imply that propensity to suicide was a sign of mental disability, accepting the intuition that drove coroners' juries' verdicts. For Scottish newspapers an accused or convicted criminal who tried to kill himself simply advertised his guilt. What did doctors say when they were asked about the connection between madness and suicide? Two forums that can be analysed are medical literature and insanity defences, offering both normative and positive angles. There were certainly medical men in England who went into print to argue that the verdict of *felo de se* was unjustified and should be abolished 'owing to insanity being present in every instance.'[91] These were the words of Forbes Winslow, writing in 1840 because, as he states in the preface to his book, a paper he gave to the Westminster Medical Society provoked 'animated discussion.'[92] The reason for this response was that most doctors flatly disagreed with Winslow, who, while a member of Royal College of Surgeons of London and with a growing public profile as an 'expert' in the field of insanity, was not a qualified surgeon and did not get his MD until 1849. In fact, most medical professionals were deeply ambivalent about the routine association made by coroners' juries – just as Winslow found himself caught between a search to understand and an impulse to condemn. Thus in 1857 the *Irish Quarterly Review* opined that a 'great difference of opinion exists among high medical authorities on the question, whether the mere act of self-destruction is in itself a proof of insanity.'[93]

What looks like evidence of a generalized association between madness and suicide may simply have been its identification in a particular case by an individual doctor. In 1784 William Hunter argued that a pregnant single woman who killed herself and her unborn child should not be held responsible because she acted 'under a phrenzy from despair.'[94] This frenzy was comparable with fever or lunacy. But Hunter had in mind a certain type of woman, who could be moved to kill herself or her child by noble feelings. He envisaged, not 'a worthless woman' who is 'insensible to infamy,' but one of 'respectable virtue' possessing 'a high sense of shame.'[95] With a distinct moral edge, Hunter's commentary is both emotive and socially selective. It drew on a revival of classical ideas of the nobility of certain types of suicide, which, while fashionable in some circles, proved deeply repugnant to others. In 1800 the Reverend Christopher Hodgson, who was also a magistrate, published a detailed refutation of the notion that infanticidal mothers were necessarily deranged, attacking William Hunter's moral judgment as well as the legal implications of such an attitude; Hunter's medical credentials were hardly considered, a sign of the status of medicine in this debate.[96]

Whatever its flaws, Hunter's article also showed a discriminating judgment about propensities towards violence. By the late eighteenth century and probably before, doctors were aware that it was mainly a certain type of deranged person, the melancholic, who killed her or himself, while in other species of insanity (except perhaps those involving delusions or hallucinations) self-destruction was quite unusual.[97] Asylum admission petitions, mostly filled out by lay people, reinforce this perception. Of 467 admissions to Glasgow Royal Asylum in the years 1815–22, 10 per cent had tried to kill themselves and 7 per cent threatened or talked about it. These figures are close to those offered for Buckinghamshire asylum entrants in the years 1853–81 but slightly higher than the 14 per cent (combining all with destructives tendencies of any kind) found for Lancaster Asylum in 1842–3.[98] Not surprisingly, medical men connected with asylums noted the same distinction. One Victorian medical superintendent, George Savage, speculated that no more than 5 per cent of entrants were 'actively suicidal,' a figure that corresponds with the 4 per cent of entrants to two mid-nineteenth-century Oxfordshire asylums studied by Parry-Jones.[99] Anne Digby has written of the nineteenth-century York Retreat, 'Suicidal propensities were frequently recorded but suicides themselves were rare.'[100] The first statement is unfortunately vague, but the second seems to hold true for most asylums. Early and mid-nineteenth-century asylum documents confirm that not all suicidal people were insane and not all insane people were suicidal.

Nearly two decades after William Hunter's article, another Dr Hunter developed court experience and was questioned before the March Assizes at York in 1803 about the state of mind of a homicidal man. He explicitly stated that the accused, Philip Samuel Maister, was 'evidently depressed in his spirits.' For Hunter, 'such a state of mind certainly often terminated in suicide, but he had never known any one in a similar situation to commit violence on others.'[101] Hunter suggested that a certain type of lunacy tended to culminate in suicide but that that sort did not usually involve doing harm to others. He rejected a necessary connection between madness and suicide or between insanity and violence. The thrust of his opinion was that Maister's insanity did not excuse his actions.

Critics of the English coroners' inquest often pointed to the fiction or 'amiable perjury' of finding a suicide *non compos mentis* in order to protect the individual's name and property.[102] Outside this domain, doctors such as Hunter had a much more robust approach to the connection between insanity and suicide that included decisions with much weightier consequences. There was none more ponderous than whether a man lived or died, yet successful insanity defences never relied solely on suicidal tendencies to indicate mental incapacity.[103] Witnesses who thought a person mad, including medical men, had to establish by other means that the person they sought to excuse was not responsible for his or her actions. In 1770 William Harries, formerly a merchant in Ayr, was tried for forgery of the banknotes of the Thistle Bank of Glasgow.[104] He escaped from custody but was recaptured, and only then did he start to behave oddly. His counsel entered an insanity defence, but Harries was found to be feigning madness and was eventually hanged. Numerous indicators of his sanity and insanity were given, but at no point was his attempted suicide mentioned in the court processes. It is cited only in newspaper accounts and then as a news item on its own.[105] Harries's sanity was proved by the testimony of three (lay) men and a woman who worked in Edinburgh's 'tolbooth,' or gaol.

However, trials where insanity defences were deployed did sometimes give physicians and surgeons the opportunity to express their scepticism about the connection between suicide and madness. When John Stewart was on trial for his life at Perth for the murder of his wife in 1833, a number of witnesses gave evidence to prove that he 'had formerly attempted to commit suicide, – that he was subject to epileptic [*sic*] fits, – and that he was insane.' However, others said the exact opposite, including Dr Ma'colm, physician in Perth and also physician to Murray's Royal Asylum there, who 'thought him perfectly sane when he first saw him, anid [*sic*] is of the same opinion still; does not hold an attempt to commit suicide an infallible proof of insanity.'[106] This was the opinion that prevailed, and Stewart was sentenced to death. There can be few more compelling indicators of the stance that doctors took on the alleged association between suicide and insanity.

This chapter offers a more restricted understanding of medicalization in the eighteenth and nineteenth century than was suggested by some of the influential authorities cited in its introduction. Professional medicine became an accepted part of everyday life, and it gained an institutional presence, at least in Scotland.[107] However, the nature of that acceptance is not what conventional interpretations of the medicalization of suicide would have us believe. Roger Smith has suggested that the relative coherence of modern psychiatry developed from very varied, often local, knowledge and usages.[108] The problem of presenting a united front was painfully evident to eighteenth- and early nineteenth-century practitioners. 'The difficulty was that medicine, doctors, and medical practice *per se*, enjoyed neither prestige nor power. At the levels of ideology, social organisation, and intellectual content, medicine was, many of its practitioners recognised, inconveniently vague, of unproven efficacy, lacking consensus, and unable to command widespread respect.'[109] Psychological interpretations had long been part of explanations of suicide, but doctors (and lawyers) continued to struggle to know how to deal with them, even in the Victorian age. As was the case with other conditions that would later become psychologized (such as homosexuality/sodomy, as Ivan Crozier has shown), medical practitioners preferred to deal in signs rather than symptoms, in the physical rather than the mental.[110]

Medicine in Scotland advanced its contribution to forensic science partly by ring-fencing the level of its involvement in the identification of suicide, confining it to corporeal pathology and to the material context in which the body was found. English doctors struggled to free themselves from a popular association between insanity and self-murder, which in turn arose from the public, participative, and broadly political nature of coroners' inquests rather than from any specifically (and certainly not any new) medical input. Arguably, doctors denied popular 'medical' (or rather, emotional, philosophical, and pragmatic) interpretations in favour of a much more discriminating association of madness and suicide based on observation. Their discourse of suicide clashed with that of their public. As Akihito Suzuki has recently put it, English psychiatric practitioners of the mid-nineteenth century 'tried hard to adapt themselves to ... the dual mastership of the family and the public [magistrate]' and were also caught between 'endorsing the old family-dependent diagnostic pattern and ... insisting that the diagnosis was a scientific one.'[111] Suzuki argues that psychiatry was profoundly 'domestic' in origins and practice until deep into the nineteenth century, incorporating rather than replacing lay information in the rendition of medical evidence.[112] This finding supports earlier interpretations of the long-established nature of 'domestic psychiatry' and of the dominance of lay and non-resident medical authentication of insanity over asylum doctors; it also pushes the origins of a professionally medicalized English psychiatry into the age of Freud and beyond.[113] Martin Weiner and others have suggested that 'from the turn of the 1880s, medical opinion coalesced around a picture of the suicide as a product of mental defect, inherited or acquired,' but in truth, debates continued into the twentieth century.[114]

In Scotland the role of medical practitioners at the bedside was much the same as in England, but their relationship to non-familial sources of authority was different. Physical medicine had gained a coherence and credibility by the end of the eighteenth century (and perhaps long before that), developing both a routine social acceptability and an institutional presence in alliance with the law. Prestigious chairs at Glasgow and Edinburgh created academic standing for the subject, while close associations with the administration of public order and public health at both a policy-making and a practical level guaranteed legal medicine's institutional and social status. For example, Robert Christison was both a professor at Edinburgh University and medical adviser to the Crown in Scotland from 1829. He was also the first chief medical officer of the Standard Life Insurance Company from 1825, and one lecture reflected his actuarial interests.[115] While still subordinated to the law (and lawyers suffered as much as other Whigs from the political dominance of Henry and Robert Dundas in the late eighteenth and early nineteenth century)[116] Scottish forensic medicine enjoyed a stronger political position and a higher social status than was the case in England. English doctors struggled to achieve that same rank – including those trained in Scotland, who may have chaffed at the structured dependence of their position after listening to lectures on forensic medicine at Scottish universities. Both Scotland and England lagged behind Continental systems of investigation, where physicians early on appropriated to forensic science issues dealt with in courts of law.[117] As these courts made provision for expert medical testimony, the medical profession developed reliable forensic tests of state of mind and mental capacity, which rested on responsibility and capability – tests not standardized until the 1840s in Britain. This chapter has suggested that for psychological medicine, as displayed in the handling of suicide, the search for standing and coherence in both Scotland and England was continuing, albeit at different paces, as late as the mid-nineteenth century.

NOTES

I should like to thank the conference participants and also Mike Barfoot, Anne Crowther, Ivan Crozier, John Weaver, and David Wright for comments on earlier drafts of this chapter. The research on which it is based is funded by a Major Research Fellowship from the Leverhulme Trust.

1 R.S. Guernsey, *Suicide: history of the penal laws relating to it in their legal, social, moral, and religious aspects, in ancient and modern times* (New York: L.K. Strouse & Co., 1883); S.A.K. Strahan, *Suicide and insanity: a physiological and sociological study* (London: Swain Sonnenschein & Co., 1893).
2 M. MacDonald, 'The secularization of suicide in England, 1660–1800,' *Past & Present* 111 (1986), 50–100.
3 M. MacDonald and T.R. Murphy, *Sleepless souls: Suicide in early modern England* (Oxford: Clarendon Press, 1990), 114.
4 Ibid., 198.
5 J.R. Watt, 'Introduction,' in Watt, ed., *From sin to insanity: suicide in early modern Europe* (Ithaca: Cornell University Press, 2004), 8.
6 G. Rosen, 'History in the study of suicide,' *Psychological Medicine* 1 (1971), 267–85, at 280.
7 H. McLeod, *Secularisation in western Europe, 1848–1914* (London: Macmillan, 2000), 1–3.
8 M. Vovelle, Mourir autrefois ([Paris]: Gallimard, 1974), 201; my translation. For another example, see T.W. Laqueur, 'The places of the dead in modernity,' in C. Jones and D. Wahrman, eds., *The age of cultural revolutions: Britain and France, 1750–1820* (Berkeley: University of California Press, 2002), 17–32.
9 M. Foucault, *Histoire de la folie à l'âge classique* (Paris: Gallimard, 1972), 108–9; my translation.
10 I.A. Burney, *Bodies of evidence: medicine and the politics of the English inquest, 1830– 1926* (Baltimore: Johns Hopkins University Press, 2000), 10; S. Sturdy, *Medicine, health and the public sphere in Britain, 1600–2000* (London: Routledge, 2002). There is a large body of writing on medicalization. See, for example, R.A. Nye, 'The evolution of the concept of medicalization in the late twentieth century,' *Journal of the History of the Behavioural Sciences* 39 (2003): 115–29.
11 P. Weindling, 'Medicine and modernization: the social history of German health and medicine,' *History of Science* 24 (1986), 277.
12 R. Smith, 'The law and insanity in Great Britain, with comments on Con-

tinental Europe,' in F. Koenraadt, ed., *Ziek of Schuldig? Twee Eeuwen foren-sische Psychiatrie en Psychologie* (Utrecht: Rodopi, 1991), 247.

13 R. Smith, 'The boundary between insanity and criminal responsibility in nineteenth century England,' in A. Scull, ed., *Madhouses, mad-doctors and madmen* (London: Athlone, 1981), 364–75.

14 W. Rowley, *A treatise on female, nervous, hysterical, hypochondriacal, bilious, convulsive diseases; apoplexy and palsy; with thoughts on madness, suicide, etc* (London: C. Nourse, 1788), 343.

15 J. C. Pritchard, *Treatise on insanity and other disorders affecting the mind* (London: Sherwood, Gilbert and Piper, 1835). J. C. Pritchard, *On the different forms of insanity in relation to jurisprudence* (London: H. Ballière, 1842). E. Esquirol, *Des maladies mentales considérées sous les rapports médical, hygiénique et médico-légal*, 2 vols. (Paris: J.B. Baillière, 1838).

16 J.P. Falret, *De l'hypochondrie et du suicide – considerations sur les causes, sur le siege et le traitement de ces maladies* (Paris: Croullebois, 1822). See B. Gates, 'Suicide and the Victorian physicians,' *Journal of the History of the Behavioral Sciences* 16 (1980), 164–74, for a valuable brief outline of medical writing on suicide and insanity in Britain, and A. Giddens, 'The suicide problem in French sociology,' *British Journal of Sociology* 16, 1 (1965), 3–18, for French approaches from the late eighteenth century, and H.I. Kushner, 'Suicide, gender, and the fear of modernity in nineteenth-century medical and social thought,' *Journal of Social History* 26, 3 (1992–3), 461–90, for British, French, and American writing.

17 R. Burton, *The anatomy of melancholy* (1621), edited in 3 vols. by T.C. Faulkner, N.K. Kiessling, and R.L. Blair (Oxford: Clarendon Press, 1989–94). T. Bright, *A treatise of melancholie. Containing the causes thereof, & reasons of the strange effects it worketh in our minds and bodies: with the phisicke cure, and spirituall consolation for such as haue thereto adjoined an afflicted conscience* (London: Thomas Vautrollier, 1586). A. Gowland, 'The problem of early modern melancholy,' *Past & Present* 191 (2006), 77–120. A. Gowland, *The worlds of Renaissance melancholy: Robert Burton in context* (Cambridge: Cambridge University Press, 2006).

18 Halbwachs, *Les causes du suicide*, discussed in Giddens, 'Suicide problem,' 6–8.

19 Giddens, 'Suicide problem,' 4.

20 A.E. Whetstone, 'The reform of the Scottish sheriffdoms in the eighteenth and early nineteenth centuries,' *Albion* 9 (1977): 61–71. V. Bailey, *This rash act: suicide across the life cycle in the Victorian city* (Stanford: Stanford University Press, 1998).

21 A.V. Sheehan, Criminal procedure in Scotland and France (Edinburgh:

HMSO, 1975), 220–1; Death and the procurator fiscal (Crown Office, 1998).

22 A. Joblin, 'Le suicide à l'époque moderne. Un exemple dans la France du nord-ouest: à Boulogne-sur-Mer,' *Revue historique* 129, 1 (1994), 89.

23 Edinburgh City Archives, McLeod Bundles, DO113, item 30 (1772).

24 R.W. Renton, 'The investigation of cases of sudden death in Scotland,' *Juridical Review* 5 (1893), 167–74, 168.

25 Ibid., 168.

26 H.M. Dingwall, *Physicians, surgeons and apothecaries. Medicine in seventeenth-century Edinburgh* (East Linton: Tuckwell Press, 1995). J. Geyer-Kordesch and F. Macdonald, *Physicians and surgeons in Glasgow. The history of the Royal College of Physicians and Surgeons of Glasgow, 1599–1858* (London: Hambledon Press, 1999).

27 National Archives of Scotland (hereafter NAS), JC4/1, 110–12 (17 July 1799). The surgeons were complaining about being routinely included on jury lists. See also R.A. Houston, Social change in the age of Enlightenment: Edinburgh, 1660–1760 (Oxford: Oxford University Press, 1994), 34.

28 NAS, SC42/23/2. The volume covers 1758–92, but the regulations are similar to those covering other aspects of the sheriff courts published in 1749. See *Regulations proposed to be observed in the sheriff and stewart courts of North Britain* (Aberdeen: J. Chalmers, 1749).

29 NAS, AD12/11–12.

30 NAS, AD12/11, p. 26.

31 J.C. Mohr, *Doctors and the law: medical jurisprudence in nineteenth-century America* (Oxford: Oxford University Press, 1993), 3–7; R. McManus, 'Freedom and suicide: a genealogy of suicide regulation in New Zealand, 1840–2000,' *Journal of Historical Sociology* 18 (2005), 430–56.

32 J.G. Smith, The principles of forensic medicine (London: T. &. G. Underwood, 1821), vi; G.E. Male, *Epitome of judicial or forensic medicine* (London, 1816).

33 Alfred Swaine Taylor, *Elements of medical jurisprudence* (London, 1836), 1.

34 Quoted in L.S. Lacyna, *Philosophic Whigs: medicine, science and citizenship in Edinburgh, 1789–1848* (London: Routledge, 1994), 83.

35 Ibid., 23.

36 M. Greenan, 'The forensic medicine archives project at the University of Glasgow archives,' *Scottish Archives* 11 (2005), 19–25.

37 Mohr, *Doctors*, 5–6.

38 J.P. Grant, *Some observations on the constitution and forms of proceeding of the Court of Session in Scotland; with remarks on the Bill now depending in the House of Lords for its reform* (London, 1807); N.T. Phillipson, *The Scottish*

Whigs and the reform of the Court of Session, 1785–1830 (Edinburgh, 1990).

39 The first edition was published in 1825; see Mohr, *Doctors*, 15–28.
40 J. Glaister, 'The evolution, development and application of modern medico-legal methods,' *Glasgow Medical Journal* 109 (1928), 417–37, at 418.
41 Edinburgh University Library (hereafter EUL) Dk.4.57, 'Asphyxia III: death by hanging' ff. 47–47v.
42 EUL Dk.4.57, 'Death from external injuries V: How to distinguish those produced by accident, by the individual himself, or by another,' ff. 15–30.
43 Ibid., ff. 15–16.
44 Ibid., ff. 17v, 20–20v.
45 EUL Dk.4.57, 'Asphyxia III: death by hanging,' f. 49v.
46 EUL Dk.4.57, 'Asphyxia IV: death by drowning,' f. 85.
47 EUL Dk.4.57, 'Asphyxia IV: death by drowning,' ff. 84–84v.
48 EUL Dk.4.57, 'Asphyxia III: death by hanging,' f. 51v.
49 EUL Dk.4.57, 'Asphyxia IV: death by drowning,' f. 90v.
50 EUL Dk.4.57, 'Asphyxia III: death by hanging,' ff. 28–30.
51 EUL Dk.4.57, 'Medical reports, medical evidence,' f. 5v.
52 EUL Dk.4.57, 'Medical reports, medical evidence,' f. 5.
53 EUL Dk.4.57, 'Death from external injuries V,' f. 27v. By the end of the 1830s medical periodicals and publications generally had begun to contain detailed accounts of forensic examinations. See J.R. Cormack, *Remarks on a case of suicide, published by Dr P.D. Handyside in CXXXIV of the* Edinburgh Medical and Surgical Journal; *intended to show that he has erroneously ascribed the cause of death to air in the organs of circulation* (Edinburgh: John Carfrae & Son, 1838).
54 S. Farr, *Elements of medical jurisprudence: or, a succinct and compendious description of such tokens in the human body as are requisite to determine the judgement of a coroner, and of courts of law, in cases of divorce, rape, murder, &c.* (London: T. Beckett, 1788).
55 Taylor, *Elements of medical jurisprudence*, 143. Taylor did hold wounds to be the medical jurist's province; see ibid., 341.
56 Ibid., 144.
57 EUL Dk4.57, 'Of Disqualifications,' 20.
58 R.A. Houston, 'Professions and the identification of mental incapacity in eighteenth-century Scotland,' *Journal of Historical Sociology* 14, 4 (2002), 441–66.
59 T.R. Forbes, *Surgeons at the Bailey: English forensic medicine to 1878* (New Haven: Yale University Press, 1985).
60 EUL Dk4.54, 'Medical reports, medical evidence,' ff. 1–5v.

61 Durham University Archives, Wharton 754.

62 Gowland, *Worlds of Renaissance melancholy*, 81.

63 R.A. Houston, 'Therapies for mental ailments in eighteenth-century Scotland,' *Proceedings of the Royal College of Physicians of Edinburgh* 28 (October, 1998), 555–68; R.A. Houston, 'Rights and wrongs in the confinement of the mentally incapable in eighteenth-century Scotland,' *Continuity and Change* 18, 3 (2003), 373–94. For a recent statement of the growing consensus around this point for England, see A. Suzuki, *Madness at home: the psychiatrist, the patient, and the family in England, 1820–1860* (London: University of California Press, 2006).

64 Cumbria Record Office, Whitehaven, D/LEC/CRI/1-139. Berwick-upon-Tweed Record Office, C14/1-15.

65 H.J. Cook, 'Good advice and little medicine: the professional authority of early modern physicians,' *Journal of British Studies* 33 (1994), 1–31.

66 J.H. Langbein, The origins of adversary criminal trial (Oxford: Oxford University Press, 2003); J.P. Eigen, *Witnessing insanity: madness and mad-doctors in the English court* (New Haven: Yale University Press, 1995); S. Landsman, 'One hundred years of rectitude: medical witnesses at the Old Bailey, 1717–1817,' *Law and History Review* 16, 3 (1998), 445–94.

67 EUL Dk4.57, 'Of Disqualifications,' 39; see also 5, 19–20.

68 M. Clark and C. Crawford, 'Introduction,' in Clark and Crawford, eds., *Legal medicine in history* (Cambridge: Cambridge University Press, 1994), 1–21, at 6.

69 M.A. Crowther, 'Scotland: a country with no criminal record,' *Scottish Economic and Social History* 12 (1992), 82–5.

70 J.H.A. MacDonald, *A practical treatise on the criminal law of Scotland* (Edinburgh: William Paterson, 1877), 479–80. This was an exception to the general rule that witnesses should speak to facts rather than give opinions.

71 Renton, 'Investigation of cases of sudden death,' 167.

72 Bailey, *This rash act*, 50.

73 O. Anderson, *Suicide in Victorian and Edwardian England* (Oxford: Clarendon Press, 1987), 36.

74 G.H.H. Glasgow, 'The election of county coroners in England and Wales circa 1800– 1888,' *Journal of Legal History* 20, 3 (1999), 75–108.

75 In 1892, 247 of 331 coroners were lawyers. Physicians or surgeons appointed as coroners had to give up private practice, but lawyers did not. See H.R. Bickerton and R.M.B. Mackenna, *A medical history of Liverpool from the earliest days to the year 1820* (London: J. Murray, 1936), 148.

76 *Newcastle Courant* 6611 (25 June 1803). At the same time the bishop of

Durham appointed Thomas Patten esq. of Ryton as coroner for Chester ward.

77 R.F. Hunnisett, 'The importance of eighteenth-century coroners' bills,' in E.W. Ives and A.H. Manchester, eds., *Law, litigants and the legal profession* (London: Royal Historical Society, 1983), 126–39, at 126.

78 Renton, 'Investigation of cases of sudden death,' 167; Crowther, 'Scotland,' 84.

79 I owe this information to Anne Crowther.

80 *The tryall of Philip Standsfield, son to Sir James Standsfield, of New-milns, for the murther of his father, and other crimes libell'd against him, Feb. 7. 1688* (Edinburgh: heir of Andrew Anderson, 1688), 12; emphasis in original.

81 S. Cooke, 'A 'dirty little secret'? The state, the press, and popular knowledge of suicide in Victoria, 1840s-1920s,' *Australian Historical Studies* 31 (2000), 304–24.

82 J. Sim and A. Ward, 'The magistrate of the poor? Coroners and deaths in custody in nineteenth-century England,' in Clark and Crawford, eds., *Legal medicine in history*, 245–67.

83 E. Cawthon, 'New life for the deodand: coroners' inquests and occupational deaths in England, 1830–46,' *American Journal of Legal History* 33 (1989), 137–47; T. Sutton, 'The deodand and responsibility for death,' *Journal of Legal History* 18 (1997), 44–55. A deodand was literally something given to God: it was the instrument of any death, deliberate or accidental, which was forfeited to the Crown for pious uses.

84 Clark and Crawford, 'Introduction,' 8.

85 P.E. Carroll, 'Medical police and the history of public health,' *Medical History* 46 (2002), 461–94, esp. 466–9.

86 B. White, 'Training medical policemen: forensic medicine and public health in nineteenth-century Scotland,' in Clark and Crawford, eds., *Legal medicine in history*, 145–63, at 149.

87 Renton, 'Investigation of cases of sudden death in Scotland,' 168.

88 R. Porter, 'Lay medical knowledge in the eighteenth century: the evidence of the *Gentleman's Magazine*,' *Medical History* 29 (1985), 138–68.

89 H. Dingwall, '"To be insert in the Mercury": medical practitioners in the press in eighteenth-century Edinburgh,' *Social History of Medicine* 13 (2000), 23–44.

90 I. Mortimer, 'The triumph of the doctors: medical assistance to the dying, c.1570–1720,' *Transactions of the Royal Historical Society* 6th series 15 (2005), 97–116.

91 F. Winslow, *The anatomy of suicide* (London: Henry Renshaw, 1840), 337.

92 Ibid., v.

93 'Suicide: its motives and mysteries,' *Irish Quarterly Review* 7 (1857), 50.

94 W. Hunter, 'On the uncertainty of the signs of murder, in the case of bastard children,' *Medical Observations and Inquiries* 6 (1784), 266–90, at 271.

95 Ibid., 270.

96 C. Hodgson, *A letter from a magistrate in the country, to his medical friend at Peterborough : occasioned by the writer's perusal of his friend's extracts from the late Doctor William Hunter's paper 'On the uncertainty of the signs of murder in the case of bastard children'* (Peterborough: C. Jacob, 1800).

97 See, for example, National Library of Scotland, ABS.4.88.14, 'Proof for the defender, in the process of declarator ... Walker v. Macadam,' p. 3. See also Anderson, *Suicide*, 383–4; Bailey, *This rash act*, 52–3; A. Shepherd and D. Wright, 'Madness, suicide and the Victorian asylum: attempted self-murder in the age of non-restraint,' *Medical History* 46 (2002), 187–9. For Ireland see M. Finnane, *Insanity and the insane in post-famine Ireland* (London: Croom Helm, 1981), 150–3.

98 Shepherd and Wright, 'Madness, suicide and the Victorian asylum,' 183, 195n, though the Surrey asylum they analysed had a higher proportion of nearly a third, and private asylums had lower at about one-seventh. See also J.K. Walton, 'Casting out and bringing back in Victorian England: pauper lunatics, 1840–70,' in W.F. Bynum, R. Porter, and M. Shepherd, eds., *The anatomy of madness: essays in the history of psychiatry*, vol. 2 (London: Tavistock, 1985), 141.

99 Shepherd and Wright, 'Madness, suicide and the Victorian asylum,' 177; W.L. Parry-Jones, *The trade in lunacy: a study of private madhouses in England and Wales in the eighteenth and nineteenth centuries* (London, 1971), 218.

100 A. Digby, *Madness, morality and medicine: a study of the York Retreat, 1796–1914* (Cambridge: Cambridge University Press, 1985), 198.

101 W.M. Medland and C. Weobly, *A collection of remarkable and interesting criminal trials, actions at law, &c.*, 2 vols (London: John Pearmain, 1808), 1: 159.

102 W.W. Westcott, *Suicide: its history, jurisprudence, causation and prevention* (London, 1885), 45.

103 D.J. Adamson, 'Insanity, idiocy and responsibility. criminal defences in southern Scotland and northern England, c1660–1830' (PhD thesis, St Andrews University, 2004).

104 NAS JC3/36.

105 *Edinburgh Advertiser* 637 (6 February 1770); *Glasgow Journal* 1489, 1501, 1502 (February 1770).

106 *[Report of trials at] Perth [Justiciary] Circuit [Court], Wednesday 17th April 1833* [n.p.].

107 J.C. Burnham, 'How the concept of profession evolved in the work of historians of medicine,' *Bulletin of the History of Medicine* 70 (1996), 1–24.

108 Smith, 'Law and insanity,' 247–81.

109 L. Jordanova, *The sense of a past in eighteenth-century medicine* (The Stenton Lecture, 1997. University of Reading, 1999), 5.

110 I. Crozier, '"All the appearances were perfectly natural": the anus of the sodomite in nineteenth-century clinical discorse,' in C.E. Forth and I. Crozier, eds., *Body parts: critical explorations in corporeality* (Oxford: Lexington Books, 2005), 65–84; I.A. Burney, 'Testing testimony: toxicology and the law of evidence in early nineteenth century England,' *Studies in History and Philosophy of Science* 33 (2002), 289–314.

111 Suzuki, *Madness at home*, 69, 183.

112 Ibid., 63–4.

113 G.N. Grob, *Mental illness and American Society*, 1875–1940 (Princeton: Princeton University Press, 1983); H.I. Kushner, 'American psychiatry and the cause of suicide,' *Bulletin of the History of Medicine* 60 (1986), 36–57; L. Zedner, *Women, crime and custody in Victorian England* (Oxford: Oxford University Press, 1991), 83–90; D. Wright, 'The certification of insanity in nineteenth-century England and Wales,' *History of Psychiatry* 9 (1998), 267–90.

114 M. Weiner, *Reconstructing the criminal: culture, law, and policy in England*, 1830–1914 (Cambridge: Cambridge University Press, 1990), 266; Gates, 'Suicide and the Victorian physicians.'

115 M. Moss, *The building of Europe's largest mutual life company: Standard Life, 1825–2000* (Edinburgh: Mainstream, 2000).

116 Jacyna, *Philosophic Whiggs*, 23.

117 French tribunals did not have to call on medical experts, and they did not have to accept their testimony. It was in Germany that the purest model of 'medical police' existed, and it was in Germany that the first lectures on legal medicine were delivered (at Leipzig in 1642). See P.N.F. Malle, *Histoire médico-légale de l'aliénation mentale* (Strasbourg, 1835); J.W.H. Conradi, *Beitrag zur Geschichte der Manie ohne Delirium* (Göttingen, 1835); E. Fischer-Homberger, *Medizin vor Gericht: Gerichtsmedezin von der Renaissance bis zur Aufklärüng* (Berne: Hans Huber, 1983); W. Cummin, 'Practice of forensic medicine as conducted in this and other countries,' *London Medical Gazette* 13 (1834), 951–2; K. Lande, 'Forensic medicine in Europe – legal medicine in America,' *New England Journal of Medicine* 215 (1936), 826–34.

5 Death by Suicide in the British Army, 1830–1900

JANET PADIAK

In the 1830s and 1840s the British army began to analyse the first collections of data on the sickness and mortality of ordinary soldiers, and it found that peacetime soldiers stationed in Britain had a mortality rate that was double that of civilian males of similar age.[1] In the cause-by-cause analysis, the statistics also showed that soldiers had a suicide rate greater than that of their civilian peers. This disparity existed despite the 'healthy warrior' effect: the fact that the soldiers were screened for superior physique and absence of signs of disease before enlistment and were therefore expected to exhibit lower mortality rates than civilian males.[2] In addition to a healthy start to their military careers, the soldiers were cared for by a system designed to keep them at a high level of fitness through superior nutrition and comprehensive medical care while in the army. During the nineteenth century, several analysts speculated on the reasons for the high suicide levels, suggesting that a combination of factors, such as dislike of military life, long length of service, drunkenness, and fear of punishment, contributed to a soldier's despair.[3] As well, the proximity of weapons allowed the unhappy soldier the means of self-destruction. This chapter is part of a comprehensive study that has investigated morbidity and mortality from all causes among British soldiers during the nineteenth century using published and unpublished army records and statistics. Suicide in the Victorian army is analysed against the total mortality burden of the time. Patterns in suicides are considered relative to changes in the terms and conditions of the soldiers' environments for the period from 1830 up until the end of the nineteenth century.

The army's approach to mortality was <u>pragmatic</u>; suicide was an unfortunate event, like any other death, but it occurred against a back-

Culture of death

ground of high mortality driven by excessive deaths as a result of infectious disease. Effective manpower was crucial for the army, and those who were incapacitated or lost because of sickness or death were considered a drain on the resources of the system. In the last four decades of the nineteenth century, the soldiers' mortality rate declined because of reductions in febrile diseases, respiratory diseases, tuberculosis, and most other causes. Suicide ranked eighth or ninth in the top ten causes, causing fewer deaths than cardiovascular disease but more deaths than cancers. But as overall mortality declined and the number of deaths resulting from injury, homicide, accident, and suicide remained constant, suicide rose in importance and ranking. With continued improvements in prevention, detection, and treatment of disease in the twentieth century, deaths from suicide remain a problem and in some modern armies suicide is now one of the top two or three causes of death.[4] However, unlike the nineteenth-century army, modern armies take positive preventative measures to reduce the potential for suicide.[5]

I

The nineteenth-century British army was a volunteer force, attracting young men between the ages of eighteen and twenty-two, largely from rural areas of Scotland and Ireland as well as England. Enlistment motivation varied. Some young men sought a life in the army because they possessed a sense of adventure and had a desire to serve their country and see the world. For others, especially those without a trade, the army offered the only way that they could ensure a roof over their heads and meat in their diet. In poor economic times, the number of men offering themselves to the army would swell, particularly with men who possessed few skills.[6] Other motives for enlistment included escape, from either family problems or debt. The regiment occupied the role of the master over a training apprentice; this meant that its rights superseded those of a soldier's wife or creditors. A man who wished to exit from an unhappy marriage could join a regiment and be free of the marriage's financial and familial responsibilities.[7] Recruits had to pass a physical examination. The exam certified that he was free of physical defects such as flat feet, poor vision, or varicose veins, showed no signs of disease, and met minimum standards such as height and chest width.[8]

Taking on the colours of the regiment did not ennoble a young man in the eyes of Victorian society; soldiering was deemed suitable only for its most undesirable members.[9] The societal aversion to the military had been reinforced by the absence of conflict at home or abroad in the decades following the end of the Napoleonic threat. Demobilization after the victory at Trafalgar had left many Peninsular War veterans penniless and disabled. Paupered old soldiers visibly swelled the number of beggars.[10] The long peace found many garrisons full of idle soldiers with little practical purpose other than occasional convoy duty and imposition of order in local affrays; their noisy after-hours pursuits increased the army's reputation for harbouring raucous and immoral men. Year after year, Parliament reduced defence expenditures. No barrack, fortification, or equipment improvements were made because substandard conditions seemed suitable for such brutish men. In 1852 the threat of Russia to the Ottoman Empire prompted a response by France and Britain. A criminal lack of planning revealed the government's and society's callousness towards soldiers. Once in the theatre of war, troops discovered that they lacked vital supplies. Parliamentary inquiries reversed the neglect, and in 1858 the Army Medical Department was created to improve the welfare of the ordinary soldier. Nevertheless, the public continued to believe that soldiers sprang from the lowest grade of people.[11]

The lack of funding was not the only basis for the view of soldiering as an unsuitable profession for a respectable young man; absence from family life was seen as a great and undesirable sacrifice. Before the introduction of shorter service in the 1870s, a soldier served a minimum of twelve years with the regiment. About half of his enlistment would be spent in colonial stations, and family leave was rarely possible. Marriage was only a distant possibility for an ordinary soldier.[12] It required the permission of the regimental commander, and when that was given, the soldier and his spouse were provided with married quarters, rations, and, in the event of children, their education. These additional domestic arrangements stretched the resources of an army that was already experiencing a shortage of habitable space. The army discouraged marriage through the imposition of regulations, and they were effective in keeping the rate of marriage well under 10 per cent of troops.[13] Despite their showy regimental uniforms and their collective attractive appearance, soldiers were not con-

Essentially Summarises my work.

sidered suitable for respectable female company; only a woman with few choices would 'go for a soldier.'[14]

Although there was widespread condemnation of soldiering, in some areas of society it was looked upon as a viable route to improving family status. Investigation of the British garrison at Gibraltar in 1878 shows a coherent community with a strong sense of identity.[15] The military census of the soldiers and their wives in the garrison at that time identifies army families by birth in garrisons abroad. A significant proportion of the soldiers had been born in colonial stations, a strong indication that between 10 and 15 per cent of soldiers came from military families. Because the army had implemented free universal education for regimental children well before that of the general British population, soldiers' boys often provided the army with its most numerate and literate troops These sons of the regiment could rise quickly through the ranks.

Motives for becoming a soldier ranged from the quasi-criminal desire to escape familial duties to a genuine wish to serve and protect. The men chose the military, rather than being randomly selected by conscription, and this is a factor when we make comparisons between civilians and soldiers. Many modern studies have shown that occupation is a factor in suicide, and soldiering is one of the professions with a positive association with higher levels.[16] One suggested explanation is that an individual who chooses the military life might have an interest in weapons and aggression. Other explanations focus on the restrictions to a man's freedom, especially for family life, as a factor. Conditions were vastly different 150 years ago and modern studies cannot be assumed to apply to the past, but consideration of recent research can help to expand the intellectual breadth that is brought to analysis of suicide in the nineteenth century. Certainly, the type of individual who chose soldiering in Victorian times could have enlisted for a number of reasons, and the regiments would have had a range of characters within the ranks.

II

The British army began keeping accurate records of regimental sickness and death as early as 1818. At first, because the aim was to ascertain the effect of climate and locale on health and mortality, accidental causes of death were omitted, thus excluding all sudden and violent deaths such as homicides, heart attacks, deaths on furlough, and sui-

Table 5.1
Suicide rate per 100,000 troops for specified periods

Period	Rate per 100,000
1830–6	78
1860–9	28
1870–9	23
1880–9	22
1890–9	22

Note: Data are for ordinary soldiers, not commissioned officers, for regiments stationed within the United Kingdom only.

cides, from the records. Suicide per se was not of interest to the army; it was a cause of death that was believed to stem from a weakness in the individual which could be aggravated by alcohol, idleness, or a tropical climate. Mortality rates for suicides were not considered pertinent when the concerns of the day were centred on the effects of the local environment, the temperature, and the diet. However, because regimental surgeons accounted for all hospital admissions and all deaths on a quarterly and annual basis, suicides and other sudden deaths had to be recorded. It is these surviving records, some of which were published as part of the series of army medical statistics in the 1830s, that give some perspective on the magnitude of suicide. From 1830 to 1836, among the Household Cavalry, the Dragoon Guards, and the Foot Guards, a population averaging 6,400 soldiers, the suicide rate was 78 per 100,000, or one suicide among every 1,390 men.[17] This rate would be considered extremely high in recent times.

Insufficient data on non-hospital deaths for the 1840s and 1850s preclude efforts to track suicide until 1859, after the Army Medical Department was created. The new department immediately paid attention to all causes of sickness and death, including those occurring outside the regimental hospital. Data amassed after 1859 showed that suicide had declined from the 1830s to levels ranging from 28 per 100,000 men in the 1860s to 22 per 100,000 men in the 1890s, or about one suicide for every 4,600 soldiers (table 5.1). Only ordinary troops, not commissioned officers, were included in calculations of rates.

There are several possible explanations for the drastic reduction in suicide levels from the 1830s. The army of that decade was much

Figure 5.1: Annual mortality rate per 100,000, 1860 to 1900, from all causes for soldiers at UK stations

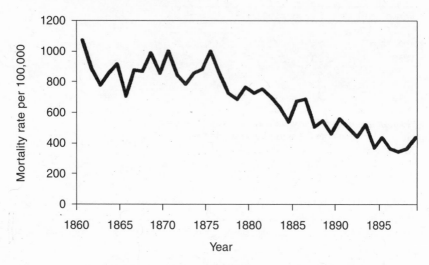

harsher, and the minimum enlistment period was much longer, fifteen years for infantry regiments and eighteen years for cavalry units. This was a lifetime to an unhappy young man.[18] Regiments were largely autonomous, and much depended on the character and education of the commanding officer. Discipline could be autocratic, and punishments were usually corporal and brutal; floggings of hundreds of lashes were not uncommon, and executions occurred in some cases. The more enlightened officers, who eschewed the lash, used cold-water immersion, prison, or hard labour as punishment.[19] Alcoholism was rampant, particularly for troops who had seen overseas duty and who had become accustomed to the fortified wines that replaced beer rations issued within the United Kingdom. For those who faced illness or pain, regimental medical care was at its nadir.[20]

In the late 1830s and 1840s some changes were instituted to make life more tolerable. Length of service was reduced by three years, and limitations were put on the number of lashes. Teetotal troops could opt out of the beer rations and receive the equivalent amount in pay; libraries were instituted, and recreational facilities authorized. Regimental medical care began to move away from the vigorous therapies of the 1830s to a more benign approach to healing in the 1840s. The

Figure 5.2: Annual suicide rate per 100,000, 1860 to 1900, for soldiers at UK stations

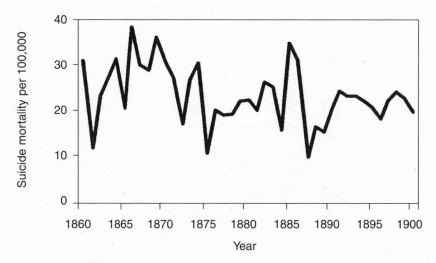

Crimean War fiasco led to changes in the king's regulations that controlled the commanding officer's authority over soldiers.

After 1860, as the focus shifted from climactic environment as a contributor to disease to the environment in the barracks, camp, and hospital, fevers commanded the most attention, particularly enteric fevers and cholera. Drains, flooring, food quality, ventilation, and hospital conditions were investigated.[21] In the 1870s the mortality rates of the soldiers were declining and by the end of the century figures show that mortality had fallen by over 50 per cent from 1860 to 1900 (figure 5.1). Mortality was declining in civilian life also, but at a slower pace. Suicide levels, however, did not decline, nor was there much year-to-year variation (figure 5.2).

A cleaner, healthier environment and better hospital care, while laudatory for controlling unnecessary deaths of other types, were unlikely to impinge on conditions that could lead a soldier to take his own life. However, policy changes could be effective in altering the potential for suicide in the army through limitations of means. In the late 1860s and early 1870s there were two changes that could affect the means of suicide. First, there was the directive requiring that firearms be stored during off-duty hours, out of reach in the case of alcohol-

Figure 5.3: Method of harm, completed and unsuccessful suicides among soldiers, 1860 to 1900

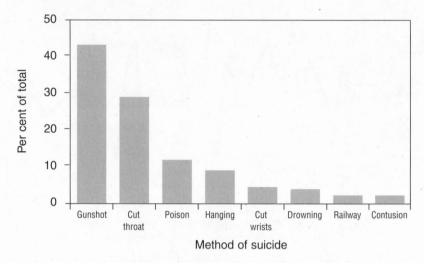

fuelled, heated arguments. This regulation was targeted to reduce homicides, but it also affected the potential for self-destruction. The second directive was one that governed the facial hair of the soldier; only in the 1870s was he permitted to remove his beard. This charge meant that the shaving razor became a common object in the barracks, available to anyone who wanted a sharp blade to cut his throat and end his life. Both of these regulations were instituted for reasons unconnected with suicides, but both affected the types of weapons of self-destruction available to a deeply despairing soldier.

However, even when properly stored, weapons are an integral part of military life, and firearms remained the primary means of death for the soldiers. Of 795 completed and unsuccessful suicides from 1860 to 1900 where the method was reported, 43 per cent were the result of gunshot wounds (figure 5.3).[22] Cutting the throat occurred in 29 per cent of the cases. Poisonings accounted for 13 per cent, and poison was often chosen by those in the Army Hospital Corps, probably because of the access to toxic chemicals.[23] Hanging, cutting one's wrists, drownings, and throwing oneself before a train were the methods in the remaining suicides. Survival was most likely in gunshot suicides (44 per cent) and cut throat attempts (30 per cent); 10 per cent of poisonings were also unsuccessful.

Figure 5.4: Age distribution for suicides from 1880 to 1900 for soldiers at UK stations

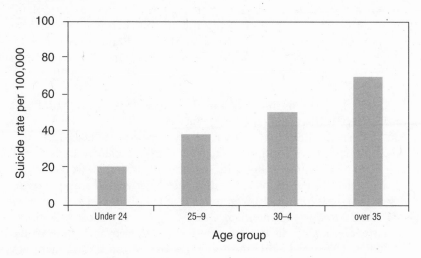

The likelihood of a soldier committing a suicidal act increased with age and service (figure 5.4). Between 1883 and 1894 the average age of a suicidal soldier was 28.9 years, and the average length of service, 9.3 years. These data are for suicides that occurred well after the introduction of six-year minimum service; so these soldiers had chosen to remain in the army beyond their required enlistment. While soldiers who killed themselves before the age of twenty-four could have been overwhelmed with dissatisfaction of military life and the seemingly endless time until their term of service expired, those in their later twenties and older had been sufficiently satisfied and sufficiently successful as soldiers to re-enlist for a second tour of duty. Furthermore, during the last decades of the nineteenth century, there were many opportunities for young men once out of the military. The growth of army infrastructure and government bureaucracy created opportunities for experienced former soldiers. Emigration also offered new opportunities for young men in the empire's settlement colonies.

The regimental surgeons recorded motivation for some of the suicides between 1883 and 1894. The attributed reasons were diverse, with depression, monetary problems, drink, and family problems foremost. Less numerous reasons included disgrace, regimental problems, fear of punishment, and disappointment in love. Two of the ninety-five known motives were from 'studying too much.' Motives were furnished for only about a quarter of the deaths, but the breadth of the known attributions is interesting. Except for 'regimental problems' and possibly 'fear of punishment,' the attributed problems were, for the most part, not unique to the military but could have been found in civil life. However, it may have been that military regulations and conventions made it more difficult to resolve problems than in civilian life.[24]

Although the army had no specific policies on suicide, conditions that have psychological bases were recognized by the regimental surgeons. Records show that many soldiers were hospitalized and sometimes invalided for conditions such as mania, melancholia, amentia, and hysteria. There was also widespread recognition of problems with physiological foundations but which were recognized to be 'nervous diseases,' conditions such as epilepsy (thousands of cases), pain in the head, inflammation of the meninges, paralysis, and chorea. Regimental surgeons had little training in the recognition and treatment of problems associated with the functions of the brain, but there was some understanding that these were illnesses requiring hospital admission and either cure or discharge.

III

While the Army Medical Department showed no interest in suicide as a cause of death for soldiers, contemporary civilian researchers published several articles that considered the issue. In 1839, in a commentary on the first published report of army medical statistics, J.W.C. Lever pointed out the high suicide rate.[25] He compared the rate of the Dragoon Guards, 1 in 1,274 soldiers per year, to those among civilians in Britain and in other countries, where about 1 in 15,000 inhabitants killed themselves. Lever acknowledged that these were not exactly equitable comparisons, as the populations were not matched for age and sex. In other words, he recognized the desirability of standardized epidemiological data in comparative populations. Despite the inadequacies of the data, Lever was the first to bring attention to the subject, and he offered possible reasons for the difference.

W.H. Millar compared the statistics of deaths by suicide among troops from 1862 to 1871 with British males between the ages of twenty and forty-five.[26] He found that soldiers had a suicide rate three times that of civilians, and this difference was even higher when regiments doing colonial duty were included. His careful study noted several interesting facts, such as the association of greater likelihood of suicide with increased length of service and the higher rates in some corps, particularly the high rate in the cavalry corps relative to the infantry. Millar was quite convinced that the reason for the high rate in the army was the abundance of possible weapons. He also used the rates from foreign armies to claim that suicide in the British army was less common than in continental armies. He reasoned that this was because the British army relied entirely on volunteers, thereby eliminating men with an aversion to the confines of military life. Millar's paper was read in the presence of other interested statisticians prior to publication, and their comments were published with the paper. William Farr's comments showed that he concurred that the presence of weapons, such as guns and shaving blades, was the aggravating factor in the military. Dr Mouat suggested the monotony of military life as a contributing factor, often exacerbated by the consumption of alcohol. Sir James Anderson felt that suicides often arose because a talented soldier who worked hard to rise in rank was frequently disappointed by the lack of challenge once his goal was achieved.[27]

A decade later William Ogle investigated suicides and occupation.[28] He used civilian death registrations where the individual's occupation was identified by close relatives and friends of the deceased and standardized these to the age and occupation information from the 1881 census. He found that the soldiers had the highest suicide rate, at 112 per 100,000, a level that is fivefold higher than that in the army medical statistics at the time. However, Ogle's rates include those up to the age of sixty-five who were identified as soldiers, rather than active soldiers, who were rarely still enlisted after the age of 45. His numbers therefore include pensioned and discharged troops; age may have had a significant effect on the level of despair of this occupational group. A fourth study, by American researcher Fred Emery, looked solely at the comparative rates of suicide in armies of several European countries in the 1870s and 1880s and concluded that while some armies had high rates (Austria, Germany, and Prussia), the British levels were comparable with the French and Belgian.[29]

All studies noted the association of higher age and increasing likelihood of death by suicide, and two found that non-commissioned and commissioned officers had higher rates. However, as both of these variables are associated with increasing age, it is difficult to identify which factor may have contributed to the great despair that would lead one to take his own life. Researchers agreed that the availability of firearms contributed to the higher levels among the military; they noted too that boredom and alcohol consumption possibly contributed. Temperature and climate, factors that were never completely absent in nineteenth-century army discussions of causes of death, were also considered as alternative explanations.[30]

IV

Suicide remains a concern for army medical personnel. It is difficult to get a consensus on its significancee as a cause of death in armies, but some consistent patterns can be seen in the studies. For example, most modern studies find that suicide levels are higher among the youngest members of the military, particularly those under twenty.[31] Basic training can be exhilarating for some young men as they expand their strength and self-confidence, but the change in circumstances and loss of freedom can be devastating.[32] This outcome is in contrast to the pattern in the historical army, where the older individuals who had re-enlisted for a second term were more likely to kill themselves. A study of the mortality of UK soldiers from 1984 to 2004 shows that annual rates during this period twice exceeded the annual rates of the previous century, although the average rate, 15 per 100,000, was lower.[33] Firearms figure prominently in methods of self-annihilation, although hanging, pharmaceutical preparations, and gases are also often used. Comparisons between civilian and army rates are inconsistent. In Finland, where there is a very high youth suicide rate, the rates for conscripts are lower. However, in the United States the civilian rate is lower. The results of the twenty-year UK study show that for those in the army under twenty, there is a higher level of suicide compared with their civilian counterparts but, among those over twenty, civilians have the higher rates. The finer level of age comparison of the UK study may explain the differences from Finnish and American findings.

Paradoxes arise when we consider suicide among nineteenth-century soldiers. The soldiers were selected from potential recruits based on their superior physique and absence of signs of ill health; they were healthy warriors who would be expected to exhibit lower overall morbidity and mortality rates than the general population. Regimental officers were entrusted with keeping the regimental troops in good health; the men were fed better than most civilian Britons, their activity levels were monitored for overexertion, and any illnesses were immediately attended to by regimental surgeons. A soldier's livelihood was steady and secure, devoid of the uncertainty faced by many labourers. However, in the early part of the nineteenth century, these advantages were offset by the brutal conditions of service: harsh discipline, long tours of duty in foreign colonies, a paucity of amenities, and high levels of sickness and death among soldiers. Until mid-century, soldiers' suicide rates were exceedingly high compared to civilians.

The reforms of the 1860s and 1870s were directed at making the army a more humane and therefore more attractive option to young men. Great attention was paid to reducing wastage from all causes, particularly infectious diseases, in the last four decades of the century. The effort was successful, and soldiers' mortality from all causes declined drastically. Although there were no policies specifically aimed at reducing suicide, deaths from this cause decreased alongside all other causes. However, after the 1880s, suicide rates remained relatively static. The result was that suicide became more prominent in the non-combat causes of death in the army.

At the close of the twentieth century, suicide remained a problem among young military men in the United Kingdom. The average levels were lower than that of the late nineteenth century, but variation in annual rates meant that there were years of similarity. In the intervening century, with the advancement of medicine, many illnesses declined to levels approaching extinction. However, despite acute awareness of the problem in the modern military, mortality from suicide remains resistant.

NOTES

1 'Statistical Reports of Sickness, Mortality and Invaliding among Troops in the U.K., Mediterranean and British North America,' Great Britain, *Parliamentary Papers*, 1839, 40: v417.

2 This term is attributed to H.K. Kang and T.A. Bullman, 'Mortality among U.S. Veterans of the Persian Gulf War,' *New England Journal of Medicine* 1996, 335: 1498–504, following the initial development of the term 'healthy worker effect' in A.J. McMichael, 'Standardized Mortality Ratios and the "Healthy Worker" Effect: Scratching beneath the Surface,' *Journal of Occupational Medicine* 1987, 131: 70–2.

3 J.W.C. Lever, 'On the Sickness and Mortality among the Troops in the United Kingdom: Abstract of the Statistical Report of Major Tulloch,' *Journal of the Royal Statistical Society of London* 1839, 2: 250–60; W.H. Millar, 'Statistics of Death by Suicide among Her Majesty's British Troops Serving at Home and Abroad during the Ten Years 1862–71,' *Journal of the Statistical Society of London* 37 (1874): 187–92; William Ogle, 'Suicides in England and Wales in Relation to Age, Sex, Season, and Occupation,' *Journal of the Statistical Society of London* 1886, 49: 101–35.

4 For example, in the United States it is second; see Elspeth Cameron Ritchie, William C. Keppler, and Joseph M. Rothenberg, 'Suicidal Admissions in the United States Military,' *Military Medicine* 2003, 168: 177–81). It is also ranked second in Finland, after accidents; see Mauri Marttunen, Markus Henriksson, Seppo Pelkonen, Martti Schroderus, and Jouko Lönnqvist, 'Suicide among Military Conscripts in Finland: A Psychological Autopsy Study,' *Military Medicine* 1997, 162: 14–18.

5 Marttunen et al., 'Suicide among Military Conscripts in Finland'; Joseph M. Rothenberg, 'Stress and Suicide in the U.S. Army: Effects of Relocation on Service Members' Mental Health,' *Armed Forces and Society* 1991 17: 449–58; 'Suicide and Open Verdict Deaths in the UK Regular Armed Forces 1984–2004,' Defence Analytical Services Agency (hereafter DASA), www.dasa.mod.uk.

6 Alan R Skelley., *The Victorian Army at Home: The Recruitment and Terms of the Recruitment and Terms and Conditions of the British Regular, 1859–1899* (London: Croom Helm, 1977); Edward M. Spiers, *The Army and Society, 1815–1914* (London: Longman, 1980).

7 Thomas Sexton and P.A. Taylor, *Speeches of Thomas Sexton and P.A. Taylor on the Army Bill 1882 with regard to the liability of a soldier for the maintenance of his wife and family* (1882), pamphlet.

8 An example of the kinds of conditions considered for rejection can be found in 'Report on Recruits Rejected in London Recruiting District, Jan. 1, 1835 to Dec 31, 1835,' National Archives of the United Kingdom (hereafter NAUK), file WO 335 2.

9 Spiers, *The Army and Society*; Gwyn Harries-Jenkins, *The Army in Victorian Society* (Toronto: University of Toronto Press, 1977).

10 Harries-Jenkins, *The Army in Victorian Society*.

11 H.W. Keays-Youngs, *On Army Re-organization and Recruiting* (Sandgate: W. Wilson, 1874).

12 Myna Trustram, *Women of the Regiment* (Cambridge; Cambridge University Press, 1984).

13 For a full discussion on marriage regulations and the effects of these reg-

ulations, see Janet Padiak, 'The "Serious Evil of Marching Regiments": ~~X~~
The Families of the British Garrison of Gibraltar,' *History of the Family: An
International Quarterly* 2005, 10: 137–50.

14 The phrase is from Henry Fielding, *A History of Tom Jones*.

15 Janet Padiak, 'Morbidity and the 19th Century Decline of Mortality: An
Analysis of the Military Population of Gibraltar 1818 to 1899' (PhD
thesis, University of Toronto, 2004).

16 Martin J. Mahon, John P. Tobin, Denis A. Cusack, Cecily Kelleher, and
Kevin M. Malone, 'Suicide among Regular-Duty Military Personnel: A
Retrospective Case-Control Study of Occupation-Specific Risk Factors for
Workplace Suicide,' *American Journal of Psychiatry* 2005, 162: 1688–96;
James C. Helkamp, 'Occupation and Suicide among Males in the US
Armed Forces,' *Annals of Epidemiology* 1996, 6: 83–8.

17 'Statistical Reports of Sickness, Mortality and Invaliding among Troops in
the U.K., Mediterranean and British North America,' Great Britain, *Parliamentary Papers*, 1852–3, 59: 1.

18 Ibid.

19 Peter Samond, 'Annual Report of the Health of the Kings Royal Rifle
Brigade 1833,' NAUK, file WO 334 10.

20 Details of regimental medical care during the 1830s, even for common
ailments such as influenza, can be found in Janet Padiak and D. Ann
Herring, 'Lost in Transition: Explaining and Treating Influenza in the
British Army in the 1830s and 1840s,' *Canadian Bulletin of Medical History*,
forthcoming.

21 'Report on Barrack and Hospital Improvement Commission on Sanitary
Condition and Improvement of Barracks and Hospitals at Mediterranean
Stations,' *British Parliamentary Papers* 1863, 13: 475.

22 Data from the 'Army Medical and Statistical Reports,' published annually in the *British Parliamentary Papers* for the years 1880–1900.

23 Millar, 'Statistics of Death by Suicide.'

24 For a fuller comparison of stresses in military and civilian life in a colonial setting, see L.A. Sawchuk, Janet Padiak, and John D. Purcell, 'Quan-
tifying the Colonized/Colonist Relationship: Suicide as a Proxy Measure
for Population Stress,' *Current Anthropology*, 2004, 45: 118–25.

25 Lever, 'On the Sickness and Mortality among the Troops.'

26 Millar, 'Statistics of Death by Suicide.' He calculated a rate of 0.34 per
1,000 for soldiers stationed within the United Kingdom and compared
this with the rate of 0.11 per 1,000 for civilian males between the ages of
twenty and forty-five. Although this current study and Millar's analysis
depend on the same regimental data, Millar's definition of troops serving

within the United Kingdom seems to have a broader base for inclusion. His annual number of troops from 1862 to 1871 averages 76,408, with 259 suicides. This study, when the same years are considered, covers 67,540 troops annually and 199 completed suicides. These latter figures give somewhat different comparative rates of 0.34 per 1,000 to 0.30 per 1,000 for these years.

27 The discussion and comments of Farr, Mouat, and Anderson are published as appendices to Millar, 'Statistics of Death by Suicide.'
28 Ogle, 'Suicides in England and Wales.'
29 Fred P. Emery, 'Suicide in European Armies,' *Publications of the American Statistical Association* 1891, 2: 387–9.
30 For example, 'Statistical Reports of Sickness,' 1852–3.
31 Marttunen et al., 'Suicide among Military Conscripts in Finland'; 'Suicide and Open Verdict Deaths,' DASA; Ritchie, Keppler, and Rothenberg, 'Suicidal Admissions in the United States Military,'; Harold E. Russell, Robert W. Conroy, and John J. Werner, 'Study of Suicidal Behavior in the Military Setting,' *Military Medicine* 1971, 136: 549–52.
32 Marttunen et al., in 'Suicide among Military Conscripts in Finland,' describe this challenge very well.
33 'Suicide and Open Verdict Deaths,' DASA.

6 Suicide and French Soldiers of the First World War: Differing Perspectives, 1914–1939

PATRICIA E. PRESTWICH

The suicide of French soldiers during the First World War remains shrouded in silence. Official statistics on military suicides exist for the pre-war and the interwar periods, but no such figures are available for the war itself. Despite an emphasis by successive French governments on the 'duty to remember' the sacrifices of those who fought for France, important military archives, particularly those of the wartime military courts, remain inaccessible. During the First World War, suicides or suicide attempts were not regularly noted in hospital records, and some death certificates were falsified to indicate the cause of death as enemy action rather than self-inflicted wounds.[1] Only occasionally have the records of military units or the diaries and memoirs of soldiers mentioned suicide.[2] Moreover, unlike the deaths of soldiers executed for desertion or cowardice, the fate of soldiers who committed suicide has never captured the interest or sympathy of the general public.[3]

Wartime conditions, with the inevitable appeals to duty, honour, patriotism, and sacrifice, made it very difficult to speak openly about suicide. Military regulations equated suicide with desertion, an act punishable by death. Soldiers who failed in their suicide attempts faced the risk of a hasty trial before military tribunals that were under pressure to impose exemplary punishments to maintain discipline.[4] The army's official attitude was harsh. Suicidal soldiers were cowards, a response sometimes captured in officers' comments in regimental or divisional records.[5] But reactions could be complex. The psychiatrist Maurice de Fleury, who defended many deserters before military tribunals, admitted that soldiers who killed themselves were, 'in a manner of speaking, deserters,' and that their actions could provoke 'anger and indignation.' Yet he himself felt only 'unlimited pity' for these 'unfortunate' men who were tormented by anguish, fear, and exhaustion.[6] In those rare instances where a soldier recorded the suicide of a comrade, the attitude seems to have been one of compassion.[7] Many comrades and many families preferred to remain silent about such events; their reticence is understandable in the face of wartime and postwar propaganda that portrayed French soldiers as unflinchingly stalwart in life and glorious in death.

Despite a recent resurgence of scholarly interest in the First World War and lively debates among French historians about how and why ordinary soldiers endured over four years of unimaginably hellish conditions,[8] only one French historian has attempted to investigate this topic. Through a painstaking and ingenious study of the records of fallen French soldiers who were not awarded the distinction of 'Mort pour la France' (Died for France), Denis Rolland has determined that there were approximately 5,000 suicides in the army from the outbreak of hostilities in August 1914 to demobilization in October 1919, or 90 per month. This rate of 23 per 100,000 is comparable to the prewar rate of suicide among the general population and slightly higher than the pre-war military rate.[9] Significantly but not surprisingly, Rolland estimates that the rates in the infantry, which bore the brunt of the fighting, were markedly higher, at 38.6 per 100,000. Suicides were most frequent on fronts where the fighting was heaviest, and they tended to peak after major offensives. Suicide appears to have been more frequent among older men, between the ages of thirty-five to forty-four, and higher among officers.[10] Both these patterns had already been observed in the peacetime army. Rolland also calculates that 49 per cent of military suicides took place away from the front – in barracks, hospitals, or when soldiers were at home on leave.[11] However, he cautions that an accurate rate of suicide will never be established because of the ease of killing oneself in the front lines simply by refusing to take elementary precautions. At a time when wartime propaganda stressed the patriotic 'self-sacrifice' and 'abnegation' of front-line soldiers,[12] the notion of suicide is inevitably blurred. How, for example, does one assess the actions of a depressed or exhausted soldier who 'ends it all' in a heroic but suicidal attack?

Given wartime circumstances and the state of military archives, those soldiers who killed themselves while on active service remain mute, anonymous figures, and historians can only speculate on their motives. However, during the war, military psychiatrists treated many men who had attempted suicide, and they also wrote about suicide within the larger context of the psychological traumas of war. Although their attitudes may seem harsh by today's standards, psychiatrists did attempt to understand suicide as something other than cowardice or desertion. In the interwar period, as the French struggled with the consequences of war, other, non-medical opinions can be heard, in particular those of veterans and the families of soldiers. Nevertheless, wartime military suicides remained a sensitive topic, evoked infrequently and discreetly but with unequivocal sympathy. Examining how people struggled to understand these acts suggests how painful and perhaps unfathomable they remained and why many preferred to remain silent.

Psychiatric Opinion and the Experience of War

On the eve of the First World War, French military psychiatrists became interested in suicide as one aspect of their larger efforts to select the fittest troops for a war that military experts assumed would be brief. They argued that selection of the fittest meant the rejection of mentally deficient (*débiles*) or mentally unstable (*déséquilibrés*) conscripts, a task that they confidently believed was within the competence of psychiatric medicine. Their arguments were based on theories of degeneration, or a hereditary predisposition to mental illness, which, for the previous forty years, had dominated French psychiatry.[13] It was assumed that the fundamental or predisposing cause of madness or any mental instability was a hereditary defect. Such a 'taint' might be immediately apparent, either in a patient's abnormal physical features or through a history of alcoholism or mental problems in the family. However, it could also be latent and would be triggered only by a specific crisis or trauma (the so-called occasional cause), such as an emotional shock, exhaustion, or alcoholism. War, military psychiatrists agreed, could not cause psychiatric disorders; it could only reveal or aggravate the pre-existing weakness. Under combat conditions, therefore, only the hereditarily damaged would be prone to psychiatric disorders, including suicide.

In the immediate pre-war years, army psychiatrists were encouraged in their efforts to improve the mental and emotional quality of troops by a number of studies on the incidence of military suicides. Although rates in the French army were higher than those in the civilian population, they were declining at a time when civilian rates were rising.[14] Even more encouraging, rates of suicide in the French army were lower than those in the German or Austrian armies.[15] However, most studies agreed that military suicides increased in wartime and that officers and non-commissioned officers had a higher incidence of suicide than the troops, a pattern that would continue during the war. Army psychiatrists stressed the importance of preventing suicide by the medical screening of recruits and by continued propaganda to warn troops of the dangers of alcohol. In fact, they emphasized that alcoholism was one of the most important causes of military suicides. They also urged officers to be concerned about the mental health of their troops and to watch for any minor mental disorders that might worsen in time of war.[16] One prominent army psychiatrist, Paul Chavigny, warned that the army was neglecting the problem of attempted suicides. In his experience, these were considerably more frequent than successful acts, and they needed to be treated as failed suicides. Such events were always taken seriously by civilian psychiatrists, he noted, as were certain forms of self-mutilation, which could be the equivalent of a suicide attempt. But the army kept no statistics on the problem, and even worse, warned Chavigny, it treated such acts as malingering (*simulation*) or an attempt to gain sympathy, especially when the soldier was facing disciplinary action.[17]

Army psychiatrists appeared confident that the psychiatric screening of conscripts would ensure the mental health of soldiers and the quality of troops in time of war; however, some civilian psychiatrists were less optimistic. They based their opinions on the reports of Russian psychiatrists on the extent of psychological trauma during the Russo-Japanese War of 1904–5. Russian psychiatrists had observed that mental disorders, especially depression, increased by 50 per cent among troops during the war. They attributed this disturbing trend in part to the increased use of older, reserve forces, but they also emphasized that many of the psychiatric problems they treated were the result of the traumatic nature of modern industrial warfare.[18] These reports prompted Professor Emmanuel Régis, a specialist in emotional trauma, to warn the French army that the fears, anxieties, and exhaustion inherent in modern combat might be more disastrous to the mental health of ordinary soldiers than any predisposition to mental illness. He urged the army to establish front-line neuropsychiatric units to treat such problems immediately,[19] but this call was not heeded by an army that confidently expected the coming war to last a matter of weeks, not years.

From the early days of combat in August and September 1914, it was evident that the young citizen-soldiers of the French army were shocked by the horrors they encountered. A lieutenant wrote of these first conflicts that 'the triumph of those who lived through the battles of Ypres was in not emerging mad or candidates for madness.'[20] There were serious problems with desertion, self-mutilation, and simulated illness among troops. The military high command countered with harsh repression, including special military tribunals and executions 'as an example.'[21] Military hospitals were flooded with soldiers displaying a range of psychological disturbances from depression and alcoholism to what would later be diagnosed as hysteria. The psychiatrist Jean Lépine, who had been mobilized along with most civilian psychiatrists, reported that men arrived in his service with diagnoses of 'mad,' 'insane,' 'nuts' or 'malingerer.'[22] By November, with the stalement on the Western Front, the potential for psychological trauma had increased. Not only did troops face the horrors of trench warfare, but the high casualty rates in this war of attrition forced the army to use older men from reserve units and those who had been rejected in 1914 as unfit for service.

It was also important to rehabilitate and redeploy as many of the wounded as possible, including those with psychiatric illnesses. By late 1914 the army had created special neuropsychiatric units at the rear. Individual psychiatrists were the first to establish front-line triage units to treat men who could be cured within two or three weeks and to evacuate the more serious cases to the neuropsychiatric units at the rear. By early 1915 two of the six armies had such units, and by February 1916 all armies had special triage and treatment formations. Equally significant, as early as the autumn of 1914, psychiatrists began to be appointed as expert witnesses to military tribunals, and by 1916 this practice had become fully established. There are no statistics on the number of French soldiers treated for mental problems either in specialized units or in regular hospitals, but the neuropsychiatric centres were the largest specialized units in the army's health service. The centre at Val-de-Grâce in Paris treated over 25,000 soldiers during the war.[23]

In these neuropsychiatric units, as well as in front-line hospitals, psychiatrists treated a large number of attempted suicides. They warned army doctors at the front of the dangers of suicide and emphasized to officers the importance of evacuating depressed or otherwise disturbed soldiers as quickly as possible. Although the war provided psychiatrists with a 'marvellously rich'[24] opportunity to study a wide range of psychological traumas in a social group rarely seen in their civilian practice – namely, healthy young men – it did not lead them to develop any new categories of psychiatric disorder. Nor did it provoke any new interest in suicide. In their voluminous writings on war trauma, suicide was discussed as one possible consequence of three specific and well-known psychiatric disorders: clinical depression, alcoholism, and the state of extreme anxiety and fear that was termed mental confusion.

Clinical depression, in its various manifestations, had been the predominant form of mental disorder in pre-war army hospitals. Not surprisingly, under the horrific conditions of trench warfare, hospital wards were filled with depressed soldiers who refused to eat, who had self-inflicted wounds, who had deserted, who asked to be shot, or who had attempted suicide. A well-established consequence of depression was suicide, and psychiatrists tried to give officers some knowledge of the warning signs, particularly as depression was more likely to be overlooked than the manic forms of mental illness, with their extravagant gestures and ravings.[25] Depression could develop slowly, and psychiatrists urged officers to look for those soldiers who became taciturn, hypochondriac, or pessimistic or who isolated themselves from their comrades. Often such men caused no trouble, but if not evacuated immediately, they would either end up before a court martial or would kill themselves. Psychiatrists also warned that suicidal depression could develop quickly, as an impulsive act that came after the shock of battle or a night of insomnia. Ironically, it seemed that depressed men could be very good soldiers. As one psychiatrist wrote, they were so convinced that they were going to die and that they deserved to die that they continually risked their lives in battle.[26]

Although psychiatrists fully appreciated the horrors of trench warfare and sometimes spoke of them in moving terms, they still concluded in their wartime publications that these depressed and suicidal men suffered from a hereditary predisposition to mental illness that was aggravated, but not caused, by the conditions of war. They could cite many examples to justify this conclusion, such as that of a forty-eight-year-old sergeant who had suffered previous bouts of depression and who had a suspicious family history. His mother was 'nervous,' and his brother had been committed to a psychiatric hospital. While instructing young recruits at the rear, the sergeant, in his own words, had suffered an attack of *cafard* (depression) and, weeping inconsolably, had tried to shoot himself. At the hospital he attempted to escape because, 'as a decorated colonial soldier,' he should have been serving at the front; in the hospital he was only taking a place away from a soldier with 'real' wounds.[27] In such cases, psychiatrists would argue that war conditions merely 'coloured' the characteristic melancholic delusions.

Psychiatrists were struck by the number of depressed soldiers who suffered from physical and mental exhaustion, notably in the latter years of the war. This finding led some to suggest that the emotions and fatigues of war might be more directly the cause of depression than any hereditary predisposition. As a consequence, these psychiatrists were often more optimistic about the success of treatment, particularly in younger men. For example, one young hospitalized soldier had volunteered for the front and had served for twenty months as the translator for a Russian unit before evacuation for severe depression. The treating psychiatrist optimistically reassured the anxious father that all his son needed was 'peace and moral comfort.'[28]

For psychiatrists, a second major cause of suicide or attempted suicide among French troops was alcoholism; it could aggravate depression or encourage impulsive acts. Before the war, France had had the highest rate of alcohol consumption in the world, and alcoholism was considered a serious social problem.[29] Both wine and distilled alcohol were part of the daily ration for combat troops, and extra rations were distributed before an attack. As well, illegal supplies were readily available in towns near the front. The widespread and excessive consumption of alcohol in the army has led some historians to argue that drink was essential to the maintenance of morale, despite the many disciplinary problems that ensued.[30] But the abuse of alcohol resulted in a serious loss of manpower. As early as 1915, army psychiatrists warned that alcoholics had become the scourge of military hospitals; one psychiatrist calculated that in his service at least one-third of his patients were there because of alcoholism.[31] In hospital records the abuse of alcohol was frequently noted in conjunction with depression and pathological anxiety. According to French psychiatric theory, alcoholism was both a cause and a sign of hereditary degeneration. Many psychiatrists were all too familiar with alcoholism from their pre-war civilian practices and had supported campaigns to reduce the consumption of alcohol. As early as 1915, both the army and the government tried to restrict its consumption.[32] Nevertheless, both wine and distilled alcohol remained widely available in the front lines, and alcoholic patients continued to arrive at military hospitals throughout the war.

From their wartime experiences, psychiatrists believed that alcoholism was more likely to appear in older soldiers who had developed drinking problems before the war. Since statistics suggest that suicide rates in both the pre-war and wartime French armies were higher among older soldiers, including many officers, alcoholism may have been one factor in these deaths. A typical case was that of a lieutenant evacuated from the trenches because he had been in a very agitated state for several days, weeping, declaring to his men that women were trying to entice him to return to the rear, and threatening to 'go up onto the plain and getting myself killed.' A fellow officer was able to calm him enough to bring him to the medical officer, who evacuated him with a diagnosis of 'mental disturbance.' Military psychiatrists attributed his condition to drinking habits acquired before the war when he was a travelling salesman, though they did add that these habits were aggravated by the 'strains and fatigue' of serving at the front.[33] In such cases, the forced detoxification of a hospital stay resulted in improvement, at least in the short term.

The most interesting aspect of wartime psychological trauma for psychiatrists was mental confusion, a condition characterized by exaggerated emotions, particularly unusual anxiety and uncontrollable fear. It could result in hysteria, desertion, self-mutilation, or suicide. Since this disorder appeared in many young soldiers with no history of mental problems, either personal or in their families, it provoked considerable medical debate. It also spawned a number of books for the general public on fear, courage, and the psychology of combat soldiers. Military psychiatrists presented case studies of soldiers obsessed with their anxieties and fears, particularly the fear of being seen as a coward. They were 'afraid of being afraid,' and since these men received little sympathy from their fellow soldiers, psychiatrists warned that they would often try to commit suicide.[34] Psychiatrists frequently identified this condition in officers, who bore a heavy burden for the morale and discipline of their troops as well as for the success of military action in their sector. In his study of fear among soldiers, Albert Brousseau, who spent over three years at the front as the medical officer for a combat unit, recounted graphic examples of terrified officers who had deserted their men in battle. He was also moved by the tragic case of one soldier who was so panicked by the idea of entering the trenches that he tried to desert to the enemy, an act for which he was executed.[35] As with clinical depression, this state of exaggerated emotion or anguish could appear suddenly, after extreme fatigue or the shock of battle, although on the battlefield these overly emotional men could be heroic.[36] Paradoxically as well, men obsessed with a fear of dying could, in the grip of such emotions, kill themselves.[37]

Psychiatrists agreed that the horrors and unremitting exhaustion of warfare triggered this severe mental confusion or anxiety, and they were optimistic about the success of treatment, especially if these men could be treated in war zones and quickly returned to service. Nevertheless, on the whole, they were unwilling to admit that war alone could cause such mental damage in apparently normal men. Rather, they concluded that these soldiers had a latent emotional fragility or predisposition to mental problems; some even argued that this could be an acquired predisposition and that in war, emotion could become a biological agent.[38] Others tried to create a type of sliding scale of predisposition to emotional shock, arguing that the trauma would have to be exceptionally strong to shatter the emotional balance of a 'normal' man, while a hereditarily susceptible soldier would need only a mild shock or limited fatigue.[39] Régis's son, a doctor who served with combat troops, claimed that he found a predisposition to emotional trauma in 60 per cent of his patients.[40] As justification for such opinions, psychiatrists could point to the apparent resilience of most soldiers and to popular beliefs that courage was acquired through will power and the practice of mastering fear.[41] Those in the grip of abnormal fear or anguish therefore simply lacked self-discipline.

Only rarely was this opinion challenged. In 1930 Dr André Fribourg-Blanc, a prominent military psychiatrist who had been wounded four times during the war, concluded after a study of 25,000 cases of war trauma that 'the strains and dangers of a war as long and as terrible as that of 1914–1918 can, without the intervention of any other aetiological factor, be the determining cause of mental troubles.'[42] Fribourg-Blanc challenged the idea that soldiers could become inured to the repeated shocks of war; rather, he argued that this experience made men more fragile,[43] a view that he had already expressed during the war. In a letter from the front, he told his wife of a 'courageous' sergeant who had suddenly developed mental trauma: 'these unfortunate men are subjected to such a continuous stress that it takes only a small incident to trigger a crisis of mental confusion.'[44] The psychiatrist Abadie, who had established one of the first front-line units to treat mental disorders, shared this view.[45] Even Albert Brousseau, who believed that fear could be overcome by will power, spend a large portion of his study of fear in the army emphasizing the many factors, such as hunger, fatigue, isolation, and poor leadership, that could engender psychological disorders in ordinary men. It may be, as the Italian historian Bruna Bianchi has suggested, that on this issue there was a difference of opinion between younger doctors who served at the front and those who treated severely traumatized men at the rear.[46]

In the light of recent research on post-traumatic stress disorder, these wartime psychiatric theories, rooted as they still were in concepts of degeneration, may appear harsh. They did, however, offer a more sympathetic view of suicidal soldiers than that of the military command. In military courts, psychiatrists could defend soldiers who had attempted suicide, had mutilated themselves, or had deserted by claiming that they suffered from a hereditary predisposition to insanity. As Maurice de Fleury concluded, 'the man who ... deserts is saved by his past.'[47] The war also forced psychiatrists to reconsider the importance of the 'occasional' causes of mental illness and to focus on the treatment and recovery of their patients. The result was a more optimistic attitude toward the treatment of attempted suicide, at least among younger soldiers.

This interest and understanding was not extended to the large number of colonial troops from North and Equatorial Africa who fought on the Western Front. Despite the fact that many such soldiers were patients in neuropsychiatric units, there was little professional interest in their mental problems, which were assumed to be uncomplicated and the result of their racial inferiority. In the limited wartime psychiatric literature on this topic, North African and colonial troops were portrayed as primitive and childlike; they were deemed more credulous, emotional, and prone to impulsive or violent actions. The rare authors who wrote on such matters occasionally tried to distinguish between Muslim soldiers from North Africa and indigenous troops from Senegal or other colonies. The former were characterized as suffering from a passivity or resignation that led them to refuse to eat or be treated but that rarely resulted in suicide because of religious prohibitions. Troops from Senegal and other African colonies were described as having a more emotionally charged childishness, with an impulsiveness that could suddenly result in desertion or suicide.[48] Only in the 1930s did one military psychiatrist begin to challenge these racist views. In an article on mental problems among France's North

African Muslim soldiers, A.-L.-D. Costedoat argued that the mental problems of North African troops 'did not differ essentially from those of our French soldiers.'[49] He attributed any perceived differences to culture not race, and he charged that French doctors often made erroneous assumptions because of their ignorance of Muslim and North African cultures. He did, however, agree with his predecessors that suicide was rare among Muslim troops. Costedoat based his opinions in part on his wartime service with a battalion of Moroccan troops, where, he noted, 'it was easy to compare their emotional reactions under fire with those of French troops.'[50] Perhaps in practice some psychiatrists took a compassionate view of their colonial patients, but their lack of interest in the topic means that the silences surrounding the suicide of colonial troops are profound.

Psychiatrists did not have a monopoly on the diagnosis of war trauma. Soldiers had their own terms for madness, and they were often the first to perceive the problem in a comrade and to alert officers. Their term for the depression and anguish that frequently accompanied warfare and could easily result in suicide was *le cafard*. Literally, the word means a cockroach, but it had been used by the nineteenth-century French poet Baudelaire to refer to melancholia or depression. Among French troops during the First World War it became the ubiquitous shorthand for the blackness of the soldier's situation. It could describe anything from the jitters to prolonged gloom, clinical depression, paralysing fear, or anguish in the face of death. Diaries often mentioned *le cafard* before an offensive, on return from leave, or at other times when soldiers were psychologically vulnerable, as in the hours after a battle.[51] Soldiers frequently used the term to explain their mental state to psychiatrists. One hospitalized soldier said simply, 'I am always sad; I always have a *cafard*,' while another explained his desertion as the result of a *cafard* and because people were treating him badly.[52] It was also a familiar condition in regular hospital wards. In his wartime memoirs the military surgeon F. Lejars recounted how 'the negro,' a decorated soldier from Martinique, attempted suicide while recovering from his wounds. Lejars explained that the man, isolated from his fellow soldiers, in a ward where no one spoke his language and where the other colonial troops called him 'the savage,' was suffering from that 'formidable disease of war, *cafard*.'[53]

Under Fire, Henri Barbusse's wartime novel, which portrays the lives of a squad of front-line soldiers, contains a good example of such a *cafard* that involved the risk of suicide and of the way in which the victim's comrades diagnosed and treated it. One soldier, Joseph, had already lost four of his five brothers in combat. His remaining brother, also a member of the squad, had been killed in the last assault, and his body lay near the trenches, buried by the explosion of a shell. His comrades, who had already discovered the body, rightly diagnosed Joseph's mental state and decided not to tell him that his brother was dead. As one soldier says, 'Joseph is the only one of six brothers to survive. And I'll tell you something else. I don't think he'll be the only one for long. That kid won't look after himself, he'll get himself bumped off. What he needs is for God to send him a lucky wound, or else he's buggered.'[54] Joseph eventually did receive his lucky wound, and a fellow soldier led him, in a dazed condition, to the first-aid post.

Some military psychiatrists tried to translate le cafard into psychiatric terminology,[55] but to do so misses the point. The concept was rooted in the reality of soldiers' lives. It allowed them to identify, discuss, and perhaps treat the emotional trauma they experienced. More important, as medical sociologists have argued, such concepts permit people to make sense of their world, to answer the broader questions of 'why me?' 'why him?' 'why here?' 'why now?'[56] Cafard was an all-encompassing, sympathetic, and democratic explanation that focused on the conditions of war, not on the nature of the individual soldier. It effectively expressed the view that the war itself, with its relentless stress and trauma, was the cause of severe mental breakdown and suicide. This was an opinion that would emerge more clearly among civilians in the postwar world.

Re-evaluations of Suicide in the Interwar Period

The psychiatric explanations for military suicide did not change markedly in the postwar period, but as the French began the long process of understanding the devastating impact of the war, other views began to emerge, albeit discreetly. Some were expressed by France's powerful veterans' associations, formed to ensure that the sacrifices and rights of French soldiers were not forgotten.[57] The complex system of applying for state pensions for disabled veterans and the families of the dead also allowed some ordinary people to express their views about suicide and the psychological devastation of war. However, as the campaign to rehabilitate the reputation of soldiers executed for desertion or cowardice illustrates, suicide remained a largely unspoken subject. Although these views on military suicide are scattered, partial, and shaped in part by postwar circumstances, they suggest a compassionate view of these anonymous men.

With rare exceptions, veterans' associations did not speak openly about the suicide of their comrades either during the war or after. But they were well aware that mental trauma and suicidal depression among veterans did not end with the war and that these conditions might be aggravated by the postwar situation. A number of men discharged as healthy in 1919 developed severe psychiatric problems several years later. With the support of their families and veterans' organizations, some claimed disability pensions from the government on the basis that their mental problems stemmed from their wartime service. The newspapers of veterans' organizations published advertisements for pills, gymnastic exercises, or even electricity to treat the symptoms of clinical depression, or what one advertisement described as 'brain anaemia, characterized by discouragement, by the tendency to see things darkly, and by a sense of helplessness.' Another advertisement counselled that these products were targeted at men 'for whom the war has wounded not only their bodies but their wills.'[58] Although some veterans were profoundly ashamed of having been treated for a psychiatric disorder during the war, they occasionally turned to their associations for understanding and support. One such man wrote in the 1950s to say that after many years of depression and three suicide attempts, he was finally stable, thanks to 'the care of a distinguished psychiatrist and the very disciplined lifestyle that I have adopted.'[59]

On occasion, veterans' associations spoke movingly of the psychological devastation of war, and they resolutely defended the rights of veterans afflicted with war trauma, including those committed to psychiatric hospitals. These illnesses, they maintained, were caused solely by the emotions and fatigue of war, and in their newspapers they frequently referred to such veterans as the *mutilés du cerveau*, the brainwounded. Soldiers, they insisted, had not been given a choice in their wounds, and therefore all disabled veterans deserved equal treatment.[60] But only in a few specific circumstances did certain organizations speak about suicide, and it was most commonly the postwar suicides of veterans who, it was argued, were driven to despair by the denial of an adequate pension or by their inability to earn a living.

By the mid-1920s, veterans' associations had become resentful about what they considered to be miserly pensions and the public's tendency to forget their sacrifices. Army pension boards were notoriously stingy in their decisions, and disabled veterans often complained bitterly that their heroism had yielded only poverty and public indifference.[61] In the early 1920s it was not unusual to find newspaper reports about the suicide of a veteran or, more rarely, of a soldier's widow because the army pension board had denied the claim or awarded an inadequate sum. The Association républicaine des anciens combattants, the left-wing, pacifist veterans' association founded by Henri Barbusse, often cited such tragedies, not only in defence of veterans' rights but as part of its anti-militarist campaigns. Officers, it suggested, had escaped the front lines during the war by claiming mental trauma, while ordinary soldiers were sacrificed or returned home with shattered minds. Other organizations were more circumspect. In 1923 the newspaper of an association for severely disabled veterans described the suicide of a member who had been denied an adequate pension and the despair of his destitute widow, who was unable to claim a widow's pension because the death was a suicide.[62] By 1925 the organization had changed its leadership, and public references to suicide disappeared. While it campaigned vigorously for the rights of its members, it preferred to remain silent about their personal distress. As one article explained, veterans knew 'how to remain dignified in their suffering and their misfortune.'[63] This was also the attitude of the association for veterans with severe facial wounds, the famous Gueules cassées. Its motto was 'Let us keep smiling nevertheless.'[64]

The most prominent veterans' group to speak openly and directly about suicide was the association for those with severe head wounds, the *blessés crâniens*. Perhaps they felt compelled to speak publicly about this painful subject because many of their members suffered from epilepsy, depression, or even severe psychiatric disorders. Often they were unable to find employment in the postwar world, even in positions reserved by the government for veterans. But their association may also have felt able to speak out because these psychiatric problems were the direct result of their physical wounds and treatment by trepanation, not of any supposed hereditary defect. The so-called trepanned syndrome, which included emotional and psychiatric disorders, was recognized by doctors and pension boards. As one psychiatrist affirmed, 'a former trepanned [soldier] is almost always physically and morally fatigued and mentally depressed.'[65] Their association's newspaper spoke openly and sympathetically of members with health problems and inadequate pensions who were driven to alcoholism or suicide: 'Who can describe their sleepless nights and nightmares or in daytime their anguish, depression, psychological misery, and constant worries. Who can describe their atrocious feeling as their reason slips away, leading some to irreparable acts.'[66] This newspaper also published a compassionate report on the attempted suicide of the president of another veterans' organization.[67]

The process of awarding government pensions to disabled veterans and the widows, orphans, and parents of deceased soldiers could involve the issue of suicide, but more indirectly. Veterans who suffered from mental illness, including depression or suicidal tendencies, were eligible for a pension as long as the condition was the result of wartime service. In the case of mental disorders, pension regulations required a police investigation to ensure that these men had been healthy before the war or that they were not feigning their illness. When questioned by the police, families, neighbours, fellow veterans, and local officials declared unequivocally that it was only the powerful shock of war that had caused the mental disorder. Overwhelmingly, they insisted that the veteran in question had been healthy and sane before he left for war but had returned a broken man. Such declarations could be influential in the awarding of a pension. Governmental pension boards usually listened to the advice of psychiatrists, who testified that the war had not caused the mental trauma; at best it had aggravated a pre-existing hereditary weakness. However, the legislation had established appeals tribunals and provided funding for veterans or families to seek the legal assistance they needed to contest the decision of a pension board. These tribunals, which included one veteran, were inclined to listen to the testimony of families and friends and to over-turn previous decisions that had awarded little or no pension.[68] It was possible, therefore, for soldiers who had attempted suicide to receive a full disability pension.

If a soldier had died when his rifle suddenly discharged, his widow could apply for a pension, as long as the death had been declared an accident, not a suicide.[69] It is probable that in some cases these deaths were suicides, and it is also probable that where the accidental death appeared suspicious, appeals tribunals might decide to overlook the ambiguous circumstances. The widows of soldiers who had clearly committed suicide were ineligible for a pension. However, some of these women did apply, possibly because they were destitute or because they believed that the war itself had caused their husband's death, leaving them as legitimate victims of war. In 1925 the Conseil d'État, France's highest court of appeal, declared that in such a case, the widow could be awarded a pension only if she could prove that her husband's suicide had been caused by military service.[70] Given the willingness of appeals tribunals to accept the popular view that the war itself was responsible for psychiatric problems among soldiers, it was at least possible after 1925 for such a widow to receive a pension, particularly if her husband had seen extensive service at the front.

The fate of soldiers who had killed themselves during the war was never directly evoked during the long campaign to rehabilitate the reputations of soldiers who had been executed by the army. During the war itself some families began to assert the innocence of individual soldiers, and their campaigns for the revision of the military judgments were supported in the 1920s by several major veterans' organizations. These campaigns focused on individual soldiers and often included photographs and a moving last letter to the family. Most often, the argument was that these men were the victims of military incompetence and injustice – executed not for what they had done but as examples to maintain discipline. Only a few men were officially rehabilitated in the interwar period, and only in 1998 did the French government officially acknowledge that these executed men were patriotic soldiers.[71] Even if families had had the courage to fight for the rehabilitation of a soldier who had killed himself, it would have been a long and difficult struggle. Moreover, since these men had not been condemned by a military court, the best that families might ask for was that these soldiers be given the distinction 'Died for France.' However, the campaigns to rehabilitate the reputation of executed soldiers and the more general discussions of an official amnesty for soldiers who had been condemned (but not executed) during the war for desertion, self-mutilation, and other acts may have promoted a more sympathetic view of suicide. Advocates for an amnesty drew on the arguments that psychiatrists had already made before the military courts, namely, that these men suffered from psychiatric disorders, not cowardice. By the mid-1930s several politicians were arguing for an amnesty for deserters on this basis.[72] In 1931 a parliamentary deputy proposed a bill that would permit the widows and children of men executed by the army to qualify for pensions. When the powerful Pensions Commission of the National Assembly discussed this bill, one member urged that the widows of those who had committed suicide be included in the legislation, arguing that 'we must be generous.'[73]

By the late 1920s in France, the First World War had become a powerful symbol of the tragedy of war. This understanding or construction of the Great War did provide some people with the opportunity to speak of suicide more openly and with a certain compassion. Nevertheless, military suicides remained isolated and tragic acts that reflected the desperation of the individual in the face of the unremitting horrors of war. In the interwar period, suicide and attempted suicide continued to be a serious problem for the French army. Perhaps soldiers who tried to kill themselves were treated with more understanding by psychiatrists, such as Fribourg-Blanc, who had fought in the war. But military psychiatrists still maintained that war trauma was in part a consequence of heredity and that the best form of prevention was the medical screening of conscripts. Only when veterans of the Algerian War, inspired by American soldiers of the Vietnam War, began to speak openly of the pathological effects of war on all soldiers, did attitudes and policies change. By the 1990s the French army had established programs to prevent and treat what is now termed the traumatic psychosis of war, or post-traumatic stress disorder. The soldiers of the First World War who killed themselves on active service remain shadowy, enigmatic figures. But as a result of the actions of veterans of later, equally horrific wars, these men are beginning to be integrated into the historical narrative, if not the historical memory, of the Great War.

NOTES

This research has been made possible by a generous grant from the Canadian Institutes of Health Research, for which I am grateful. I also wish to thank Mme Nadine Rodary of the Sainte-Anne library, Paris, and M. Bernard Le Ferran of the Fédération nationale des plus grands invalides de guerre for their assistance in this research.

1 Denis Rolland, 'Le suicide aux armies en 1914–1918: Une première approche quantitative globale,' in *La Grande Guerre: Pratiques et expériences*, ed. Rémy Cazals, Emmanuelle Picard, and Denis Rolland (Laon, 2005), 272.

2 Thierry Hardier and Jean-François Jagielski, *Combattre et mourir pendant la Grande Guerre, 1914–1925* (Paris, 2004), 63.

3 For the campaigns to rehabilitate the reputation of executed soldiers, see Nicolas Offenstadt, *Les fusillés de la Grande Guerre et la mémoire collective (1914–1999)* (Paris, 1999).

4 See Andé Bach, *Fusillés pour l'exemple, 1914–1915* (Paris, 2003). Bach estimates that in 1914–15, 2,400 French soldiers were condemned to death and 600 were executed (ibid., 9).

5 Ibid., 580.

6 Maurice de Fleury, *L'angoisse humaine* (Paris, 1925), 240.

7 Rolland, 'Le suicide aux armées,' 269.

8 An excellent introduction to the debates and recent scholarship can be found in Frédéric Rousseau, *La guerre censurée: Une histoire des combattants européens de 14–18* (Paris, 2003), 7–23.

9 Rolland, 'Le suicide aux armées,' 278. However, the wartime rate was higher than that of the pre-war rate for young men. For details see note 14.

10 Ibid., 275–7.

11 In his sample, 18 per cent committed suicide at home; see ibid., 274.

12 See, for example, Louis Huot and Paul Voivenel, *Le courage* (Paris, 1917), in which the patriotic self-sacrifice of combat soldiers is glorified.

13 Ian Dowbiggin, *Inheriting Madness: Professionalization and Psychiatric Knowledge in Nineteenth Century France* (Berkeley, 1991).

14 Army rates were difficult to calculate because France's North African army, which was fighting in Morocco, had consistently higher rates of suicide than the metropolitan army. The most interesting statistics come from Georges Botte, who tried to compare the army rate, not with the rate in the general population, as did other writers, but with a comparable civilian group: young men between the ages of sixteen and twenty-nine. The rate for the civilians in the period 1896–1900 was 20 per 100,000 or 18 per 100,000 for unmarried men in this age group, while the army rate was 23 per 100,000. Botte concluded that suicides would always be higher in the army but that these rates were declining, while civilian rates were rising. See Georges Botte, 'Le suicide dans l'armée: Étude statistique, étiologique et prophylactique' (Medical thesis, University of Lyon, Bordeaux, 1910), 27–8.

15 Des Cilleuls, 'Le suicide dans l'armée,' *Annales d'hygiène publique et de médecine légale*, 13, no. 6, 1910, 512; Jean-Claude Chesnais, *Histoire de la violence* (Paris, 1981), 305.

16 Cilleuls,'Le suicide dans l'armée,' 515.

17 P. Chavigny, 'Suicide et suicide manqué dans l'armée,' *Annales d'hygiène publique et de médecine légale*, 13, no. 6, 1910, 483, 486, 491.

18 Ernest Montembault, 'Contribution à l'étude des maladies mentales chez les militaires pendant la guerre actuelle' (Medical thesis, Faculty of Medicine, University of Paris, 1916), 18–20.

19 Jacques Baruk and René Bessière, *Quelques considérations sur la neuro-psychiatrie de guerre (Service de Sainte-Gemmes 1914–1919)* (Angers, 1920), 2.

20 As cited in Louis Huot and Paul Voivenel, *Le courage* (Paris, 1917), 218.

21 Bach notes that the largest number of executions occurred in the first year of the war, from 1914 to 1915. Bach, *Fusillés pour l'exemple*, 15.

22 Jean Lépine, *Troubles mentaux de guerre* (Paris, 1917), 4.

23 *Science et dévouement: Le service de Santé-La Croix rouge–Les oeuvres de solidarité de guerre et d'après-guerre* (Paris, 1918) 207–11; A. Fribourg-Blanc and A. Rodiet, 'L'influence de la guerre sur l'aliénation mentale à Paris,' *Annales médico-psychologiques*, 1, January 1930, 7–8. This article was based on an analysis of the 25,000 files.

24 *Science et dévouement*, 201.

25 A.-L.-D. Costedoat, 'Les troubles mentaux des militaires indigènes musulmans de l'Afrique du Nord,' *Archives de médecine et pharmacie militaire*, 2, no. 2, April 1934, 248.

26 Fribourg-Blanc and Rodiet, 'L'influence de la guerre,' 16.

27 Montembault, 'Contribution à l'étude des maladies mentales chez les militaires,' 44–5.

28 Service historique de l'armée de terre (hereafter SHAT), Archives hospitalières, Limoges, Braqueville hospital, file no. 343.

29 Patricia E. Prestwich, *Drink and the Politics of Social Reform: Antialcoholism in France, 1870–1970* (Palo Alto, 1988), 37–74.

30 Rousseau, *La guerre censurée*, 195–200.

31 Lépine, *Troubles mentaux de guerre*, 7–8.

32 Prestwich, *Drink*, chapter 5, 'The Enemy Within,' 143–78.

33 SHAT, Archives hospitalières, Limoges, Hospital 58A, case no. 7137.

34 A. Léri, *Commotions et émotions de guerre* (Paris, 1918), 95–6.

35 Albert Brousseau, *Essai sur la peur aux armées 1914–1918* (Paris, 1920), 109–10.

36 Huot and Voivenel, *Le courage*, 186, 348.

37 André Fribourg-Blanc, 'Le role du médecin catholique dans le soulagement de l'angoisse humaine' (unpublished presentation, 1940), 4. I am grateful to M. Noël Fribourg-Blanc for this material and for the permission to cite it.

38 A. Porot and A. Hesnard, *Psychiatrie de guerre* (Paris, 1919), 14.

39 Ibid., 18.

40 Louis-Joseph-André Régis, 'Les amnésies de guerre' (Medical thesis, University of Bordeaux, Bordeaux, 1920), 22.

41 See, for example, Fleury, *L'angoisse humaine*, 217, and Huot and Voivenel, *Le courage*.

42 Fribourg-Blanc and Rodiet, 'L'influence de la guerre,' 17.
43 A. Fribourg-Blanc and M. Gauthier, *La pratique psychiatrique dans l'armée* (Paris, 1935), 110.
44 Noël Fribourg-Blanc, 'Le médecin-général André Fribourg-Blanc (1888–1963)' (unpublished manuscript), 3. I am grateful for the permission of the author to cite this passage.
45 *Science et dévouement*, 211.
46 Cited in Rousseau, *La guerre censurée*, 209.
47 Fleury, *L'angoisse humaine*, 255.
48 Porot and Hesnard, *Psychiatrie de guerre*, 66–9; Fribourg-Blanc and Gauthier, *La pratique psychiatrique*, chapter 19, 'Les psychopathies chez les militaires coloniaux,' 485–9. See also Richard C. Kellar, *Colonial Madness: Psychiatry in French North Africa* (Chicago and London, 2007) 129–32.
49 Costedoat,' Les troubles mentaux,' 231.
50 Ibid., 232.
51 See 'cafard' on the website www.aphgcaen.free.fr.1418; Gaston Esnault, 'Le français de la tranchée, *Mercure de France*, 126, March-April 1918, 428.
52 SHAT, Limoges, Archives hospitalières, Hospital 58A, files no. 7401, 7044.
53 F. Lejars, *Un hôpital militaire à Paris pendant la guerre: Villemin 1914–1919* (Paris, 1923), 331.
54 Henri Barbusse, *Under Fire*, trans. Robin Buss (London, 2003), 217.
55 Fribourg-Blanc and Gauthier, *La pratique psychiatrique*, 489. *Cafard* included simple depressive states, some types of alcoholic confusion, and impulsive reactions.
56 C. Herzlich, 'Modern Medicine and the Quest for Meaning: Illness as a Social Signifier,' in *The Meaning of Illness: Anthropology, History and Sociology*, ed. Marc Augé and Claude Herzlich (Chur, Philadelphia, 1995), 160.
57 For the history of these associations, see Antoine Prost, *Les anciens combattants et la société française, 1914–1939*, 3 vols. (Paris, 1977).
58 These advertisements ran regularly in *La Voix du combattant* in the 1920s.
59 Fédération nationale des plus grands invalides de guerre, file no. 6705
60 *La Voix du mutilé*, October/November 1924, 3.
61 *La Voix du mutilé*, March 1924, 8–9.
62 *La Voix du mutilé*, July 1923, 9. This was one of several such reports.
63 *Le Grand Invalide*, December 1925.
64 See Sophie Delaporte, *Les gueules cassées: Les blessés de la face de la Grande Guerre* (Paris, 1996.)
65 See A. Fribourg-Blanc, 'A propos des séquelles tardives des blessures du crâne: Considérations cliniques et medico-légales,' *Société de médecine légale*, 1927, 61.

66 *Le Blessé crânien*, July 1934, September/October 1937.
67 *Le Blessé crânien*, November 1937.
68 For details, see Patricia E. Prestwich, '"Victims of War"? Mentally-Traumatized Soldiers and the State, 1918–1939,' *Proceedings of the Western Society for French History*, 31, 2003, 243–354.
69 See Joseph Caperan, *Commentaire de la Loi du 31 mars 1919 sur les pensions militaires, suivi des barêmes et des tableaux officials* (Paris, 1919), 51–2. I wish to thank Dr Michael Lanthier for this reference.
70 Decision of 29 July 1925, no. 82,444.
71 For details, see Offenstadt, *Les fusillés de la Grande Guerre*.
72 For example, the deputy Félix Brun, who was vice-president of Barbusse's association, the Association républicaine des anciens combattants. See *Réveil des combattants*, July 1934.
73 Archives nationales, carton 14907, Assemblée nationale, Commission des pensions, 9 December 1931.

7 'This Painful Subject': Racial Politics and Suicide in Colonial Natal and Zululand

JULIE PARLE

> We have given the remarks of the Protector on this painful subject in full, and we cannot help expressing our surprise that it has been dismissed so light-heartedly. Suicides among indentured Indians have become a feature year after year, and we think that the cause ought to be probed to the bottom. And it is hardly an answer coming from the Protector of Indians that he cannot arrive at even a probable cause if those who are supposed to know decline to give any information. There is enough in the Protector's statement to shew that there must be something wrong.
>
> Editorial, *Indian Opinion*, 4 June 1904[1]

In June 1904 in Natal, South Africa, *Indian Opinion*, the newspaper begun by Gandhi a year earlier, published a commentary on the annual report of the colony's protector of immigrants, which testified to the unacceptably high death rate among Indians, especially those who had come to the colony as indentured workers.[2] The newspaper's editorial drew particular attention to the 31 deaths that had occurred in the previous year as a result of suicide. It went on to call upon the colonial government to institute a commission of inquiry into 'this painful subject.' No such inquiry into the rate of suicide in Natal was ever held; instead, the settler state sought to blame the epidemic of self-inflicted deaths amongst Indians in the colony on 'the nature'– the character and the culture of – 'the Indian himself.'

Suicide amongst South African Indians, whether under colonialism or during the segregationist era of the 1910s to the 1940s or the apartheid regime of the late 1940s to the 1990s has been written about by several important sociologists and historians, and the picture that has come down to us, both statistical and sociological, is that indentured and later 'free' Indians in Natal and Zululand had not only higher rates of suicide than Africans and whites in the region but also perhaps extraordinarily elevated rates in comparison to indentured worker populations elsewhere in the British Empire. These scholars have interpreted the high rate of suicide amongst Natal Indians as a form of social protest against their extreme exploitation as workers. It has also been interpreted as an expression of alienation, both from the settler society that subjected them to such conditions and denied them the rights accorded to citizens and to some extent also from the majority African population.[3] South African Indian suicide has, then, been politicized as well as being pathologized.

The ample evidence of Indian suicides in the period before the First World War is not matched by that for other residents of Natal and Zululand, however. For while both the colonial state and its critics had good reason to document Indian suicides, there was neither the will nor the means to do so for whites or Africans. Indeed, until the second decade of the twentieth century, settler suicide was regarded as extremely shameful and therefore seldom noted in official records. Moreover, it can be argued that self-killing by Africans has only received significant coverage since they have become citizens of the 'new South Africa,' moving away from a supposedly traditional, conservative, and rurally based life where suicide was rare, if not unthinkable. In this view, it is the stresses, strains, and conflicts of modernity that are to blame for escalating rates of suicide amongst Africans.

This chapter is a distillation of a wider history of mental illness and suicide in colonial Natal and Zululand, where I have argued that archival research shows that segregating the history of self-murder by race has both reflected and contributed to racialized record-keeping and that these separate narratives of suicide fit too neatly into a view of South African history that served the needs of apartheid.[4] My intention in this chapter is to foreground the argument that it was the different subject positions of Africans, whites, and Indians in colonial Natal and Zululand that influenced the ways that suicide did or did not come to the notice of the state and was recorded thereafter. In other words, subjects' political, legal, and social status influenced the response of the state to the painful subject of self-murder.

Indenture, Suicide, and Statistics

'The result of these enquiries proved beyond doubt that no blame could be attached to anyone but the Indians themselves.'[5]

By 1904, indentured workers had been coming to Natal from India for four decades. They worked mostly on Natal's sugar estates but also on the railways, in the coal mines, and as domestic servants. Their labour was necessary because of the failure of the emerging settler capitalist state to force Africans off the land and into permanent wage labour. Their presence in the colony was not intended to be permanent, but many indentured workers declined to take up the free return passage to India at the end of their contract. Instead, they entered into further periods of indenture or became market gardeners, fishermen, hawkers, and small-scale traders. By 1911, after which no further indentures were contracted, there were approximately 133,000 Indians resident in Natal and Zululand, of whom nearly 70,000 were classified as 'free Indians,' that is, those who had served out their contracts or their descendants. Around 44,000 persons were still serving out their indenture. To the growing alarm of colonists, Indians now outnumbered whites.

Most of the indentured workers had come from southern India, and the majority were Hindu, speaking a variety of languages: Tamil, Telegu, and Urdu. There was a second category of immigrants from India, the 'Passenger Indians,' who had at no stage been indentured and who in 1911 numbered just under 20,000 persons; they had come of their own volition to Natal as immigrants. They were usually Muslim, and many became successful traders.[6] From the late nineteenth century, these 'Arab' traders began to compete with white Natalians, who from 1893 enjoyed greater political autonomy from Britain under responsible government. It is no coincidence that from this time hostile rhetoric against a supposed 'Asiatic menace,' invoking commercial as well as public health concerns, was voiced by white traders, politicians, and workers.[7] From the late 1890s the rights of full citizenship that had originally been guaranteed to Indians who remained in the colony after indenture were systematically stripped away, and a variety of pressures were brought to bear to push them into leaving the colony. After 1896, payment of an annual licence fee of £3 was enforced; this proved especially crippling, forcing many workers to reindenture or to return to India. It was against this backdrop that Gandhi had begun his political career, drawing up petitions, calling mass meetings, and finally initiating the momentous *satyagraha* movement, which was largely focused against the compulsory registration of and denial of citizenship rights to Indians in the Transvaal and, after 1910, the Union of South Africa.

Gandhi returned to India in 1914. While his legacy in South Africa is complex and increasingly contested, it seems certain that for many he embodied aspirations for political rights and for better conditions for Indians in the region.[8] Certainly, by the early twentieth century, these were being pushed for by the nascent Natal Indian middle class, such as those who wrote for and read *Indian Opinion*. It was also this newspaper which drew repeated attention to the unsanitary conditions on many of the sugar estates, collieries, and barracks where Indians lived and worked, and which reacted with alarm and indignation to the high incidence of suicide, especially amongst indentured Indians. In its editorial of 4 June 1904 the newspaper noted that according to the protector's report for 1903, 'Out of the free Indian population of 51,259, there were 8 suicides. Out of 30,131 indentured Indians, there were 23.'[9] The paper went on to add that the highest rate of suicide in the world was to be found in Paris, where 422 suicides per million inhabitants occurred. In Natal, however, calculations revealed that the comparative figure amongst indentured workers was 741 per million. The editorialist commented: 'These figures are sufficient to give cause for very serious reflection.'

It is perhaps ironic that of all the people of the region at the time, it was Indians coming to Natal as indentured workers who were most thoroughly, even forcibly, brought within the ambit of Western biomedicine. For even before they embarked on their voyage to Natal, they were subjected to a level of state-sponsored medical scrutiny and surveillance that exceeded that of whites and Africans. At the Indian ports, Natal emigration agents in India (primarily based in Madras and Calcutta) engaged medical officers to check the health of the prospective migrants before they embarked on one of the ships specially chartered to transport them. Since the Natal government had to pay the cost of transporting the workers, it was anxious to ensure that their health was good and that they were capable of manual work when they arrived.[10]

A long list of undesirable physiological and behavioural defects was issued to the medical officers, instructing that applicants be rejected if they showed signs of contagious disease (including smallpox and syphilis) or physical abnormality (including being one-eyed or having enlarged testes), and men who had formerly worked in trades such as shopkeeping or weaving were as unwelcome as beggars or 'users or opium and ganja.'[11] On the sea voyage the ship's medical officer combined medical and moral oversight and kept a 'daily record of medical treatment, rations provided, any punishments, and any special weather condition likely to cause sickness.'[12] After landing in Durban and before they could be allocated to employers, the indentured immigrants were lodged in a depot, where they were subjected to another medical examination. Anyone found to be seriously unhealthy or undesirable was either successfully treated or returned to India 'on the next ship.'[13]

The first phase of Indian indentures in Natal had been halted in 1866 after returning workers complained of the harsh conditions of life and labour in the colony. Clawing its way out of a deep economic recession and still too weak to force Africans into the labour market, Natal desperately needed cheap labour, and a new phase of indenture had begun in the mid-1870s. Natal law no. 12 of 1872 established the Office of the Protector of (Indian) Immigrants. This officer was to administer the civil affairs of indentured workers as well as to safeguard the interests of both workers and their employers. As time went by, the holders of this office would often find themselves in an unenviable position, caught between the interests of settlers and indentured and, later, free Indians. In attempting to investigate the subject of Indian suicide as well as in trying to bring about sanitary reforms on the estates, the protector would be lambasted in the press but hamstrung by the colonial judicial authorities, especially under responsible government.

The law of 1872 also stipulated that medical treatment for indentured workers should be provided. The districts in which Indians were employed were divided into medical circles, each with an appointed medical officer whose duty it was to visit the estates and other employers of Indians in the district and to ensure the health of Indian employees. After the establishment of the medical circles, a number of small hospitals were built specifically for the care and treatment of Indians.[14] Employers were required to subsidize the provision of these medical facilities by paying a shilling a week for each indentured labourer. State-appointed doctors were to visit each estate within their circle once a week and to provide a regular update of data to the protector on housing, sanitation, water supplies, food rations, the health of workers, and illnesses and injuries. The protector was also to be notified immediately on the death of an indentured worker, and investigations and autopsies were carried out if any death was deemed to be due to unnatural causes.

Suicides amongst indentured workers were recorded from 1880. Beyond the bald stating of numbers, however, the first official comment on suicide by Natal Indians appeared in 1886, when the protector noted that of the deaths of 392 Indians that year, nearly half children under ten, 45 were from unnatural causes, and there had been a 'marked decrease' in suicides, with the number dropping to 6 from 17 in the previous year. He made no further comment. In 1894 the protector stated that the majority of the 16 male suicides which had occurred in the previous eighteen months were 'new or comparatively new arrivals in the Colony.'[15] This pattern was confirmed the following year. It may be no coincidence that it was recently arrived indentured labourers who also laid the greatest number of complaints of assault and mistreatment against Indian and European overseers.[16]

In his annual report for 1903, the protector emphasized that he was obliged to investigate suicides personally, but he noted that of his inquiries into the 31 suicidal deaths of that year, only 1 had suggested that the fault may have lain with anyone other than the deceased, and that the underlying reasons were 'a mystery yet to be explained.' The *Indian Opinion*, however, effectively accused the colonial government, including the protector, of a genuine lack of interest in establishing the root cause of the 'staggering figures.' 'There is a homely English proverb,' it went on to say: 'Where there's a will, there's a way, and if the Protector would only feel as we feel, having the powers of an autocrat, he should have not the slightest difficulty in tracing the cause.'[17] A call for a commission of inquiry went unheeded.

In 1906 there was further comment by the same newspaper on the topic; this time attention was drawn to the different proportions of suicide by burning between free and indentured Indian women:[18] 'Such frightful mortality from self-immolation, being almost three times as great amongst indentured Indians as amongst free Indians, says very little in favour of the treatment that is meted out to Indians on the estates. Again, we find that, as against one free woman who committed suicide, there were three indentured women, or, if we

correct the figures, there are six times as many suicides amongst indentured women as amongst free women. Can there be any occult reasons
for this astonishing discrepancy? Is *all* well on the estates?'[19]

Both these reports singled out James A. Polkinghorne, then protector of immigrants, for criticism, virtually accusing him of a cover-
up. However, correspondence between Polkinghorne and the Colonial Secretary's Office shows that the protector was sincerely
concerned about the suicide statistics. His efforts to establish with
any degree of certainty where the blame lay were frustrated. In 1904
or 1905 – the documentation is unclear as to the exact date – Polkinghorne had written to the attorney general suggesting that 'the
Deputy Protector might assist in the enquiries' by magistrates into
unnatural and accidental deaths. The attorney general rejected this
as an 'improper suggestion,' regarding it as unwarranted interference in his department's jurisdiction.[20] In 1906 Polkinghorne once
more wrote to the colonial secretary that 'the suicides are excessive,'
and referring to the attorney general's resistance to any perceived
interference in the judicial process by his office, he added that 'all
that can be done now is for me to read through the depositions and
if there are any suspicious circumstances then to make further
enquiries.' By now he was unequivocal in identifying 'treatment by
the Employer [as] a contributory factor' in the case of at least 3 of the
20 suicides officially recorded for 1905. He ended his report with a
request for greater supervisory powers for his office, stating that this
would 'probably tend to lessen the suicides among Indentured
Indians in this Colony.'[21]

Once more Polkinghorne was denied further powers to explore the
causes of what he was now referring to as an 'epidemic of suicide.' In
late 1906 he pointed out that this epidemic gave the colony the
dubious distinction of having one of the highest rates of self-killing by
indentured workers in the British Empire. He himself noted that the
local rates were higher than those of Mauritius, Fiji, and Jamaica but
lower than those in Demarara (British Guiana). This analysis stands in
contrast to the figures quoted by Surendra Bhana and Arvinkumar
Bhana, who produced probably the most thorough study of suicide
amongst Natal's indentured Indians to date. They state that Natal's
rate 'far [exceeded] the rates in other British colonies,' being second
only to that of indentured workers in Fiji.[22]

No matter which colony ranked first in the statistical stakes, the
figures for Natal are startlingly high. The statistical tables that estab-

lished deaths as unnatural, suicidal, or accidental initially detailed only indentured Indian labourers, noting the (first) name, official number, sex, age, and cause of death. The earliest entry for suicide was in 1880. In surveying the records of the protector, as well as these tables, for the thirty-six years between 1875 and 1911, Bhana and Bhana identified 363 deaths by suicide of indentured Indians. They also note, however, that because of discrepancies between the protector's records and their own archival searches, which revealed some 'individual suicide reports' of persons not listed by the official records, 'it is doubtful that the actual number of suicides will ever be known.' For instance, they found that a further 44 Indians who had killed themselves might also have been indentured workers, but their status was not clearly marked in the records.[23] By my own calculations, in Natal's published colonial records between 1880 and 1916, the deaths of more than 670 Indians were officially recorded as intentional suicide.[24] It is likely that the actual number of suicides was somewhat higher than these figures since some deaths determined as accidental could have been suicides. Intent is difficult to establish. In 1885, for example, at least 6 deaths – 2 from burns, 2 from drowning, 1 by gunshot, and another by swallowing poison – could have been intentional.[25] Even so, the number of suicides as a proportion of deaths recorded as being due to unnatural causes is astonishingly high for Indians, ranging in the years between 1880 and 1906 from 8 to more than 50 per cent. On average, a quarter of deaths of Indians in Natal from other than natural causes in these years were self-inflicted.

The social and economic pressures experienced by indentured Indians in the late nineteenth and early twentieth centuries, as identified by *Indian Opinion*, have formed the basis for recent explanations of the high rates of self-killing at the time. As a number of detailed histories have shown, the experience of indentured workers in Natal was harsh. Employers exercised substantial powers of control under the terms of contracts.[26] Capitalist owners of sugar plantations and mines sought to ensure profits by minimizing production costs, and it was not uncommon for the conditions of the indenture to be flouted by employers. On the large estates especially, the picture of indentured life that emerges from the documentary evidence is one of frequent brutality, overwork, squalid housing, poverty, and malnourishment. Alcoholism and excessive use of cannabis were common. It had proved difficult to persuade Indian women to emigrate to Natal, and the imbalance in the ratio of males to females, combined with the strictures of life on the estates and mines, rendered a reasonably settled family life practically impossible to create or sustain in the early years. Indeed, the situation in Natal exacerbated the vulnerability of Indian women within wider patriarchal structures, often leaving them the victims of violence at the hands of men and neglected by employers and authorities.

It is with this background in mind that Bhana and Bhana argue that 'the high incidence [of suicide between 1875 and 1911] is attributable to the conditions under which indentured Indians lived and laboured.'[27] Drawing on insights that flow from Émile Durkheim's seminal study of suicide from the late nineteenth century, they add that 'the narrow confines of an estate constituted a mini-laboratory in which alienation and acculturation co-existed.'[28] Overwork and employer callousness, illness, lack of family support, and grinding poverty with few means of relief, combined with religious ambiguity on the issue of self-killing and an overwhelming sense of despair, were likely to lead to a phenomenon rooted in both psychological and material circumstances.

This is not a line of argument with which I disagree. The economic and political context of Natal at this time does much to account for the increasing incidence of self-inflicted deaths of indentured Indians, as well as of some recently qualified free Indians. Suicides began to rise consistently from the early 1890s, peaking later that decade and again in 1905, 1906, and 1907. This pattern coincided, as already noted, with the granting of responsible government to Natal in 1893. All this suggests a general context for the increase in suicide amongst indentured workers from the 1890s and through the first decade of the next century.[29] On the larger estates, in particular, the need to maximize worker productivity would have been even greater during these years, with a concomitant possibility that the pressures under which Indian workers lived and laboured would have intensified.[30]

Henry S.L. Polak, editor of *Indian Opinion* on the eve of Union, vividly portrayed the increased misery of Indians in the colony, linking 'the state of squalor in which those people are compelled to live who just manage to scrape together the annual tax' and a number of poverty-related diseases, such as malaria, hookworm, tuberculosis, and dysentery. In his impassioned but ignored submission to the Commission into Indian Immigration into Natal (1909), he drew a direct line between the £3 licence fee – which was extended in 1903 to girls over thirteen and boys over sixteen – and 'the depression caused by these diseases that the greater number of suicides amongst the "free" Indian population is due.'[31] Marshalling an impressive array of comparative statistics, Polak urged the commission to take the suicide rates seriously. He compared the rates amongst 'covenanted workers' in Natal to those for India as a whole (fourteen times higher) and to free Indians in Natal (between two and five times higher). Attempting to drive his point home, he highlighted the contrast between the number of suicides per indentured Indians – 585 per million – to that amongst whites in the colony – 168 per million – and in Johannesburg – 370 per million. 'Again and again,' he said, 'the Indian communal leaders' have 'sought an explanation for these figures, but none has been forthcoming. Again and again an inquiry has been pressed for, but without avail. It is submitted the Commission should give the figures supplied the closest examination.'[32] As with the previous calls in 1904 and 1906, Polak's plea fell on deaf ears.

From the 1890s, then, in the colonial records of Natal, the incidence of unnatural death, including by suicide, amongst Indians was meticulously recorded and used on occasion to challenge the authority of the state. Moreover, there were divisions within the state's bureaucracy over suicide. By the early twentieth century, the protector of Indian immigrants gained an ally in the colony's first chief health officer, Ernest Hill, who embarked upon a campaign to compile the 'vital statistics' of the colony. Marcia Wright has commented that although Hill made no direct comments on the policies of the Colony of Natal, from the perspective of the twenty-first century, 'the findings were devastating.' These 'vital statistics' she argues, were used to challenge prevailing racial orthodoxies and to advance public health measures that led to improvements in the living and working conditions of arguably the most exploited labourers in the region.[33]

The significance of the statistics concerning suicides collected by the protector of immigrants is more difficult to establish. Despite a large and detailed body of facts and knowledge, amassed and tabulated by colonial authorities from district surgeons to resident magistrates and the protector's officials, the underlying motives for Indian suicides remained a mystery. In 1906, for instance, the protector investigated 20 suicides. In his opinion, the causes 'in so far as can be ascertained' were depression (6), nostalgia (5), various (2), and unknown (7). While he identified the employer as a 'contributory factor' in 3 of the cases, he also thought that an epidemic of malarial fever might have been the cause of several suicides.[34]

Hindered by estate owners and others in his efforts to get testimony from indentured workers about specific complaints that they might have, the protector also found it nearly impossible to establish the state of mind of the victims of suicide immediately prior to their final act, even when he could freely interview the surviving family members or co-workers of an Indian who had killed him or herself. In the official annual reports, the testimony of witnesses to suicide or of family members was seldom noted, but it does seem that when questioned, they too were often at a loss to explain the reasons for the suicide or declined to do so.[35]

Witnesses commonly blamed excessive consumption of alcohol or abuse of cannabis for suicides. Nor was the protector immune from the tendency to place the blame for disease, illness, and suicide on the proclivities of the persons concerned, rather than on the conditions of their lives under indenture or, as free Indians, often in grinding poverty. For instance, in 1886, despite the deaths of 153 children under the age of ten and 45 unnatural deaths of adults, the protector stated: 'There is not, I believe, a Colony having Indian immigrants as part of its population that can show such favourable statistics, taken as a whole, of births and deaths, as can Natal. There can be no doubt of the suitability of this climate for Indians, and this is proved by the favourable reports of the physical condition of Indians who, after completing their term of residence in Natal, return to their native country, as furnished from time to time by the authorities in India.'[36] The reports echoed the sentiment baldly expressed in 1891: 'There can be no question about it. Natal is a perfect Paradise for these people, and they know it.'[37] By implication, and sometimes by accusation, illness and mortality were represented as being in some way the fault of the individual.

Similarly, explanations for suicides were sometimes provided by reference to 'the character or temperament of some Indians ... as this ... is such that quite trivial circumstances are sufficient to cause them to threaten to take their lives – à threat too often put into execution.' Even in the cases of the 'many suicides of the beggar class,' people were regarded as ultimately responsible for their own demise. In 1886 the protector's report commented that 'such men will not accept work although they might readily obtain it, and seem to prefer the unsettled life, with its attendant miseries of begging. Eventually apparently, they tire of the existence they have made so little effort to render useful or happy, and put an end to it in some isolated bush or deserted hut.'[38]

The causes of Indian suicides were not infrequently regarded as being 'frivolous' and inexplicable. In 1900, commenting on the 13 suicides that had occurred during the previous year, the protector opined, 'The majority of the suicides that take place amongst the Indian population here are attributable, directly or indirectly, to jealousy, domestic troubles, or disappointments of some or other kind.'[39] This interpretation of the ultimate cause of suicidal acts by indentured workers echoed that stated six years earlier: 'The result of these enquiries [has] proved beyond doubt that no blame could be attached to anyone but the Indians themselves.'[40]

Death in Black and White:
Suicide, Civilization, and Citizenship

In the early twentieth century, Indians were not citizens of the colonial state in Natal but were entitled to its protection. In the case of abuse, infringements of rights, and direct physical harm by employers and settlers, the rule of law was enforced by the state, albeit sometimes with reluctance. There was little, or so the most powerful colonial administrators claimed, the government could do to save suicidal Indians from themselves. Charged with the responsibility for subject peoples and unable to ignore suicide amongst Indians in Natal, officials located the impulse to suicidal acts within the individual or the innate nature of 'the Indian.' This way, colonial responsibility for exploitation, alienation, and oppression could be evaded. Instead, 'race' served as a self-evident explanation for behaviours and acts that might otherwise have required closer investigation and intervention by the state.

What form that intervention might have taken in the context of the times is a matter of some contention, since views about the causes of and appropriate response to suicide still mixed criminality, morality, and mental derangement. In Natal and Zululand before 1918, suicidal acts by Indians received no special comment from the colony's emerging psychiatric profession. The perception of suicide as belonging in the medical domain, rather than that of the magistrate, grew only slowly and unevenly in this region. Unsurprisingly, this gradual shift in attitude involved an alleged relationship between race and mental

capacity. Whites' supposed greater vulnerability to nervous prostra-
tion and neurasthenia was connected to their more highly 'civilized
state' characterized by refined mental and emotional capacities, while
Africans' apparently low rate of self-inflicted deaths was thought
indicative of their lack of fitness for civilization, which in part
stemmed from their very mental make-up.

The colonial government of Natal and later the Union of South
Africa had, of course, a different relationship to whites, whom it
regarded as its legitimate citizens. In the late nineteenth century and
early twentieth centuries, whites who killed themselves were a source
of family and social shame, but more than that, their deaths challenged
the facade of enlightened civilization that imperialism sought to
present. Hence, suicide amongst whites was initially ignored and went
largely unrecorded. I was able to find only two instances in the thirty-
three-year period 1870 to 1903 where completed suicides by 'Europeans' (to use the terminology of the time) were noted and published
in the colony's records,

At a time when suicide not only was an offence but also carried substantial social censure, district surgeons, magistrates, and police probably shared a reluctance to stigmatize colonists with the shame of a
verdict of suicidal death. Yet from newspapers and anecdotal and sec-
ondary sources, we know that many whites deliberately took their
own lives. Moreover, committal papers from 1916 show that in that
year the Pietermaritzburg Mental Hospital admitted at least one-third
of 'European' patients for acts suspected as 'suicidal.' It was not until
after the establishment of the Office of Public Health in 1901 that a
formal channel was created for the compilation of statistics concerning
'European' self-inflicted deaths, and this occurred at the same time as
a softening of attitude towards whites who attempted suicide. From
the early twentieth century, both popular and administrative opinion
began to favour the mental hospital rather than the jail as the appropriate place for suicidal whites.

The medicalization of suicide took several more decades for South
Africans of Indian descent, perhaps even a century for Africans. Even
for 'Europeans,' the move towards a medico-psychiatric framework of
response to suicide occurred unevenly. For instance, in South Africa, as
around the world, the early twentieth century was a time when race,
heredity, and the dangers of degeneration entered popular and scientific thought and practice. It appeared that the 'burdens of civilization'
which whites were believed to carry made them vulnerable to nervous

strain and possible collapse, including suicide. Some whites, especially middle-class colonists, intent on self-destruction began to receive more sympathetic responses to their suicidal impulses and to obtain treatment at asylums and mental hospitals. Poorer-class white patients, on the other hand, were viewed with increasing suspicion, along with the perceived threat that they, in the words of Dr J.T. Dunston, South Africa's first commissioner for mentally disordered and defective persons, 'posed to the white race' through 'the propagation of the unfit' by the 'feeble-minded' and by those whom he said 'spread insanity by being discharged [from psychiatric facilities] unrecovered.'[41] Sanity and suicide were therefore linked to state responsibility for providing psychiatric facilities for mentally vulnerable citizens and to its role in protecting subjects from themselves and from each other.

Alternatively, Africans, while subjects of the colonial state, were never intended to be full citizens. The extremely restricted ability of the small numbers of settlers and the state to observe, let alone to police, the African population of both Natal and Zululand meant recourse to indirect rule. The majority would stay on the land, and migrant labour would be regulated. Some forms of authority were devolved onto local rulers, who governed in certain matters according to 'customary law.' Indirect rule meant that the colonial state relied on chiefs and headmen to report births and deaths. In Natal and Zululand, chiefs were, on pain of a fine, required to report unnatural deaths, including suicides, to the local resident magistrate, and in some instances heavy fines were imposed when it became apparent that they had failed to do so. Sporadic accounts of investigations and post-mortems into cases of suspected suicide surface in magistrates' and district surgeons' records. However, there was no systematic reporting on African suicides as there was for indentured Indians. In part, this was because the process of reporting and registering a death would be laborious, and it seems safe to surmise that the colonial authorities were not informed of many incidents of voluntary death that Africans themselves had recognized as such. Consulting official records today thus endorses what appears to be a picture of a very low occurrence of African suicides, or at least completed suicides; the statistics show a significant number of African men being charged with and punished for attempting suicide.[42]

As Mahmood Mamdani has eloquently explored in his book *Citizen and Subject:. Contemporary Africa and the Legacy of Late Colonialism,* central to the rationale that underpinned the ideology of indirect rule was the set of beliefs – from popular and political discourse alike – that Africans were not only 'uncivilized'; they were in some ways unique. More specifically, Africans were childlike, underdeveloped psychologically and emotionally, and incapable of experiencing self-reflection, depression, or unhappiness. South African prime minister and international statesman Jan Smuts, in his Rhodes Memorial Lectures at Oxford in 1929, described 'the African as the only happy human I have come across.'[43] Given this essentialized nature, Africans were thought not to be given to suicide except in unusual, even perverse, circumstances. Elsewhere in this volume, Andrew Fearnley explains that it was only after the Second World War that those who studied suicide in the United States began to recognize that black people 'do kill themselves.'[44] The alleged motivation for their suicide, however, continued the long-established trope of 'black people commit[ing] suicide principally out of frustration and rage, rather than introspection and depression, [in] ... a particularly obvious use of the longstanding associations of blackness and violence.'[45] As late as 1952, anthropologist and colonial administrator M.D.W. Jeffreys suggested that Africans were prone to a different type of suicide, which he termed 'Samsonic.'[46] Death was intentionally sought because of the belief that the suicide's 'ghost' could take revenge on living persons.

Archival research challenges both the recorded incidence of African suicide and the supposed impulses that drove people to self-destruction. A reading of the inquests scattered through the colonial archives attests that Africans who attempted or completed suicide came from various backgrounds and took their lives for a variety of reasons. A few examples will suffice. Chief Manqamu of the Mbonambi in Zululand was arrested after setting fire to his hut and apparently threatening to commit suicide by drowning himself in the sea.[47] In 1909 the 'kraal head, Mqatshelwa Nqaiyana, in the Lower Umfolozi' region, reported to the resident magistrate that one of his wives, the thirty-five-year-old Xotshwasi, had hanged herself from a tree the morning after refusing to 'sleep in my hut.'[48] 'Mavili, of the kraal of Chief Ngokwana' in Zululand, hanged himself after murdering his wife, Nogusa, in early 1915.[49]

These accounts give us a glimpse into African suicides, but we can be sure that there were many more. Serendipitously, in a search of a single box in the remaining records of Lower Umfolozi, for example, I came upon two probable suicidal deaths that had not been specifically noted. In May 1909 a young woman named Nqobokazana died as a result of stabbing herself with an assegai. Six months later Banonile, wife of Mhlanhlo, died in a similar way, insisting as she died that 'her "heart" had directed her to cut her throat and accordingly she did so.' Chief Manqamu kaSomelomo reported Banonile's death to the resident magistrate. Although not a medical doctor, let alone a psychiatrist, Turnbull pronounced, 'I am of opinion that deceased must have been suffering from puerperal fever and consequent hysterical mania to have acted as she did.'[50]

After the death by hanging of Xotshwasi, her husband, her stepson, and the chief wife all testified that they 'could not account for her actions.' This was a constant refrain in recorded testimony. Officials did not, however, make overt connections between suicides by Africans and race. When Bafikile kaMpepo, wife of Putili kaNomageja, was found hanging by her neck, Resident Magistrate Turnbull decided that, despite discrepancies in the testimonies of various witnesses, including that of her husband, her suicide had little or nothing to do with a row she had had with Putili or the favour he had shown to another woman. Instead, the magistrate expressed the verdict that 'the mere fact of her adorning herself with her beadwork before committing suicide indicates that she must have been of a jealous and selfish disposition, and ... her whole action was premeditated. In the opinion of the court, temporary insanity cannot be advanced.'[51] His chauvinism has been shared by many commentators on female suicide the world over, but his comments are not racialized.

Nor were African suicides uniquely driven by the need for 're-venge.' Instead, testimony often revealed a history of troubled behaviour and relationships, sometimes accompanied by an apparent abuse of alcohol, and intra-familial interactions fraught with tensions and violence, especially between husbands and wives and brothers and sisters. 'Look at this gun, and look at me for the last time, see how I finish myself off,' said Umkonjiswa after repeatedly beating his sister and threatening to kill her, and shortly before stepping outside their hut and fatally shooting himself in the face. Often the act of suicide seems to have been precipitated by an argument like many others. Officials and those closest to the deceased were usually unable to comprehend the final thoughts and actions of the suicidal person.

In part, it is because records of African suicide were not systematically kept that most studies of suicide stressed the *absence* of self-
destruction by Africans until an apparent marked and rapid increase
in very recent times. While there may have been some cultural
restraints on African suicide that kept its incidence in check, I would
put forward two points: first, we cannot know this with any certainty,
given the paucity of records; and second, the absence of these records
is in part a consequence of an ideological bias that has rendered
African suicide largely invisible in the records which do exist.

To admit to Africans sharing a common mental – psychological and
emotional – landscape with 'Europeans' (including a capacity for
suicide as well as for depression, alienation, and inner conflict) was to
undermine the justifications for colonial rule and to open the door to
the recognition that Africans could and should share equal rights with
whites and enjoy equal protection from the state – in other words, to
be recognized as citizens as well as subjects. It perhaps, then, not surprising that suicide amongst black Africans in South Africa has only
recently become recognized as a serious matter. Unfortunately, understanding these patterns of self-destruction is hampered by the inadequate and racially skewed statistics of the past.[52]

Conclusions

In nineteenth- and early twentieth-century Natal and Zululand, as
elsewhere, suicide had not yet become an issue of mental health.
Instead, it could be perceived of as being primarily a personal failure
in the face of circumstances that were trying but not unbearable. Or, as
for the editorialists of *Indian Opinion* in 1904, the high incidence of self-
killing could be regarded as a tragic response to intolerable conditions
that robbed people of hope and dignity. In the apartheid era, suicide
amongst South African Indians was regarded, at least in part, as a form
of protest against racial discrimination and the social pressures of a
newly forming cultural and class subjectivity. For black South
Africans, suicide went largely unrecorded and unremarked, supposedly a 'taboo surrounded by silence.' Each of these separate stories of
suicide was imbued with beliefs about the relationship between race
and culture. Each was influenced by the subjects' relationship to the
state.

From the perspective of the twenty-first century, we might also think
about suicide as being tied to not only to notions of citizenship and the

right to representation but also to the broader principles of a citizen's right to protection by the state. On the one hand, in South Africa today the toxic combination of post-apartheid social upheavals, escalating poverty, violent crime, and, above all, the devastation of HIV/AIDS means that the relationship between suicide and the broader context of public health provision is perhaps more significant than ever before. On the other hand, suicide results from a profoundly complex interaction between individuals and the society in which they live, and I do not wish to overemphasize the role that the state can play in preventing such deaths. Indeed, as a U.S. government response to three simultaneous suicides at Guantánamo Bay in mid-2006 revealed,[53] for detainees in prisons and other places of detention today – and as this chapter has shown, for indentured Indians in colonial Natal in the nineteenth and early twentieth century – it is possible to be subjected to intense medical and other forms of state surveillance but denied essential human rights. In such circumstances, then, it becomes possible for self-killing to be officially treated, not as a result of intolerable circumstances, but as simply 'this painful subject.'

NOTES

My sincere thanks to David Wright and Barbara-Ann Bartlett at McMaster University for assisting me in the arrangements to travel to Canada to participate in the International Conference on the History of Suicide, August 2006, and to UKZN Press for permission to reproduce portions of this chapter. Unless otherwise stated, all archival references are to the Pietermaritzburg Archives Repository, South Africa.

1 Quoted in S. Bhana and B. Pachai, eds., *A Documentary History of Indian South Africans* (Cape Town and Johannesburg: David Philip, 1984), 18–20.
2 Today South Africans of Indian descent form a significant demographic, cultural, economic and professional sector of the population of KwaZulu-Natal: according to the 2001 census, they comprised circa 8.5 per cent of the population of the province, with whites at 4.7 per cent; of the population of Durban, the percentages were Indians as just under 20 and whites at a fraction under 10. The use of racialized terminology in this chapter is regrettable but unavoidable.
3 For suicide amongst Indians in Natal in the colonial period, see S. Bhana and A. Bhana, 'An Exploration of the Psycho-Historical Circumstances

Surrounding Suicide among Indentured Indians, 1875–1911,' in *Essays on Indentured Indians in Natal*, ed. S. Bhana (Leeds: Peepal Tree Press, 1990), 137–89. For suicide under apartheid, see F. Meer, *Race and Suicide in South Africa* (London: Routledge and Kegan Paul, 1976); and for current analyses, see various works by Lourens Schlebusch, the most recent of which is *Suicidal Behaviour in South Africa* (Pietermaritzburg: University of KwaZulu-Natal Press, 2005).

4 J. Parle, *States of Mind: Searching for Mental Health in Natal and Zululand, 1868–1918* (Pietermaritzburg: University of KwaZulu-Natal Press, 2007), especially chapter 5, 'Death in Black and White: Race, Suicide and the Colonial State.'

5 'Annual Report of the Protector of Immigrants for the Year Ending June 30, 1894,' Indian Immigration Department, II, 8/4.

6 For an accessible history of South African Indians, see U. Dhupelia-Mesthrie, *From Cane Fields to Freedom: A Chronicle of Indian South African Life* (Cape Town: Kwela Books, 2000).

7 M.W. Swanson, '"The Asiatic Menace": Creating Segregation in Durban, 1870–1900,' *International Journal of African Historical Studies*, 1983, 16, 3, 401–21.

8 For Gandhi in South Africa, see especially M. Swan, *Gandhi: The South African Experience* (Johannesburg: Ravan Press, 1995); and V. Jagarnath, 'The South African Gandhi: A Critical Historiographical Review,' unpublished paper presented at the History and African Studies Seminar Series, Department of History, University of KwaZulu-Natal, 7 June 2006. Available at http://www.history.ukzn.ac.za; accessed 7 December 2006.

9 *Indian Opinion*, 4 June 1904, quoted in Bhana and Pachai, eds., *A Documentary History*, 20.

10 J. Brain and P. Brain, 'The Health of Indentured Indian Migrants to Natal, 1860–1911,' *South African Medical Journal*, 1982, 62, 6, 739–42, 740.

11 Ibid., 741.

12 Ibid.

13 Ibid.

14 M. Palmer, *The History of the Indians in Natal* (Cape Town: Oxford University Press for the University of Natal, 1957), 39–41.

15 'Annual Report of the Protector of Immigrants for the Year Ending June 30, 1894,' II 8/4.

16 'Report of the Protector of Immigrants for the Year 1896,' Natal Colonial Publications (NCP), 8/1/10/5/6.

17 *Indian Opinion*, 4 June 1904.

18 The gendered patterns of suicide in Natal and Zululand at this time are

discussed in Parle, *States of Mind*, chapter 5. Briefly, of the officially recorded suicides of Indians, the overwhelming majority were men between the ages of twenty and forty, though suicide by hanging was recorded for the deaths of persons as young as ten and a half and twelve. The most commonly used method by both sexes was hanging, which probably reflected both the availability of means and preference. Other forms of self-destruction involved gunshots, stabbing and cutting (usually of the throat), burning, drowning, and later, as Natal's transport infrastructure expanded, by intentionally lying in front of an oncoming train.

19 'Second Thoughts on the Protector's Report,' *Indian Opinion*, 15 September 1906, together with correspondence between James A. Polkinghorne, protector of Indian immigrants, and the colonial secretary, 8 October 1906, II I/146 3491/1906; emphasis in original.

20 'Attorney-General to Protector, 5 November 1904' and 'Copy of Attorney General's Minute to Colonial Secretary,' 4 April 1904,' II I/130 I2409/04.

21 Polkinghorne to colonial secretary, 8 October 1906, II I/146 3491/1906.

22 Bhana and Bhana, 'An Exploration,' 137 and 151. For suicide amongst indentured Indians in Fiji, see Brij V. Lal, 'Veil of Dishonour: Sexual Jealousy and Suicide on Fiji Plantations,' *Journal of Pacific History*, 1985, 20, 3, 135–55. There are many parallels between the discourse of blame that held indentured Indian women responsible for male suicide in Fiji and colonial Natal. Thanks to John Weaver for pointing me to this reference.

23 Bhana and Bhana, 'An Exploration,' 139.

24 These and the following figures have been extrapolated from the annual reports of the protector of immigrants, found in II 8/3–8/5 and NCP 8/1/10/5/1–8/1/10/5/11.

25 Annexure A, 'Deaths of Indian Immigrants from Other than Natural Causes, Natal, 1885,' in 'Annual Report of the Protector of Immigrants for the Year 1885,' II 8/3, 21–4.

26 B. Freund, *Insiders and Outsiders: The Indian Working Class of Durban, 1910–1990* (Pietermaritzburg: University of Natal Press, 1995), 2.

27 Bhana and Bhana, 'An Exploration,' 137.

28 Hinduism, the religion of the majority of indentured Indians, condemned suicide, but there were special circumstances where it was considered acceptable.

29 The indenture system was abolished in 1911, largely at the behest of the Indian government, and the £3 was tax dropped in 1914, but thereafter, with the Immigration Act of 1913 and repatriation schemes from 1914 in particular, the state actively limited opportunities for Natal's Indians. See

J. Brain, 'Natal's Indians, 1860–1910: From Co-operation, through Compe-
tition, to Conflict,' in *Natal and Zululand from Earliest Times to 1910: A New
History*, ed. A. Duminy and B. Guest (Pietermaritzburg: University of
Natal Press and Shooter and Shuter, 1989), 249–74.

30 Suicides and threats of suicide were not restricted to the large estates,
however, and archival evidence shows that threats of suicide were sometimes made by Indians in an effort to lever for themselves a better form
of employment.

31 Unnumbered eleven-typed-page document 'Indian Indentured Immigration into Natal,' signed by H.S.L. Polak and placed with the testimonies
before the (Clayton) Commission into Indian Immigration into Natal,
1909, Colonial Secretary's Office, 2783.

32 Ibid.

33 M. Wright, 'Public Health among the Lineaments of the Colonial State
in Natal, 1901–1910,' *Journal of Natal and Zulu History*, 2006–7, 24, and 25,
22.

34 James A. Polkinghorne, protector of Indian immigrants, to the colonial
secretary, 8 October 1906, II I/146 3491/1906.

35 'Report of the Protector of Immigrants for the Year 1903,' NCP
8/1/10/5/9.

36 'Report of the Protector of Immigrants for the Year 1886,' NCP
8/1/10/5/3.

37 'Report of the Protector of Immigrants for the Year 1891,' NCP
8/1/10/5/4.

38 'Report of the Protector of Immigrants for the Year 1886,' NCP
8/1/10/5/3.

39 'Report of the Protector of Immigrants for the Year 1900,' NCP
8/1/10/5/8.

40 'Annual Report of the Protector of Immigrants for the Year Ending June
30 1894,' II 8/4.

41 Memorandum, presumably authored by J.T. Dunston, to the acting secretary for the Interior, Pretoria, 'Public Health: Expansion of Asylum
Accommodation, 22 December 1912,' 12, Prime Minister's Office,
1/1/322 184/2/1913, National Archives Repository, Pretoria.

42 This is more fully explored in Parle, *States of Mind*, chapter 5. In the magistrates' courts of Natal and Zululand every year between 1895 and 1909,
at least a dozen such cases were heard. In 1903, 36 Africans – 29 from
Natal and 7 from Zululand – were tried for attempting to commit suicide.
In the following year, of the 52 formal charges on the grounds of
attempted suicide heard by magistrates, 37 were concerned with

Africans. In 1904 there were 11 cases of attempted murder and 18 of culpable homicide, making the number of persons charged with trying to
kill themselves greater than those tried for killing others. Figures extrapolated from 'Return of Crimes and Offences Tried by the Magistrates
during the Year,' Colony of Natal, *Statistical Yearbooks*, 1895–1909, NCP
7/3/23–7/3/16, and 'Bound Departmental Reports, 1899–1905, Summary
of Crimes and Offences Committed by Natives and Tried in the Courts of
Magistrates for the Year,' *Blue Book on Native Affairs*, NCP 8/2/13–8/2/6.

43 M. Mamdani, *Citizen and Subject: Contemporary Africa and the Legacy of Late
Colonialism* (Princeton: Princeton University Press, 1996), 4.

44 Andrew Fearnley, 'Race and the Intellectualizing of Suicide in the American Human Sciences, circa 1950–1975' in this volume, 251.

45 Ibid.

46 M.D.W. Jeffreys, '"Samsonic" Suicide or Suicide of Revenge among
Africans,' *African Studies*, 11, 3, 1952, 118–22, quoted in *African Homicide
and Suicide*, ed. Paul Bohannan (New York: Atheneum, 1967), 9–10.

47 'Depositions charging Manqamu (lately Regent of the Mbonambi tribe)
with the crimes or offences of Incendiarism and Attempted Suicide, while
in a state of temporary Insanity, 10 March 1902,' 1/EPI 3/2/7, LU
154/1902, Durban Archives Repository (hereafter DAR).

48 'Death of Xotshwana, 19 April 1909,' EPI/1 3/2/13, LU 197/09, DAR.

49 Magistrate, Mtunzini Division, to district native commissioner, Zululand,
2 January 1915, Chief Native Commissioner 191, 1915/16.

50 'Death of Nqobokazana by stabbing herself with an assegai, 26 May
1909,' EPI/1 3/2/13 198/1909, and 'Medical Certificate and Report on
Suicide, at Mhlalilo's kraal, Chief Manqamu's ward, Reserve IV, of a
native woman, Banonilie Mhlahlo, 23 November 1909,' EPI/1 3/2/13, LU
727, DAR.

51 'Depositions with regard to the suicide of one Bafikile kaMpepo, a native
woman, the wife of Putili kaNomageja, of the chief Bejane's tribe, 16 July
1897,' 1/EPI 3//2/4, LU 381/1897, DAR.

52 Schlebusch, *Suicidal Behaviour in South Africa*, 2.

53 'Guantánamo Triple Suicide is Good PR for Terrorists, says America,'
http://www.telegraph.co.uk; accessed 12 June 2006 at 6:45 a.m.

8 Medico-legal and Popular Interpretations of Suicide in Early Twentieth-Century Lima

PAULO DRINOT

This chapter examines the history of suicide in early twentieth-century Lima. It explores how elite and popular interpretations of suicide coincided, cross-fertilized one another, and, on occasion, collided. It does so by looking at, on the one hand, medical and legal discourse on suicide as it was recorded in professional journals, treatises, and university theses and, on the other, popular views on suicide recorded by police officers, journalists, court registrars, relatives, and the suicides themselves, when they left notes. It is concerned, in particular, with what different interpretations of suicide can tell us about Limeño society in the first two decades of the twentieth century, a period often referred to as the Aristocratic Republic.

An examination of elite and popular attitudes towards suicide must be considered within a broader discussion of the changing structural and cultural landscape of Lima in this period. Fuelled by a buoyant national export economy, the Peruvian capital expanded both physically and in terms of population, largely as a result of internal migration. Soon the city boasted many of the trappings of 'progress,' including wide boulevards, public buildings, electricity, textile mills, trams, and automobiles, while its population, increasingly cosmopolitan and multi-ethnic, increased from 120,276 in 1897, to 154,617 in 1908 and to 203,381 in 1920.[1] New spaces of socialization, such as theatres, cinemas, bars, and restaurants, as well as exclusive salons and grimy alleyways, contributed to the emergence of new urban cultures.[2] The capital also witnessed the emergence of new social and political actors, particularly an increasingly unionized working class and a large and diverse middle class with growing demands of its own.[3] Soon the city developed a class-based spatial demarcation, as the rich began to move to the southern districts while the poor congregated in high-density housing in the central districts, which became breeding grounds for elite anxieties about the disease-spreading masses, whether these diseases were biological (plague) or political (anarchism). As elsewhere in Latin America, these anxieties were shaped by notions of class and racial (as well as gender) difference.[4]

From 1895 to 1919 Peru was ruled by a small oligarchy, which, though less cohesive or powerful than is sometimes claimed, controlled the dominant Civilista party and key economic sectors and drew from scientific racism the justification for its rule over, and the political exclusion of, what it considered to be a socially and racially degenerate population.[5] Defeat in the War of the Pacific (1879–84) had called into question Peru's viability as a nation-state, which came to be seen as depending on rebuilding the country on the basis of its supposedly vast and largely untapped natural resources and on increasing and, following the failure of campaigns to draw European immigrants, 'improving' its population.[6] Such views informed the thinking of a growing corpus of university-trained professionals, who found in positivism (briefly) the basis for a new national project. In early twentieth-century Lima, ordinary people's lives came under increasing scrutiny; how people lived and died and how they worked and played became the subject of numerous university theses and scholarly articles written by young lawyers and physicians, who saw themselves as the stalwarts of a new civilizing mission. With few exceptions, these studies painted a sombre picture: the population of Lima was not only suffering from racial degeneration as a result of increasing racial mixture; it was also afflicted by social and moral degeneration, a product of ignorance, unsanitary practices and licentiousness. However, although these professionals despaired at the wretchedness of Lima's population, they believed that it could be overcome if a corrective environment was provided. These findings influenced the campaigns led by public health officials, or *higienistas*, backed by a fledgling state apparatus, to inculcate 'modern' and sanitary customs in the city's poor. Although these campaigns had laudable objectives, such as eradicating diseases like the bubonic plague, and found support among sectors of the population, they reproduced the authoritarianism and racial prejudice that characterized the broader interaction between elite and popular sectors.[7]

Both medico-legal and popular understandings of suicide were shaped by this context. Physicians and lawyers in early twentieth-century Lima interpreted suicide through the lens of modern scientific and legal thought and came to challenge the traditional interpretations of the church, which insisted that it was a voluntary act. For these groups, suicide, almost invariably an act of madness, was essentially a modern phenomenon, both product and evidence of Lima's growing 'modernity,' as well as a social disease that could be combated by adopting adequate policies. However, though they opposed the church's insistence on the responsibility of the suicide, physicians and lawyers viewed the propensity to suicide as evidence of moral and racial degeneration and shared its condemnation of suicide as a shameful and immoral act. For ordinary people, medico-legal discourse on suicide provided an additional explanation for self-death. In particular, the idea that suicide was caused by forces over which no one had any real control, especially forces that were a product of the perceived 'modernization' of Lima, helped in the need to dilute blame and guilt. But although medico-legal and popular understandings of suicide cross-fertilized each other, attempts by ordinary people to apportion certain meanings to the phenomenon, particularly those that constructed it as a voluntary act, were perceived by the medico-legal community – and, indeed, more broadly – as threats to society.

Madness, Neurasthenia, and the Secularization of Suicide

Initially, much of the local debate on suicide was based on European examples. Legal journals and medical journals such as *La Gaceta judicial* or *La Crónica médica* reproduced articles on suicide published in European journals, which described the phenomenon abroad. Soon, however, Peruvians also began to write on suicide. Two approaches dominated. On the one hand, the study of suicide became an important component of the specialization in 'legal medicine' or 'medical jurisprudence.' On the other, the interest in suicide coincided with the growing attention to illnesses of the mind and the development of psychiatric treatment.[8] Together these two approaches produced the dominant medical and legal discourse on suicide in the late nineteenth century, which held that it was an act of madness and could not therefore be considered a crime.[9] This interpretation corresponded to the process of secularization of suicide which began with the Enlightenment and which implied a dilution of responsibility for suicide into social and psychological factors. It was a process that still, in early twentieth-century Peru, generated debate between liberals and con-

servatives, as well as among scientists, lawyers, and religious authorities, and was part of a broader process of secularization that included
the laicization of cemeteries (1888), the introduction of civil matrimony
(1897), and the adoption of religious tolerance (1915). According to the
medico-legal discourse on suicide, though there were a number of
'predisposing' and 'determining' causes, both physical (poverty,
illness, alcoholism) and moral (jealousy, vanity), suicide was first and
foremost an act of madness. In his 1899 thesis, physician Neptalí Pérez
Velásquez noted that 'everyone experiences poverty, tragedy, bank-
ruptcy and the death of loved ones ... but not everyone commits
suicide; one needs to be mentally ill in order to commit suicide.'[10] If
suicide was an act that resulted from a loss of reason, it followed that
the suicide could not be considered responsible for his or her death.
Modesto Silva Santisteban, another physician, argued that 'the homicide is a criminal, the suicide is just a poor soul broken by mental
disease.'[11] In particular, physicians contended, punishment was point-
less. Pérez Velásquez criticized 'the devout, the conservatives who are
and have been the ardent defenders of the responsibility of the suicide'
and who insisted on denying burial to suicides.[12] Indeed, punishment
for suicide was increasingly seen as ineffective. According to Sabino
Ríos, the author of a 1920 thesis on suicide in Lima, laws that stipulated the incarceration of failed suicides or the confiscation of the property of suicides served no purpose, as had been recognized by more
developed countries such as the United States.[13]

These views were challenged by the church. An article in *La Revista
católica* from 1894, for example, suggested that the rise in the suicide
rate in France, reported in local medical journals, was the result of lax
religious ideas.[14] As it had done since the Middle Ages, for most of the
nineteenth century the church still refused sanctified burial to suicides
(and in at least one case, refused to marry a person who had tried to
commit suicide).[15] When a suicide was buried either by mistake or,
more often, as a result of pressure from municipal authorities, the
ecclesiastical authorities went out of their way to exhume the body
since the presence of a suicide in the cemetery made it unfit for Christian burial.[16] In fact, it was the exhumation of one suicide (and a
Freemason to boot) in 1888 that sparked a parliamentary debate which
resulted in the creation of laic cemeteries.

In spite of such criticisms, the scientific position of non-responsibil-
ity of the suicide was reflected in Peruvian criminal law, which, in contrast to canon law, established no punishment for suicide or attempted

suicide. As José Viterbo Arias, a lawyer, noted in his commentary on the 1863 Penal Code, 'it makes no sense to punish the suicide.'[17] In contrast to Victorian Britain, where attempted suicide was an indictable offence, liable to up to two years' imprisonment, in Peru only those who assisted or instigated suicides were considered criminals.[18] Both the 1863 and 1924 Penal Codes established severe sanctions, including imprisonment for those who either provided the means for others to commit suicide or helped in the execution of the suicide.[19] Therefore when a suicide took place, a criminal investigation followed to determine, first, if a suicide had indeed taken place and, second, if anyone apart from the suicide victim had had a part. In practice, however, police authorities often treated failed suicides as criminals, subjecting them to interrogations and, at least in some cases, arresting them and transferring them to one of Lima's hospitals.

In refining their thinking about the links between mental illness and suicide, physicians gradually turned to the concept of neurasthenia. The medical profession conceived of neurasthenia as a growing susceptibility to fatigue, not unlike the *tedium vitae* of the classical age or modern-day chronic fatigue syndrome, but more generally as the incapacity to deal with a modern and fast-changing world.[20] As early as 1906, an article in the *Gaceta de los hospitales* noted that what drove those afflicted with psychastenia, a condition related to neurasthenia, to suicide was not a 'systematized obsession,' as in the case of manias, or a 'moral absence,' as in the case of epilepsy, but rather, a state of 'despondence, of moral solitude,' which led them to feel lost and abandoned and to seek to end their lives.[21] As happened with the question of the responsibility of the suicide, the scientific explanation for neurasthenia was challenged by a religious and moral interpretation. For the church, neurasthenia was a form of divine retribution for those who opted for a life of indulgence and carnal pleasure. According to P. Gorena, writing in *El Buen Consejo*, a weekly Catholic magazine, in 1926, 'No doubt about it; the root of all these physical disorders and anomalies lies principally in sloth and gluttony, in dishonest pastimes, in sin; much as a healthy disposition results from work, abstinence, fasting, and Christian precepts, neurasthenia is almost always preceded by a slovenly existence, which, unfortunately, because of the laws of heredity, is transmitted from father to son. The most powerful and proper cure for neurosis is virtue. Repress your passion, crucify your evil instincts, and you will obtain a healthy body and soul.'[22]

Gorena's views on neurasthenia echoed the church's position on suicide more generally. For some, then, neurasthenia was a by-product of excessive work, of a modern and accelerated world. For others, it was a by-product of not enough work, lassitude, immorality, and lapsed religiosity. Significantly, Gorena incorporated scientific notions of heredity into his analysis. L.A. Barandarián, in the same periodical, backed up his argument that suicide was voluntary by reference to scientific knowledge: 'man has principles and instincts whose function is to preserve life. Physiology will tell us of the role played by kidneys, the lymph, the lymphatic ganglion, the bile, the antitoxins, saliva etc.'[23] As I will suggest below, in the same way that Gorena and Barandarián could reconcile their religious dogma with scientific knowledge, early twentieth-century physicians and lawyers combined scientific interpretations of suicide with a religious or moral outlook.

'Modernity' and Degeneration

By the late 1920s the concept of neurasthenia had become debased as a result of overuse. Hermilio Valdizán, one of the leading figures in Peruvian psychiatry and the director of Lima's mental asylum in the 1920s, noted in 1929 that neurasthenia was no longer diagnosed as frequently as before as a consequence of the tendency to use this psychiatric label even in cases where there was no real evidence of nervous exhaustion.[24] Valdizán's comments raise the question of why neurasthenia was so easily adopted as a diagnostic for nervous illness and, in particular, for suicide, and why physicians and lawyers were so particularly concerned about suicide in the first two decades of the twentieth century. Most commentators accepted that suicide in Lima had not achieved the proportions that it had in 'modern' societies. According to Sabino Ríos, in Lima 'our "young village" life does not possess the many complications characteristic of big conglomerations; we do not witness the titanic "struggle for life" of modern cities.'[25] Nevertheless, there was a sense that the rate of suicide was rising. In an article entitled 'The Bane of the Century,' published in 1915, a young journalist called Juan Croniqueur pointed to the perceived increase in the suicide rate: 'suicides take place day after day, and leave on these tragic statistics the bitter impression of disillusionment, despair, and wretchedness.'[26] The following year, Carlos Enrique Paz Soldán, the pioneer of Peruvian social medicine, published an article in La Crónica in which he suggested that Lima was suffering a suicide epidemic: 'There have been few weeks as tragic as the last one for our capital; six suicides in less than ten days. A true epidemic, full of social unease and public anxiety.' Paz Soldán urged newspapers to refrain from reporting at length on suicides, which, he argued, were contagious: 'a suicide takes place: two short condemnatory lines in the newspapers, and end of story.'[27] Significantly, the concern with the reporting of suicides and with acts of violence more generally, whether in the newspapers or, increasingly, in the cinema, became a common theme in the press around this time. In 1918, for example, *La Prensa* pointed to a supposed rise in violence and criminality in the city and urged moderation in the reporting of such acts, arguing that such stories 'push abnormal beings to seek similar experiences of pain.'[28]

The belief in a suicide epidemic – or, indeed, in the rise in criminality – and the adoption of neurasthenia as an explanation for suicide fitted well with the sense that the world, and even backward and parochial Lima, was accelerating at a faster pace than ever before. As José Carlos Mariátegui had remarked in 1912, 'Lima is modernizing! ... The calm, beatific placidity of the old Lima has become a bewildering effervescence, a continuous coming and going; a crazy nervousness.'[29] Suicide was seen as a product of this accelerated world rhythm increasingly experienced in the capital. To the extent that suicide and neurasthenia were perceived as essentially modern phenomena, their growing occurrence gave a boost to the belief (or desire) that Lima was indeed becoming a more 'modern' city: 'The maelstrom of this hectic life that makes us ill, the electricity that gradually sensitizes our nerves, the telephone that gently generates mental breakdowns, the dizzying confusion of automobiles that whiz past with howling horns, all become fertile seeds of neurasthenia. The man who committed suicide yesterday was a neurasthenic... The neurasthenia invaded his body and made him a slave. Once she had taken over his strength, she led him to suicide.'[30]

Whether suicide was effectively on the rise is, in a sense, irrelevant (and the available evidence hardly supports such a rise). It was not the process of 'modernization' that produced a suicide 'epidemic' in the early twentieth century.[31] Rather, the suicide 'epidemic' that Paz Soldán and others diagnosed was more likely a product of, on the one hand, the growing popular awareness of suicide as a result of increasing discussion of it in the press, which in this period experienced a boom in terms of titles and circulation, and, on the other, a growing preoccupation among the medico-legal community regarding suicidal death. This preoccupation was shaped by broader currents in local scientific thought, which were intimately linked to contemporary debates on the social and racial degeneration of the *gente del pueblo* and on the need to 'improve' the population.

As we have seen, physicians had taken a stance against the church's views by insisting on the suicide's lack of responsibility. However, though they opposed the church's insistence on responsibility, most still viewed suicide as a product of a moral and religious degeneration, of a sick society. According to Modesto Silva Santisteban, for example, suicide was a by-product of 'the lack of religiosity ... and therefore of the vulgar straying towards philosophical ideas. Licentiousness, celibacy and onanism are all factors that produce men who frequently end up killing themselves.'[32] Viterbo Arias, a lawyer, argued that life was a duty to God: 'All men have a duty to carry out on earth, and he who shirks his duty, when he is not called elsewhere, fails in his duty to remain where he was put in the first place.'[33] Physicians and lawyers agreed that those who committed suicide were not criminals as far as the law was concerned, but they were criminals from a moral and religious perspective. People who committed suicide shirked their responsibilities. The implications of such views are clear: suicide was shameful and immoral and deserved some form of moral punishment. To kill oneself was to subvert the natural order of things, to undermine divine authority or, indeed, authority *tout court*.

Significantly, some physicians viewed suicide not only as a product of social or moral degeneration but also of racial degeneration. Andrés Muñoz, for example, called for a ban on interracial marriages because he saw them as conducive to hereditary diseases such as 'illness of the nervous system, madness, epilepsy, alcoholism, and particularly suicide, which, as is well known, is transmitted with great ease.'[34] Sabino Ríos, meanwhile, suggested that suicide functioned as a social safety valve of a biological origin: 'Suicide is simply a sort of human safety valve that protects us from the restlessness of future generations and that leads neuropaths to eliminate themselves voluntarily, thus reducing the number of diseased elements and transforming suicide into a kind of involuntary death.'[35] In Ríos's analysis, the usual definition of suicide became totally inverted: from his perspective, a suicidal person had no control over his or her death, which is naturally predetermined. Such a person was a degenerate being who had been programmed to self-destroy for the benefit of society.

This extreme form of biological determinism was rare. Most physicians believed, in characteristic neo-Lamarckian style, that suicide could be prevented if a corrective environment was provided: suicide, they believed, could be fought on the social field, by rooting out the causes of social and moral degeneration and strengthening those institutions, such as the family and work, which would avert suicide.[36] Andrés Muñoz suggested that young people should be taught 'to love work, order, and freedom, in order to reduce poverty and laziness, which, sooner or later, will have disastrous consequences.'[37] According to Pérez Velásquez, a prophylaxis against suicide necessarily involved 'the provision of work, to combat laziness, hospices for habitual drunks, the closure of taverns and gambling parlours, the regulation of prostitution, and the obligatory medical examination of those who are to marry, in order to prevent the transmission of the seeds of illnesses that may later flourish.'[38] Despite the biological determinism of his thesis, Sabino Ríos too called for an improvement in primary and technical education, alcoholic temperance campaigns, a strengthening of the family by making marriage easier, allowing divorce for 'unequal unions,' and punishment for 'seduction followed by abandonment,' as well as 'a thorough system of protection for the working man,' including guaranteed work and the provision of hygienic housing.

The Experience of Suicide

This chapter now examines how suicide was experienced both by the people who committed suicide and by those around them. Statistical evidence on suicide in this period is scarce and not very reliable. Some sense of suicide rates can be gleaned from the yearly 'Memorias' of the Lima municipality. Some of the medical theses dealing with suicide written at this time contain statistical information, although the authors are quick to admit that the data presented are unreliable. The most complete series for this period appears in Sabino Ríos's 1920 thesis, which includes a sample, based on morgue documents, of 121 suicides for the years 1904–19.[39] A brief analysis of these data shows that suicide in Lima was, to a considerable degree, shaped by local circumstances. For what they are worth, these figures would suggest an overall suicide rate of around 0.04 per 1,000, considerably lower than Buenos Aires (where, according to one estimate, the suicide rate at the time was about ten times higher).[40]

One of the most compelling conclusions that emerge from these data is the extremely high gender imbalance in suicide rates. According to this sample, only 6 women committed suicide between 1904 and 1919. This is considerably lower than the average: around 3 male suicides per female suicide. Certainly, female suicide appears to have been considered rare. When a young woman called Matilde Saavedra shot herself in 1901, *El Comercio* noted that 'female suicides are rare, particularly those that are committed using the method employed by Miss Saavedra.'[41] It is likely that some female suicides were reported as accidents, either because the methods used (such as poison, drowning, or jumping under a train) made it difficult to determine whether there had been intent or, more likely, in order to protect the reputation of the women and, more often, their families. In a highly patriarchal society such as Lima, as Christine Hunefeldt notes, 'women's social and moral duties gave them no right to be unhappy.'[42]

A second compelling conclusion is the high number of foreigners, 42 out of 121. This figure produces a suicide rate of around 0.2 per 1,000 for foreigners in Lima, a rate that is not too dissimilar from that of immigrants in Buenos Aires (0.3 per 1,000 for Italians and 0.6 per 1,000 for other immigrants).[43] Of the 42, the Chinese (13) and Italians (7) form the largest groups, although we also find a variety of European nationalities, as well as other South Americans and Japanese. As well, the sample includes information on the 'races' of the suicides, although naturally we must be wary of such classifications. For what it is worth, these data point to an over-representation of Asians and, marginally, of Indians and an under-representation of blacks.[44] One possible explanation for the over-representation of foreigners may be the absence of social networks of support, which could lead to social isolation, considered by many to be one of the key contributors to suicide. However, the social isolation argument should not be taken too far. As a number of studies show, immigrants, whether Europeans or Asians, in early twentieth-century Lima were quick to set up social networks and institutions to provide support for their fellow nationals.[45]

Other data seem to reflect more closely the structure of Lima's population. According to the sample, most suicides were classified as being of a 'humble' social condition (97), followed by those of 'medium' social condition (28). Only 2 suicides were judged to be of a 'high' social condition. These numbers broadly reflect the structure of the city's social pyramid, but admittedly, we do not know what criteria were used in this classification. It seems likely that there was a greater degree of concealment among the elite.[46] The quality of the data makes it difficult to establish a correlation between certain professions and suicide, although some physicians suggested that 'businessmen, accountants, bankers, and soldiers account for the bulk of the suicides, and this makes sense when we consider that they are the ones most at risk from a turn in their fortune or from a mental disequilibrium arising from excessive work.'[47] Despite the prevalence of poor people in Ríos's sample, there were more literate suicides (39) than illiterate ones (11), although in the case of 21 people, no data on their literacy were available. Again, this outcome reflects the fact that the people of Lima enjoyed a high level of literacy, particularly when compared to the very low national average. In 1908 only 18.3 per cent of Lima's population was classified as illiterate. This figure fell to 9.6 per cent in 1920 and rose marginally in 1931 to 11 per cent, a reflection of the inflow of illiterate provincial migrants.

If we examine suicide across the life cycle, we find that most suicides, 46 out of 121, took place during the 'prime of life' between twenty-six and forty years of age; followed by 'early old age,' forty-one to sixty (31); the period of 'early transitions,' sixteen to twenty-five (28), and 'late old age,' sixty plus (10). Unfortunately, the data do not allow a more detailed analysis of suicide across the life cycle of the type that Bailey has done for Victorian Hull. However, as discussed briefly below, a qualitative appraisal of the data shows, perhaps naturally enough, that the dominant motives for suicide changed across the age groups.[48] Finally, it is worth noting that as many as 70 per cent of suicides were committed using a firearm, usually a revolver.[49] The high incidence of firearms may be linked to the wide availability of guns in Lima at this time, left over from recent wars, including the War of the Pacific and the 1895 civil war. It was certainly higher than in Victorian Hull, where most suicides were committed using a rope.

Despite their limitations, Sabino Ríos's data provide a useful perspective on who committed suicide in early twentieth-century Lima and how. But we need to turn to other sources in order to understand how ordinary people 'interpreted' suicide or, as Bailey suggests, how suicide was constructed socially; that is, how those who committed suicide and those close to them, as well as the police and other authorities who had to deal with suicides, explained the phenomenon, and in so doing, apportioned meaning to self-death. In order to do so, this chapter examines the motives that were given for suicides in a variety of documents, including police files, court records, newspaper reports, and suicide notes. Establishing a motive for a suicide served a number of functions. At one level, it was purely a legal requirement: a probable motive was necessary in order to rule out the possibility that the death was not in fact a homicide or an accident. Although suicides were not considered criminals, when a suicide failed, the man or woman was almost always placed under arrest and sent to one of Lima's hospitals or, in some cases, to prison. How long they remained there is unclear, but available evidence suggests that once the wounds healed, the individuals were allowed to go home. Although physicians viewed suicide almost always as an act of madness, it would seem that those who survived were not automatically sent to Lima's mental asylum, as indicated by the fact that when Magdalena Morón's daughter, Petronila Castillo, who was described as 'mentally ill,' survived a suicide attempt, Morón had to plead with the authorities to have Castillo interned.[50] As a number of cases reveal, the police's job was made harder because the stigma attached to suicide meant that in most cases of failed suicide, the survivors tried to claim that they had not attempted suicide at all or that they had been victims of an attempted homicide.[51]

At a broader level, establishing a motive corresponded to the need to rationalize self-destruction, to give it a logic. The motives can be read as a product of social perceptions of what led a man or a woman to commit suicide. As MacDonald and Murphy suggest, the motives given serve as windows into the fears, and therefore longings, of the people whose lives were affected by suicide: 'The motives that observers and suicides gave for self-killing are an index of what contemporaries were most afraid to lose. They demonstrated the importance of the nuclear family, the precariousness of economic life, and the importance of honor and shame.'[52] Although this comment refers to early modern England, it seems perfectly applicable to early twentieth-century Peru. According to Sabino Ríos's sample, the motives most often given were unrequited love (17 cases), physical illness (16), alcohol (13), financial problems (10), mental illness (9), business problems (5), being 'tired of living' (5), family problems (4), other motives (2), fleeing from punishment (1), and, significantly, 'unknown' (37). Such motives made suicides rational and therefore understandable and acceptable; by establishing a motive, people apportioned an acceptable meaning to self-death. Indeed, to refuse to give a motive for suicide was considered almost subversive, as can be seen from the baffled tone of the police report on the attempted suicide of Sergio Lama y Ossa, an employee of the Chamber of Deputies, in 1899, which noted that Lama y Ossa 'has refused to explain to me the cause of his fatal decision, he has only said that he had simply "decided to take his own life," and that he regretted that he had failed to do so.'[53] As I will discuss below and as this example suggests, though apportioning meaning to suicide was considered necessary, some meanings, and also the absence of meaning, were seen as unacceptable.

When a suicide attempt failed, the survivors were almost always asked to explain why they had decided to kill themselves. When the suicide was successful, however, indirect evidence was needed to establish a motive. In a few cases, suicide notes were left. As Bailey suggests, 'by a suicide note the deceased had an opportunity to turn an act of self-destruction into a form of self-expression: a private act into a public statement.'[54] Suicide notes could serve as a will or testament; they helped to explain the suicide to loved ones or, sometimes, the authorities. In most cases, they were left to reassure those who knew the deceased that they were not to blame. When Juan de la Cruz, a sixty-four-year-old Spaniard who owned a bakery on Zavala Street, shot himself in the mouth in 1899, he left two notes, one addressed to the Spanish consul, indicating that the contents of his trunk were to be distributed among his creditors, together with a list of debtors, whom he forgave, and the other a letter to the police chief in which he urged the officer not to 'bother anyone regarding my death. I have killed myself with my own hands.'[55] For other suicides, the notes served as a form of revenge, apportioning blame for the suicide on others, as was subtly implied in the note that Luis Salinas y Rávago wrote to his soon-to-be widow in 1915: 'Forgive me, your mother and brothers are not to blame.'[56] In yet other cases, the notes were not written with anyone in mind; they can be read as tragic and final personal comments. This is the case in the note left by Felicita Olartegui, a woman who abandoned her husband in Pomabamba to escape to the city with her lover, who then in turn abandoned her when she became pregnant, leading her to throw herself down a ravine: 'Goodbye! I say farewell to this world and I hope that those who remain in it will enjoy it. What a wonderful afternoon for me! Darkness beckons. *May man be damned a thousand times.*'[57]

However, suicide notes were rare. More often, motives were established following police interrogations of close relatives, neighbours, or friends. Suicide brought shame and guilt to the family of the deceased and sometimes to his or her whole entourage. As politician and literary critic Luis Alberto Sánchez recalls in his childhood memoirs, the suicide of Ramón Beltroy in 1916 'was a tragedy for the whole neighbourhood.'[58] The motives given were therefore intended to help to explain the suicide or attempted suicide, to render it acceptable in the face of society's otherwise condemnatory stance on suicide. This was the case with alcoholism, which, as Ríos's data suggests, was seen as one of the main causes of suicides. In 1904, for example, Francisco Huapaya, an employee in a piano store, drank nitric acid but survived. According to his employer, 'every time he gets drunk he develops suicidal tendencies.'[59] Similarly, the suicide of Guillermo Cerrun, a gendarme, in June 1918 was blamed on the fact that 'he was very often drinking alcoholic beverages.'[60] One physician, Alberto García, went so far as to argue that all deaths by alcohol should be considered suicides: 'conscious suicides most of the time, unconscious sometimes, but always suicides.'[61] Suicide was also blamed on economic hardship, whether it came about because of unemployment or because of debt. In 1904, for example, Griceldo Gutierrez, a twenty-four-year-old, jumped off the Salta bridge into the murky waters of the Rímac River. He survived to explain that he had tried to kill himself because he was 'tired of life because he had no work.'[62] In 1911 Florencio Matienzo killed himself in a tavern. The police reported that the motive for Matienzo's suicide was 'the fact that he had outstanding debts and that he was afraid that he would be found out.'[63]

Economic hardship, particularly when it resulted from losing one's employment, and the dishonour attached to debts are likely to have been factors for suicide among the better-off element of Lima society. The poor were mostly self-employed and had little access to credit. Physical illness was also often invoked in explanations of suicide. The wife of Nicanor Merino, who killed himself in August 1907, declared that Merino 'told her repeatedly that he wished to end his life because of the pain cause[d] by his grave illness.'[64] Such explanations are particularly common among older people such as Bernardo Rueckner, a fifty-two-year-old German who in 1898, after failing to kill himself with a bullet to the head, told the Intendente de Policía that 'he had taken such an extreme decision because he could no longer stand being alive or the mortification caused by his lack of sight.'[65]

Love or, more often, unrequited love was also a common explanation for suicide, particularly among younger people. In a number of cases, young men killed themselves because they were scorned and therefore, in their eyes, humiliated and dishonored by the women they loved. Leoncio F. Nuñez, a student at the Escuela Técnica de Comercio, surprised everyone when he committed suicide in 1902. According to his uncle, Nuñez was well behaved and went to bed early, and his frank and merry character had never wavered. However, as three letters found on the corpse revealed, 'Nuñez has taken his life under the influence of an amorous passion.'[66] In some extreme cases, men tried to commit suicide after killing the women they loved or desired. In 1915, for example, Honorio Márquez Valderrama, an eighteen-year-old man from Cajamarca shot the twenty-year-old Julia Vargas twice, killing her, and then turned the gun on himself. According to the police report, Márquez 'had been in love for a year or so.'[67] Although women also committed suicide because of unrequited love, for some women it was a tragic way out of a violent relationship. In March 1918, for example, Faustina Lucero tried to throw herself under a tram but was saved just in time by a police officer. She later claimed that she had tried to kill herself because 'she was tired of the life of suffering that she led, and that her husband beat her all the time for no reason.'[68] A week later Carmen de Bustamante, a nineteen-year-old woman described as 'young and beautiful,' tried to poison herself but survived. Under interrogation, she revealed that she 'she wished to die because her husband abused her.'[69]

The social construction of suicidal death also incorporated the dominant scientific interpretation: that suicide was brought about by mental illness. In 1900, for example, Rodolfo Decher, a sixty-six-year-old German, threw himself off the roof of his house. He had previously tried to kill himself by jumping in front of a train. According to the police report, Decher had killed himself because 'he suffers from a mental disorder.'[70] The following year Isidro Reyes, an agricultural labourer, killed himself. His wife explained that Reyes 'had been mentally ill for some time.'[71] However, in popular perceptions of suicide, the relationship between mental illness and suicide was sometimes ambiguous. One attempted suicide illustrates this. In March 1910 Miguel Huertas and his wife, Eusebia Rivera, were crossing the Puente de Piedra when suddenly Huertas threw himself in the river. Several policemen and passers-by attempted a rescue. Two men jumped in and managed to tie a rope around Huertas's chest, despite his opposition, and dragged him out. The police report noted: 'we conclude [...] that: Huertas, 58 years old, is mentally ill and that he recently left the mental asylum, which leads us to believe that *what led him to jump off the bridge was not an attempt to commit suicide but rather the fact that he does not possess all of his mental faculties*, given that when this happened he was returning from receiving treatment in the pharmacy of the

"Colegio Real."'[72] In this case, therefore, suicide and mental illness were seen as incompatible. Suicide required intent, and mental illness implied that intent was impossible.

Like mental illness more generally, neurasthenia also filtered through to society as one of the dominant interpretations of suicide. In March 1917 Juan V. Brown, an Englishman, shot himself because, according to the police report, 'he suffered from an acute neurasthenia, which led him to take this fatal decision.'[73] Similarly, the cause of Eduardo Pedro Mena's suicide in November 1918, according to the police report, was 'an acute neurasthenia that the deceased has suffered from for some six years.'[74] Significantly, even those who committed suicide cited neurasthenia as a cause: when Luis Salinas y Rávago shot himself in 1915, he left a note to his wife which explained that 'a terrible neurasthenia takes me to the other world.'[75] Neurasthenia became synonymous with a death wish. In April 1917, for example, Melecio Moreno was arrested because he was suspected of intending to commit suicide. He had been seen walking around the police station for some fifteen minutes, and his suspicious behaviour had led the police chief to believe that Moreno 'would in a moment of despair or as result of neurasthenic impulse, throw himself on the tracks or commit a crime.'[76] According to El Comercio, the suicide of Otto Silvestry, an employee of the Ministerio de Hacienda who threw himself down a ravine in 1905, was, as the title of the short article noted, 'a suicide by neurasthenia.' According to the article, Silvestry led a life that was bound to end in misery: 'Silvestry had no family and he lived the melancholic life of those people who have no home and live from hotel room to hotel room.'[77]

As these examples suggest, the social construction of suicidal death largely echoed scientific understandings of the phenomenon. It combined predisposing causes, such as alcoholism and unrequited love, with the dominant medico-legal explanation that suicide was an act of madness and that suicide was brought about by neurasthenia. This cross-fertilization of medico-legal and popular discourses suggests that ordinary people were keen to incorporate scientific interpretations into their understanding of suicide. In this sense, this analysis fits well with interpretations of the medicalization of Latin American societies that stress both top-down and bottom-up processes.[78] Medico-legal explanations gave ordinary people the tools to explain suicide. For the police, medico-legal discourse provided an expedient and authoritative explanation of suicidal death. For relatives, who almost always felt shamed by a suicide in the family, and for the suicides themselves, medico-legal explanations helped to dilute guilt and responsibility by apportioning blame to forces of a psychological nature over which no one had real control.

Conclusion

What do these interpretations of and attitudes towards suicide tell us about Limeño society during the Aristocratic Republic? On the one hand, scientific and popular interpretations of suicide reveal the need felt by both the medico-legal community and ordinary people in early twentieth-century Lima to frame suicide within a logic that made it acceptable, both socially and morally. Doing so meant, to a considerable extent, diluting blame. This rationale may explain the degree to which medical discourse on suicide permeated popular interpretations. If suicide was an act of madness, then those who committed suicide and those who felt they had either precipitated or failed to avert a suicide could not be guilty: suicides were led to kill themselves by forces, some social, others psychological, and yet others biological, over which they had no control. The suicide's agency was therefore removed. People who killed themselves became victims, to be pitied rather than blamed, shunned, or punished. In early twentieth-century Lima, neurasthenia was widely accepted as one of the dominant causes of suicide precisely because it offered an explanation that not only diluted blame but also fitted in well with the belief (or desire) that Lima was becoming a 'modern' city.

On the other hand, although medico-legal and popular interpretations of suicide often cross-fertilized one another, they also sometimes collided. When Julio Guerrero Ortwald, a sergeant in Lima's 5th regiment, killed himself in 1916 after having suffered from acute stomach pains for many years, he left a note that was published in one of Lima's newspapers. The note was addressed to his regiment: 'The pain will not ease; I can bear no more suffering. My footsteps are needles that pierce my gut. I am demoralized and physically defeated. I have therefore resolved to kill myself. Do not call me a coward ... Think. You have witnessed my suffering. Blessed are you who remain to serve the Fatherland ... I am a wretched creature. Destiny has taken me from the army, but, I, who have loved my Fatherland so dearly, dedicate my last words to it: long live Peru!'[79] Guerrero Ortwald inscribed his suicide within a logic of patriotism: in his mind, his death was justified because he could no longer carry out his patriotic duty. Moreover, he dedicated his death, as he had his life, to his country. In this way Guerrero Ortwald gave specific meaning to his death, which, he hoped, would appear in the eyes of his regiment to be a rational, honourable, and patriotic act.

The publication of this suicide note provoked Carlos Enrique Paz Soldán, one of Peru's most eminent physicians, to publish an article a few days later in the same newspaper in which he condemned the reporting of suicides (as noted above) and attempted to demolish the meaning that Guerrero Ortwald had apportioned to his suicide and to replace it with the dominant scientific interpretation: suicide was an act devoid of logic, an act of madness. According to Paz Soldán, 'To boast of love for his country, to write a series of platitudes aimed at, in the author's mind, glorifying what recollection we have of him, and then to shoot himself is evidence of the most complete absence of logic.'[80]

As I suggested earlier, although physicians rejected the church's insistence on responsibility for suicide, they shared its condemnation of suicide as a shameful and immoral act. It is fair to speculate that what irked Paz Soldán and prompted him to write his rebuke was the reference to patriotism: if physicians saw suicide as a shameful and immoral act, an interpretation of suicide as honourable and patriotic that came from a soldier (of all people) represented a palpable threat to the role of physicians in preserving life for the greater glory of, if not necessarily God, then at the very least the nation. Paz Soldán's letter, I would suggest, should be seen as an attempt to control the meaning of suicide.

As this example suggests, the medico-legal community in early twentieth-century Lima accepted that people were (legally) free to kill themselves but not to imprint their own meaning on their death. Suicides such as Guerrero Ortwald's were seen, for good reason, as threats both to the medico-legal discourse on suicide and to society more broadly because they suggested that suicide could be voluntary and even honourable. We should not underestimate how subversive this proposition was in the context of the Aristocratic Republic, when, as I have suggested, the viability of the Peruvian nation-state was seen by many as dependent on the increase and improvement of the population. As Georges Minois has pithily noted, 'How ... can anyone rule people who are not even sure they should remain alive? What hold can anyone have on subjects or citizens who have full liberty to leave life as they please? How can anyone inspire them with confidence if every day a certain number of them manifest their defiance and despair by preferring death to life?'[81]

NOTES

This essay, which appears here in an abridged and revised form, was first published as 'Madness, Neurasthenia, and "Modernity": Medico-legal and Popular Interpretations of Suicide in Early Twentieth-Century Lima,' in the *Latin American Research Review* 39:2, 89–113; copyright 2004 by the University of Texas Press; all rights reserved.

1 Gabriel Ramon Joffré, *La muralla y los callejones: Intervención urbana y proyecto político en Lima durante la segunda mitad del siglo XIX* (Lima: SIDEA, 1999). Although Lima was not a major recipient of immigrants like Buenos Aires or São Paulo, according to the 1908 census, about 10 per cent of the city's population were foreign-born. The majority were Europeans (6,113), followed by Asians, mainly Chinese and Japanese (5,494), and those from other countries in the American continent (1,694). Among the Europeans, Italians (3,094) constituted by far the biggest group, but almost all other European countries were represented. In addition to various nationalities, Lima also was characterized by great racial diversity. According to the same census, the city was home to 66,750 whites (38.6 per cent), 55,831 mestizos (32.3), 32,842 Indians (19.0), 9,400 blacks (5.4), and 7,694 'yellows' (4.4).

2 See Alicia del Aguila, *Callejones y mansiones: Espacios de opinión pública y redes sociales y políticas en la Lima del 900* (Lima: Fondo Editorial PUCP, 1997); Carmen Mc Evoy, 'Entre la nostalgia y el escándalo: Abraham Valdelomar y la construcción de una sensibilidad moderna en las postrimerías de la "República Aristocrática,"' in Carmen Mc Evoy, *Forjando la nación: Ensayos de historia republicana* (Lima: Instituto Riva-Agüero, 1999), 247–313; Fanni Muñoz Cabrejo, *Diversiones públicas en Lima, 1890–1920: La experiencia de la modernidad* (Lima: IEP, 2001).

3 Peter Blanchard, *The Origins of the Peruvian Labor Movement, 1883–1919* (Pittsburgh: University of Pittsburgh Press, 1982), 153–78; Augusto Ruiz Zevallos, *La multitud, las subsistencias y el trabajo: Lima, 1890–1920* (Lima: Fondo Editorial PUCP, 2001); D. S. Parker, *The Idea of the Middle Class : White-Collar Workers and Peruvian Society, 1900–1950* (University Park: Pennsylvania State University Press, 1998).

4 D. S. Parker, 'Civilizing the City of Kings: Hygiene and Housing in Lima,
   Peru,' in *Cities of Hope: People, Protests, and Progress in Urbanizing Latin
   America, 1870–1930*, ed. Ronn F. Pineo and James A. Baer (Boulder: West-
   view Press, 1998); Marcos Cueto, *El regreso de las epidemias: Salud y
   sociedad en el Perú del siglo XX* (Lima: IEP, 1997).

5 Manuel Burga and Alberto Flores Galindo, *Apogeo y crisis de la República
   Aristocrática* (Lima: Rikchay Perú, 1984); Gonzalo Portocarrero, 'El funda-
   mento invisible: Función y lugar de las ideas racistas en la República
   Aristocrática,' in *Mundos interiores: Lima 1850–1950*, ed. Aldo Panfichi and
   Felipe Portocarrero (Lima: Universidad del Pacífico, 1995), 219–59.

6 See Mario Marcone, 'Indígenas e inmigrantes durante la República Aristocrática: Población e ideología civilista,' *Histórica* 19:I (1995), 73–93.

7 See Parker, 'Civilizing'; María Emma Mannarelli, *Limpias y modernas:
   Genero, higiene y cultura en la Lima del novecientos* (Lima: Ediciones Flora
   Tristán, 1999); Juan Fonseca Ariza, 'Antialcoholismo y modernización en
   el Perú (1900–1930),' *Histórica* 24:2 (2000), 327–64.

8 Augusto Ruiz Zevallos, *Psiquiatras y locos: Entre la modernización contra los
   Andes y el nuevo proyecto de modernidad: Perú, 1850–1930* (Lima, Instituto
   Pasado y Presente, 1994).

9 These two approaches can already be gleaned in a couple of articles published as early as 1861 in *La Gaceta médica de Lima* by José Casimiro Ulloa
   and Domingo Vera. See *La Gaceta médica de Lima*, año 6, no. 123, October
   1861, 345–53.

10 Neptalí Perez Velásquez, 'El suicidio como entidad neuropatologica'
    (Thesis, Faculty of Medicine, Lima, 1899).

11 Modesto Silva Santisteban, 'Homicidio y suicidio – sus caracteres
    medico-legales' (Thesis, Faculty of Medicine, Lima). Published in *La
    Gaceta médica*, año 5, no. 10, 31 October 1878, 305–7.

12 Pérez Velásquez, 'El suicidio.'

13 Sabino Ríos, 'El suicidio en Lima' (Thesis. Faculty of Medicine, Lima,
    1920).

14 *La Revista Católica*, año 15, no. 661, 29 September 1894.

15 Archivo Arzobispal de Lima (hereafter AAL), Comunicaciones 35:39, case
    of Liborio Paz Burbano, 3 March 1891.

16 AAL, Notas de Supremo Gobierno XA: 220, Fernando Cavero to director
    de la Beneficencia pública, 3 August 1867; XIIIA:254A, Fernando Cavero
    to obispo de Lima, 5 August 1888; Comunicaciones, XXXIX:121, parish
    priest of San Mateo to archbishop, 1 June 1903.

17 José Viterbo Arias, *Exposición comentada y comparada del Código Penal del
    Perú de 1863*, vol. 3 (Lima, 1902): 36.

18   Victor Bailey, *This Rash Act: Suicide across the Life Cycle in the Victorian City* (Stanford: Stanford University Press, 1998), 130.

19   República del Perú, *Código penal* (Lima, 1924), 48 (Ley no. 4868).

20   On neurasthenia, see Marijke Giswijt-Hofstra and Roy Porter, eds., *Cultures of Neurasthenia: From Beard to the First World War* (Amsterdam and New York: Rodopi, 2001).

21   M.O. Tamayo, 'Un caso grave de psicastenia,' *Gaceta de los hospitales*, año 3, no. 65, 1 August 1906, 141–50.

22   P. Gorena, 'Causas de la neurastenia,' *El Buen Consejo*, año 5, no. 2, 1926.

23   Barandarián, 'El suicidio,' *El Buen Consejo*, año 2, no. 2, 1923, 61.

24   Hermilio Valdizán, *Elementos de jurisprudencia médica* (Lima: Empresa Editora 'Excelsior,' 1929), 43–4.

25   Ríos, 'El suicidio.'

26   Juan Croniqueur was José Carlos Mariátegui's pen name. See 'El mal del siglo,' *La Prensa*, 29 April 1915; cited in José Carlos Mariátegui, *Escritos juveniles (La edad de piedra)* (Lima: Empresa Editora Amauta, 1991), 235.

27   Carlos Enrique Paz Soldán, 'El inquietante problema del suicidio,' *La Crónica*, 25 June 1916.

28   *La Prensa*, 31 March 1918.

29   *La Prensa*, 7 August 1912; cited in Mariátegui, *Escritos juveniles*, 2: 20.

30   Croniqueur, 'El mal del siglo,' 236.

31   In this sense, I disagree with Ruiz Zevallos's analysis; see *Psiquiatras y locos*, 97–8.

32   Silva Santisteban, 'Homicidio y suicidio,' 306.

33   Viterbo Arias, *Exposición comentada*, 36.

34   Andrés S. Muñoz, 'El estado mental del suicida,' *La Crónica Médica*, año 3, no. 32, 31 August 1886, 297–301.

35   Ríos, 'El suicidio.'

36   On neo-Lamarckism and, more generally, eugenics in Latin America, see Nancy Leys Stepan, *The Hour of Eugenics: Race, Gender, and Nation in Latin America* (Ithaca and London: Cornell University Press, 1991).

37   Muñoz, 'El estado mental,' 301.

38   Pérez Velásquez, 'El suicidio,' n.p.

39   Although we know that Ríos constructed his suicide statistics from morgue records, and for that reason, we can assume that they reflect the total number of suicides registered by the morgue during the 1904–19 period, these figures are clearly far from accurate and do not reflect all suicides in this period. Indeed, suicide statistics included in yearly

municipal reports would suggest that Ríos's data underestimate the real rate of suicide.

40 See Eugenia Scarzanella, *Ni gringos ni indios: Inmigración, criminalidad y racismo en Argentina, 1890–1940* (Buenos Aires: Universidad Nacional de Quilmes Ediciones, 1999), 50.

41 *El Comercio*, 6 July 1901 (evening).

42 Christine Hunefeldt, *Liberalism in the Bedroom : Quarreling Spouses in Nineteenth-Century Lima* (University Park: Pennsylvania State University Press, 2000).

43 Scarzanella, *Ni gringos*, 50.

44 According to the data, the sample included 39 whites, 1 black, 36 Indians, 29 mestizos, and 16 'yellows.'

45 Janet E. Worrall, *La inmigración italiana en el Perú 1860–1914* (Lima: Instituto Italiano de Cultura, 1990); Giovanni Bonfiglio, *Los italianos en la sociedad peruana* (Lima: SAYWA ediciones, 1994); Jorge Bracamonte, 'La modernidad de los subalternos: Los inmigrantes chinos en la ciudad de Lima, 1895–1930,' in Santiago López Maguiña et al., *Estudios culturales: Discursos, poderes, pulsiones* (Lima, 2001), 167–88.

46 On elite attitudes to death, see Felipe Portocarrero, 'Religión, familia, riqueza y muerte en la élite económica. Perú: 1900–1950,' in Panfichi and Portocarrero, *Mundos interiores*, 131–8.

47 See Pérez Velásquez, 'El suicidio.'

48 Only one person under fifteen years of age committed suicide (in the case of three people, it proved impossible to determine their age). I take these categories, with small modifications for the age groups, from Bailey, *This Rash Act*. It is worth bearing in mind that in 1940 the average life expectancy was estimated at just below 40 years.

49 Less common forms included hanging (15 per cent), the use of knifes or razors (13 per cent); poison (11 per cent); jumping from heights (3 per cent), and lying under trams or trains (1 per cent).

50 Archivo General de la Nación (hereafter AGN) /3.9.5.1.15.16.15, Intendente to prefecto, 25 May 1904.

51 See AGN/RPJ, Causas criminales, Legajo 83, 'De oficio contra Tomas Fuentes por intento de suicidio.'

52 Michael MacDonald and Terence R. Murphy, *Sleepless Souls: Suicide in Early Modern England* (Oxford: Oxford University Press, 1990), 298.

53 AGN/3.9.5.1.15.116.12, Intendente to prefecto, 11 October 1899.

54 Bailey, *This Rash Act*, 56.

55 AGN/República Poder Judicial [RPJ], Causas criminales, legajo 680, 1899, 'Oficio para descubrir las causas de la muerte de Juan de la Cruz.'

56 AGN/RPJ, Causas criminales, legajo 75, 1915, 'Seguidos con motivo del suicidio de Don Luis Salinas y Rávago.'

57 *La Crónica*, 11 July 1916.

58 Luis Alberto Sánchez, *Testimonio personal*, vol. 1 (Lima, Ediciones Villasan, 1969), 66.

59 AGN/3.9.5.1.15.1.16.15, Intendente to Prefecto, 9 May 1904.

60 AGN/3.9.5.1.15.1.16.35, Intendente to Prefecto, 7 June 1918.

61 See Alberto García, 'Alcohol y alcoholismo,' in *La Crónica médica*, año 18, no. 295, 15 April 1901, 103–6.

62 AGN/3.9.5.1.15.1.16.15, Intendente to prefecto, 7 June 1904.

63 AGN/3.9.5.1.15.1.16.25, Intendente to prefecto, 10 July 1911.

64 AGN/3.9.5.1.15.1.16.19, Intendente to prefecto, 6 August 1907.

65 AGN/3.9.5.1.15.1.16.12, Intendente to prefecto, 6 December 1898.

66 AGN/3.9.5.1.15.1.16.13, Intendente to prefecto, 17 September 1902.

67 AGN/3.9.5.1.15.1.16.29, Intendente to prefecto, 1 June 1915.

68 *La Prensa*, 19 March 1918 (evening).

69 *La Prensa*, 27 March 1918 (evening).

70 AGN/3.9.5.1.15.1.16.12, Intendente to prefecto, 13 July 1900.

71 AGN/3.9.5.1.15.1.16.13, Intendente to prefecto, 26 December 1901.

72 AGN/3.9.5.1.15.1.16.12, Intendente to prefecto, 10 March 1910.

73 AGN/3.9.5.1.15.1.16.33, Intendente to prefecto, 8 March 1917.

74 AGN/3.9.5.1.15.1.16.34, Intendente to prefecto, 27 November 1918; my emphasis.

75 AGN/RPJ, Causas criminales, legajo 75, 'Seguidos con motivo del suicidio de Don Luis Salinas y Rávago.'

76 AGN/3.9.5.1.15.1.16.32, Comisario to subprefecto, 11 April 1917.

77 *El Comercio*, 10 April 1905 (evening).

78 See Diego Armus, ed., *Disease in the History of Modern Latin America: From Malaria to AIDS* (Durham: Duke University Press, 2003).

79 *La Crónica*, 22 June 1916.

80 Paz Soldán, 'El inquietante problema del suicidio.'

81 Georges Minois, *History of Suicide: Voluntary Death in Western Culture* (Baltimore: Johns Hopkins University Press, 1999), 325–6.

9 Violence against the Collective Self: Suicide and the Problem of Social Integration in Early Bolshevik Russia

KENNETH M. PINNOW

The categories used by the Bolshevik Party to study suicide look very similar to our own and do not differ greatly from the work of other Europeans during the early twentieth century. Its investigators broke down the numbers according to such personal indicators as class, sex, age, occupation, and marital status; such environmental determinants as date, time, and season; and to such causal factors as unrequited love, fear of punishment, incurable illness, degenerative conditions, material want, family squabbles, and the ubiquitous 'disappointment with life.'[1] Like their contemporaries elsewhere, they too believed that suicide was an entry point into a deeper understanding of the individual and his or her relationship to society. As a consequence, the facts of Soviet suicide (as with so many other aspects of Soviet society and social knowledge) appear easily transposable to our sociological framework of interpretation, seemingly affording us a clear window into ennui, anomie, and other facets of subjective experience under socialism.[2]

The historian of suicide, however, faces certain interpretative challenges in trying to discern the meaning of suicide under the Soviet regime. Specifically, our conceptual categories of analysis are not fully applicable to a regime where the boundaries between the 'individual' and 'society' were blurred. Any historical study of suicide must confront the problem of how the Bolsheviks conceptualized the self when dealing with instances of this phenomenon among their ranks. It clearly was not the autonomous liberal self but, rather, an individualized 'social body' that was understood through and against the larger collective (*kollektiv*). The direct application of such analytical categories as the 'individual' and 'society' is therefore problematic and demands a different approach to the sources.[3]

This chapter contends that suicide, as a form of violence committed against the self, is best used to examine the way that the individual and society – and the relationship between them – were constructed within Bolshevik Party discourse during the 1920s. Instead of using suicide to measure socialization, resistance, and other structural processes that have occupied social historians, it employs the phenomenon to explore how the Bolsheviks themselves conceptualized human relationships and sought to transform the quality of subjective experience. In this respect, my approach builds upon the work of scholars who have emphasized the historically and culturally contingent nature of suicide's significance.[4] The aim here is to uncover the ways that the Bolsheviks put the idea of social integration into practice and to demonstrate that official responses to suicide must be interpreted within the context of the regime's efforts to build a collectivist social order.

My investigation suggests that within Bolshevik discourse the individual was understood to be the collective's greatest resource and its greatest threat. The act of suicide violated conceptions of the *kollektiv* as a space in which the individual would have the opportunity to achieve genuine self-fulfillment as a member of the group. Party investigators and theoreticians argued that a person could not commit suicide because the self belonged, not to him or her, but to the collective. Acts of self-destruction therefore did harm to the group as well as to the individual. In response, both the civilian and military wings of the Bolshevik Party used the language and methods of social investigation, gathering statistics and other types of information about suicide in the belief that these data were telling of social integration and organizational well-being. They also encouraged a number of distinct practices around the suicide, all of which aimed at integrating the remaining individuals more strongly within the collective. Central to these practices were the joint creation of a 'collective opinion' and the promotion of mutual surveillance as a means of fostering communal relations, strengthening both group and individual accountability, and preventing future acts of suicide.

Suicide as Symbol of Social (Dis)Integration

The cultural meaning of suicide reflects broader understandings of the individual and his/her place in the world. Historically, violence towards the self has figured prominently in the debates surrounding such existential questions as the problem of free will, the possibility of human immortality, and the connection between the individual and God. These debates in turn have shaped the meaning of suicide, as well as policy towards the person who commits or attempts suicide. For example, conceptions of 'man' as a part of God have justified religious and legal proscriptions against the act of violence toward the self, since the individual ultimately belonged to his/her Creator, who solely had the power to determine the individual's ultimate fate.[5]

During the nineteenth century, researchers and social commentators increasingly understood suicide as a symbol of social disintegration. In particular, they connected it to the breakdown of traditional social bonds and to the alienation, nervousness, and pressures of modern life. The axiomatic link they established between suicide rates and 'civilization' helped to explain why suicide seemed to be on the rise across Europe as the century moved forward. It also seemed to explain why levels of suicide were greater among more 'civilized' nations as compared to 'backward' peoples, among city dwellers as compared to rural villagers, among men as compared to women, and among the upper classes as compared to the masses.[6] Suicide thus became associated in the popular mind with the dark side of progress, signalling the destruction of the self amid the quickening pace and materialistic tendencies of the modern world.

The meaning of suicide is also closely linked to those disciplines that defined the individual as a 'social body' whose condition was representative of the larger 'social organism.' Moral statistics, for example, helped to make individual actions significant for the rest of society and thus the business of investigators who professed an interest in knowing and maintaining its well-being. What seemed to be deeply voluntary or individualistic acts, determined solely by the actor's personal whims, were increasingly seen in the nineteenth century as the product of 'social laws' or forces outside the individual. In fact, suicide statistics played a critical role in the construction of 'society' as an entity that could be studied – and ultimately regulated – by the state and various experts.[7] It is no coincidence that Émile Durkheim chose suicide as the vehicle through which he sought to establish the 'new science' of sociology as a distinct field with its own object of inquiry.[8]

I contend that the advent of the Soviet regime in 1917 marks the first time in Russia that the state and various 'experts' could fully participate in this broader discourse about 'society.'[9] To be sure, medical doctors, journalists, and other investigators in pre-revolutionary

Russia engaged in the European debates about suicide and the social order, especially during the era of the Great Reforms; furthermore, their view of suicide as an indicator of social 'illness' suggested a unitary understanding of the population.[10] Nevertheless, their efforts to translate ideas into practice were continually thwarted by an auto-cratic regime that made a holistic conception of the empire's people difficult. Students of suicide in imperial Russia particularly decried the absence of reliable statistics and other governmental technologies needed to intervene in the population. Their primary obstacle was a state and populace that could not see suicide as an injury to the society at large, since individuals were defined by their relationship to their estate (*soslovie*), to the sovereign, or to God and not by their relation-ship to society as a whole.[11]

In sharp contrast, the Bolsheviks emphasized the inherently social nature of the individual, believing that human potential and freedom could only be realized once the false dichotomy between the public and private self was destroyed. Specifically, they assumed that social-ism promised enlightenment, salvation, and immortality by allowing for the complete harmonization of inner being and outer function.[12] The emphasis on the *kollektiv* therefore did not negate the development of the individual, if by this we have in mind distinct persons rather than the liberal notion of autonomous agents. In fact, the Bolshevik regime actively fostered self-awareness and self-discovery as part of its revolutionary project. Public confession, autobiography, and diary-writing were all tools by which men and women would become truly conscious of themselves and their relationship to the *kollektiv*.[13]

These beliefs and practices help us to explain the character of Soviet investigations – both their intent and their usage – into suicide. The abundant statistics, questionnaires (*ankety*), and political reports (*svodki*) relating to suicide during the 1920s reflect in part the triumph of a modern ethos that made the study of human behaviour essential to the governmental regulation of the population. However, the trans-formational goals of the regime gave these efforts a distinctive edge. Soviet social investigation aimed not simply to describe the objective state of affairs in the country but also to reveal the subjective state of affairs inside the individual.[14] In particular, its practitioners were con-cerned with establishing levels of belief and consciousness within the Bolshevik Party and the Red Army, two of the primary locations for attempts to create the new socialist society on a micro-level.

This overview returns us to my opening observations regarding the difficulty of using our own sociological definitions to establish the historical meaning of Soviet suicide. If we instead interpret the sources within the regime's larger transformational agenda, they suggest that suicide provided an opportunity for individual and group formation inside the Bolshevik Party. Although party investigators and theoreticians read suicide within the explanatory framework of social integration, in particular using it as a sign and source of 'illness' within the collective, their notions of suicide – what it meant and what it did violence to – were based on their specific conception of the individual as a collective, rather than autonomous, being. As a result, their understanding of suicide placed comparatively greater emphasis on the social elements of the self and promoted a much more extensive application of government power in the personal affairs of the individual. These inclinations in turn gave rise to a set of practices – in particular, the formation of a 'collective opinion' and the active promotion of mutual surveillance – that conveyed a distinct vision of civic responsibility and social solidarity.

Suicide and the Creation of a 'Collective Opinion'

To commit suicide is to hand over one's self and story to others. Although suicides often try to shape how people will read their life and death by leaving behind a suicide note or choosing a particular method of self-destruction, death effectively robs them of control over their body and their biography. This inherent loss of control was sensed by the pre-revolutionary Russian physician Grigorii Izrailevich Gordon, who wrote that suicide notes 'cease to be private property and become public property [obshchestvennoe dostoianie] from the moment when those who wrote them cease to exist.'[15] Death, it seems, provides a new life for suicides, as their end becomes the object of others' fascination, imagination, and need for explanation. Both their body and their history are taken over and reinterpreted by the broader culture.

The making of suicide into 'public property' achieved one of its ultimate expressions inside the Bolshevik Party. During the 1920s suicide became everyone's business within a revolutionary regime that deemed the kollektiv as possessing interests that superseded but ideally harmonized with those of its individual members. In fact, many rejected suicide as a valid form of self-expression under Soviet power precisely because it contradicted the ideal of complete unity between the part and the whole. Not surprisingly, this understanding of suicide received its fullest articulation in the Bolshevik Party, which was understood to be an 'organism' that was giving birth to the conventions and relationships – the new 'everyday life' (*byt*) – of the future socialist society.[16]

Party leaders proclaimed that membership in the Bolshevik Party was the first step towards the development of a fundamentally new form of individual. In a speech delivered at the Sverdlov Communist University in 1924, the university's rector, Martyn Nikolaevich Liadov argued that those who joined the party were learning how to freely accept limitations on their personal 'will' (*volia*) for the sake of the party as a whole. 'For us,' Liadov proclaimed, 'the interests of the party are becoming more important than our own ... We envisage the future society to be a society in which every person will feel that his interests coincide with the interests of the entire collective.'[17] However, in the same speech Liadov warned that in the near term suicide and other forms of unbridled individualism could result from this difficult transition. Gone were the old restraints on personal behaviour – notions of sin, fear of social reproach, and internalized codes of morality – while new ones had yet to take their place. Without such 'restraining centres,' there was nothing to hold back egoistic impulses and desires, including those that led the individual towards self-annihilation.[18]

Liadov's portrayal of the new relationship between the individual and the collective reflected broader currents of revolutionary thought and tradition, while at the same time expressing the special concerns regarding party youth as the bearers of the new culture. For example, he echoed Marxist conceptions of the proletariat as the source of universalistic, rather than particularistic, values. His discussion of the new human being emphasized that the workplace – the large-scale factory or enterprise – was another site where the 'collective psychology' was being cultivated in Soviet Russia. Here the workers laboured together and learned to place the 'we' over the 'I.'[19] This concept partly explains why Soviet investigators maintained that workers were less likely to kill themselves than were members of the intelligentsia and the white-collar classes.[20] It also explains why the Bolsheviks emphasized the importance of factory work experience and grew increasingly anxious during the 1920s about the large number of party members, such as students, who either lacked such experience or no longer had living ties to the industrial workplace. Isolation from the factory was seen as a key ingredient in the growth of individualism and in the ideological and moral disintegration of the collective's constituent elements.

Such emergent orthodoxies in Bolshevik thought on the individual helped to define understandings of suicide. Violence against the self could have no place in the party because it was an act of individualism that put personal concerns over group interests. By definition, suicide was a 'vestige' of bourgeois society and an act committed by someone who lacked true knowledge of him or herself as a social being with responsibilities that extended beyond the individual's immediate realm of existence. For example, P. Tsel'min, a member of the Red Army's Political Administration (PUR) and Conflict Commission (KK), contended, 'He who is a conscious Communist or a conscious worker cannot become a suicide because he does not belong to himself and is not his private property. Rather, he belongs to his party and to his class.'[21] In a similar vein, party declarations frequently characterized the act of suicide as a violation of collective norms; killing oneself was a form of 'desertion' that showed weakness, pessimism, and egoism in the face of personal difficulties or frustrations about the delayed advent of socialism.[22] Responding to the 1924 suicide of the Red commander Sukhanov, the collective of the Seventh Communications Regiment adopted a resolution condemning Sukhanov's behaviour as unbecoming a true proletarian. It emphasized the responsibility of every individual to participate in the messianic cause of the revolution and proclaimed, 'Our lives do not belong to us, but to the working class and all the oppressed of the world.'[23]

This line of reasoning made suicide – indeed, every personal act and thought of the party member – the business of the collective. To kill oneself was to violate the notion that a distinction could be made between one's personal and social life, since the suicide had displayed autonomy by taking the fundamental question of life and death into his or her own hands.[24] Death in the cause of communism was possible, even welcomed by some as form of heroic martyrdom, but as P. Tsel'min concluded in his article on party suicides, 'life and death cannot be decided on one's own.'[25] Even Vladimir I'lich Lenin could not escape this ethos after his death in early 1924. During the intraparty discussions about whether to embalm Lenin's corpse, several prominent Bolsheviks argued that the body should be preserved because Lenin belonged to the people and to the larger cause of the Revolution and not to himself or to his family. After all, they maintained, during his lifetime Lenin had renounced any personal or private life in order to give himself over completely to the revolutionary struggle.[26]

Taken to their furthest extreme, such understandings implied that in the Bolshevik Party suicide was essentially a form of murder, since it involved an act of violence perpetrated by one actor (the individual) against another (the self, which belonged to the collective). In this respect, Bolshevik attitudes echoed early Christian theology, which branded suicide a sin committed against God the Creator, and secular Petrine law, which defined suicide as a crime against the state. However, in Soviet Russia the suicide transgressed against society, which had endowed him or her with consciousness and purpose, rather than God or the sovereign. This substitution of society for God is clearly evident in one of the most unequivocal denunciations of suicide that I have uncovered from the early Soviet period. In 1930 the physician Vladimir Ivanovich Velichkin vigorously disputed the idea that the individual had complete control over his body and was therefore free to choose when he would die. 'No one,' he argued, 'has a right to die according to his desire ... Reproduced by society, a person belongs to it, and only society, in the interests of the majority, can deprive him of life.'[27] Velichkin's severe attitude towards suicide denied 'free will' in the sense of the individual as a fully autonomous being separate from the rest. Instead, it gave society a claim on the individual, who committed a kind of sin against his creator by killing one of its progeny – himself. The collective therefore had a right to punish or sanction the 'murderer' for his misdeeds.

The conflation of the individual with the collective helps to explain one of the Bolsheviks' primary responses to suicide – the formation of a 'collective opinion' (*obshchestvennoe mnenie*)[28] around the problem. In the event of a suicide, local party leaders were instructed to convene a special meeting of the organization that had suffered the loss.[29] Directed at both the collective and its individual members, these gatherings of the faithful emphasized the 'social' nature of the individual in Soviet Russia. On one level, they provided a venue where the group negotiated questions regarding how the individual should think, feel, and behave under Soviet power. On another, they involved the diagnosis of the 'health' or condition of the collective as a whole. Since the suicide once helped to constitute the larger whole, and thus contained part of it within him or her, this person's separation from the group could never be treated as a purely private matter.

Suicide was in this respect a form of individuation that highlighted the significance of the individual for the well-being of the collective.[30] By killing themselves, suicides set themselves apart from the group and forced others to deal with them separately. Their behaviour placed the question of the individual directly before the group, and it made their personal life (as well as their death) the object of study and contemplation. Indeed, one of the striking aspects of the party discussions is the emphasis given to the individual qualities of the suicide. Emel'ian Iaroslavskii, who carried out a special investigation of party suicides in 1924, concluded that there existed no 'general' set of causes applicable to all party suicides; rather, he argued that each case must be examined 'on an individual basis' (*individual'no*).[31] More broadly, the party's military wing was emphatic in its recommendation that each and every instance of suicide undergo a thorough investigation. The information gathered from such studies was later used to create an aggregate or holistic picture of suicide and the party's 'health.' However, behind each number there was to be a careful study that explored the history of the party member and the circumstances that led to his/her suicide.[32]

Within the political meeting, the suicide functioned like a 'text' that could be interpreted and studied by the group, often under the tutelage of a trained political officer. Political workers dissected the life and death of the suicide in order to teach the cadres the 'Soviet line' on suicide, including the kinds of people likely to kill themselves, the causes of self-destructive behaviour, the warning signs of suicidal intent, and the implications of taking one's own life in a socialist society. The point of this exercise was to establish the significance of suicide in terms of the collective. We must therefore regard such gatherings as part of the larger effort to get people to see themselves, and not just suicide, as inherently 'social.'[33]

Discussions of suicide followed a pattern, with the party expressing its 'collective opinion' in verbal and non-verbal form. After the open discussion of the suicide, the party cell or commission would usually adopt a resolution containing its diagnosis of both the individual and the collective. These resolutions were generally 'negative' in tone and content, as the group highlighted the particular mistakes or weaknesses of the deceased that contributed to his/her disintegration. In addition, the collective also communicated its 'opinion' through a number of symbolic gestures, including the posthumous expulsion of the suicide from the party or the refusal to accord the body any ceremonial honours, such as a funereal escort. By committing suicide, the deceased had placed his/her own interests above those of the collective; in response, the collective purified itself and formally recognized this separation by invoking the ultimate punishment for a social being – excommunication from the group.[34]

In this concern for maintaining – indeed, actively constructing – a collective opinion among the communist faithful, we see that social investigation was essential to individual and group formation in Soviet Russia. Fostering a single voice around the question of suicide was an expression of the idealized convergence of the part and the whole. It broke the 'silence' around suicide and forced the group to confront the problem or 'illness' within it. Moreover, the point of the exercise was not simply the achievement of a common interpretative framework, but also adherence to the 'correct' (*pravil'nyi*) one. Thus the creation of a collective opinion implied unity in thought, feeling, and cognition, as the party member spoke for the organization, which in turn spoke for him/her. The part and the whole ideally came together in a single voice around the suicide.[35]

As a practice of group formation, the ritualistic creation of a collective opinion also involved collective self-diagnostics and self-therapeutics. Acts of suicide were a catalyst for introspective examinations of both the political 'health' of the membership and the general conditions prevailing within the organization. This self-reflexive impulse was readily apparent in the stated goals of the meeting convened to discuss the death of Evgenii Funt, a military commissar who shot himself in 1924. The gathering set the following tasks for itself: '1) to elucidate the general condition of the party organization in connection with the incident, and [to establish] whether it is the result of amoral deviations among the members of our organization; 2) to outline a range of measures, having explained the essence of this suicide.'[36] The idea here and at similar gatherings was to create a controlled environment where the question of suicide and other party 'illnesses' (*bolezni*) could be discussed in an edifying manner that would strengthen relations between the membership and decrease the likelihood that others would commit similar 'crimes' against the collective.[37]

Party cells of the Red Army routinely examined the social background, character, medical history, and service record of the suicide in order to identify those factors that might explain his 'degeneration.' The political meeting held to discuss the suicide of Evgenii Funt began with a reading of various documents from his personnel file, which included a biographical questionnaire (*anketa*) as well as letters of reference and attestations. On this basis, several members in attendance concluded that Funt, the young son of a baker who 'stood close to trade,' failed to develop into a 'firmly seasoned communist' and therefore never became a 'stable member of the RKP.' In other words, the suicide lacked the political consciousness needed to correctly understand his personal problems within the larger context of the Soviet Union's difficult transition to socialism; instead, he 'fell under the influence [*vliianie*] of difficult material circumstances and deserted in a disgraceful manner from the ranks of the RKP(b).' This diagnosis apparently made Funt's death more comprehensible to the rest of the group; comrade Burmakin, for example, stood before the gathering and stated that 'one can expect such faint-heartedness and such acts from these [unseasoned] party members.'[38]

Funt's questionable social background, in addition to his flaws as both an individual and a political figure, were deemed sufficient explanation for the organization to absolve itself of any direct culpability in the suicide. The 'collective opinion' organized around his suicide stated this view explicitly:

> The political meeting, having thoroughly examined the question of comrade Funt's suicide on the basis of the available materials, establishes that this incident is in no way connected to the overall condition of the party organization as a consequence and result of its moral decomposition and instability. On the contrary, the divisional party organization is completely healthy, morally stable, and the line taken by the organization in relation to individual members is correct and requires no changes ... The political meeting calls on the organization to categorically denounce the phenomenon of suicide in the ranks of the party as one of the greatest crimes before the working class.

By declaring Funt a 'temporary fellow-traveller of the party,' the collective suggested that his 'crime' did not reflect fully on the condition of the 'party organism.' He could not stand for the larger group or collective because he was never truly part of it in the first place.[39] As the author of another investigation declared, the suicide of the Komsomol Schesnovich demonstrated that he 'was a communist on paper but not in his outlook [*mirovozrenie*].'[40]

This separation of the individual body from the collective was expressed literally in the case of Filatov, who killed himself in early

1924. Following his suicide, the party cell of the Lenin Command School in Tashkent determined that Filatov's suicide was the product of 'romanticism,' a state of mind that had no place within the ranks of the Communist Party, and it labelled his death a 'weak-willed' act of 'cowardice' that 'absolutely contradicts the principles of the Red Commander and communist ethics.' Moreover, the party cell concluded that Filatov had revealed his true self by destroying it. His choice of death had exposed his intrinsic 'petite-bourgeois *intelligent* psychology,' as well as his underlying devotion to 'tsarist, junker, and medieval traditions.' The cell therefore sought to break with Filatov. It posthumously expelled him from the organization, resolved to forgo any funereal escort of his body, and literally ceased referring to him as 'comrade' during its discussions. The message was clear: in death, as in life, the suicide never achieved full integration in the group.[41]

Even in this instance, however, the diagnostic performance of the party cell meeting was not restricted to the individual. Although the collective pronounced Filatov's deed completely inexcusable, it nevertheless drew a connection to general conditions prevailing inside the school and its political organs. When the cadet Petunin called on the command staff to spend more time getting to know each cadet personally, he intimated that the suicide was somehow related to the failure of school authorities to pay sufficient attention to the needs and concerns of individual students. For this reason, the group urged the leadership to be more 'sociable' with the students and to conduct 'intimate and concrete talks with the cadets.' Similarly, the collectively diagnosed cause of Filatov's action – 'romanticism' – was also addressed within the context of everyday life at the Command School. Members passed a resolution calling for a new direction in the party cell's 'club work.' Dances, parties, and other 'romantic settings,' which were said to foster 'romanticism' and strengthen 'bourgeois-philistine' ideology among the cadres, were no longer to be organized. The banning of such activities, it was argued, would help to 'prevent these acts we find so offensive.'[42]

The creation of a collective opinion always possessed this prophylactic intent. In fact, the notion of fostering a collective opinion around suicide and other forms of deviance had a strong disciplinary character. Party leaders conceived of the practice as a means of inoculating the collective and its members against ideological 'infection,' an organic metaphor that stood for the active formation and internalization of norms and beliefs. In other words, it involved the creation of the new individual 'restraining centres' foreseen by Martyn Liadov in his discussion of everyday life. Through the story of the suicide, the party cadres would come to understand that suicide was an illegitimate response to personal difficulties or disappointments. They would develop a cognitive awareness of dangerous places, harmful literature, or even threatening social groups that should be avoided. Moreover, they also would learn to recognize the 'signs' of suicide that foreshadowed individual breakdown. Ideally, the group exercise in analysis would produce an individual who would see him or herself and others as 'social bodies' whose actions had meaning and consequences that extended beyond their immediate experience.

Mutual Surveillance and the Integration of the Individual

Suicide unsettled the party leadership because it represented the breakdown of collective bonds that were exercised through mutual surveillance. A successful suicide suggested that the formation and presence of a suicidal individual had gone undetected for days, weeks, or months until the person finally made her or himself known to others in the most horrific and irreversible manner. Only after the fact did the people who lived and worked alongside the suicide really get to know this person. As suggested above in the discussion of the collective opinion, the very act of suicide forced others to ascribe certain significance to actions, words, or gestures that now, in retrospect, indicated emotional or mental instability on the part of the individual. This was certainly the case in the death in 1927 of the regimental party bureau secretary, who reportedly committed suicide on the grounds of his non-communist lifestyle. The summary narrative of his suicide read: 'He [the suicide] approached his party duties formally and spread his demoralizing influence to individual members of his organization, dragging them into bouts of drinking and an alien [social] environment. Having embarked on a path foreign to the party, he shot himself. Neither the party organization nor the political department anticipated it, and the full extent of his disintegration [*razlozhenie*] only became clear after he committed suicide.'[43] In many respects, what most disturbed the political leadership was not so much the suicide of a degenerate party member as the lack of comradely (*tovarishcheskii*) relations within the collective, which had allowed the individual to break away in the first place.[44]

Bolshevik explanations of this collective breakdown were a variation on the narrative of alienation and failed transition that dominated the modern discourse of suicide. Within the above diagnoses, for example, suicide clearly signalled the fact that a party member had somehow developed a life and sense of him or herself outside the collective. This theme of separation from the group ran throughout other explanations of suicide. In his description of suicides in the party's military wing, P. Tsel'min used the metaphor of 'digestion,' the process by which something is broken down and absorbed into the body, to account for instances of self-destruction. Suicides were, in his opinion, individuals who had never been fully 'digested' (*ne perevarilis'*) by the organization.[45] Several years later the authors of an investigation into suicides in the Moscow organization used a similar metaphor, arguing that suicides were often young people who had not been fully 'cooked in the cauldron of the party [*ne perevarennyie v partiinom kotle*].'[46] In both instances, the metaphors of 'digestion' and 'cooking' conveyed the idea of the party as an organic whole composed of individuals whose qualities had been transformed and blended together in something greater than themselves; consequently, isolation from the collective (*otryv ot kollektiva*) equalled social, political, and in some instances, physical death.[47]

From such understandings arose the imperative to 'envelop' (*okhvatit'*) the individual more fully within the collective as a way to prevent additional acts of violence against the self. Political activists framed this goal as a matter of *vliianie*, or 'influence,' a concept that emphasizes the environmental determination of human behaviour and figures prominently in Bolshevik notions of social integration. Both individuals and milieux were thought to exert an 'influence' on the human mind and body, thereby shaping the self. Depending on the particular class nature of its source, as well as the condition of its object, an influence could have a positive or negative effect. A 'healthy' milieu, such as a factory or a party collective, helped to foster political consciousness and a spirit of collectivism, while 'morbid' influences emanating from social aliens or from a work of decadent literature produced antisocial attitudes and degenerate morality.[48] Amid the transition to socialism, the Bolsheviks understood the fate of the individual's development as part of this struggle between the forces of good and evil. The weakest and least developed party members, especially those young people who lacked sufficient 'tempering' in the crucible of revolution or the factory workplace, were considered the most vulnerable to 'unhealthy' influences. They lacked the inner strength necessary to overcome obstacles and the will power to resist corruption.[49]

A suicide signalled the strength of 'unhealthy' influences and, conversely, the weakness of the collective. In 1926 the political meeting of the Central Asian Military District drew a direct connection between the command staff's 'susceptibility to its surrounding petit-bourgeois milieu,' its isolation from the troops, and the increase observed in suicides among the Red Army men under its command. The political meeting contended that drinking and relaxing with 'hostile elements' had gradually distracted the officers from their custodial responsibilities. The resulting inattention increased the likelihood that soldiers gripped by 'suicidal moods' would not be detected in time to prevent their deaths. In other words, there was no healthy 'counter-influence' on the part of the collective and its leadership.[50]

This understanding raised questions about responsibility. The political authorities recognized that in some instances the suicide was fully to blame; he had willfully masked or hidden his inner thoughts and feelings from those around him.[51] However, the reports summarizing instances of suicide in the Red Army were most frequently critical of commanders, political officers, and Red Army men for failing to recognize the tangible signs of suicide in time to prevent the tragedy from occurring. As early as 1924, the district political administration of the Turkfront concluded, 'Certain individuals, who are weak-willed, who lose heart under the influence of the environment and other attendant circumstances, who have hit bottom [opuskaiushchiesia], do not find timely support, influence, and assistance from their social [obshchestvennyi] and party milieu.'[52] Several years later the political meeting of the Moscow Military District suggested that suicides came as a surprise only when commanders did not bother to know the everyday life of the soldiers in their unit. It concluded:

> The insufficient knowledge of every Red Army man as an individual, the lack of interest in this knowledge on the part of the most immediate commander (the platoon commander) leads to the fact that the suicide most of the time takes the unit by surprise and seems completely unexpected. However, the inquiry [later] shows that the causes which provoked it were in view of the command staff and political instructor, and that they ignored them, not having attached any significance to them. By not knowing the moods of the Red Army man, it is impossible through educational work to strengthen those impulses which hold them back, in order to counteract these moods with the firm grounds for eradicating them.[53]

In essence, suicide signalled that the web of mutual surveillance which bound the collective together was not in full effect. The apparent inability or unwillingness of people to carefully observe others meant that those servicemen who were in a state of personal crisis often remained unnoticed until it was too late to help them.

The importance attached to these cognitive lapses surfaced in the very statistical categories used to arrange and compare suicides according to motive. Failures on the part of commanders, political workers, and servicemen to realize when others were in trouble became formalized as a distinct group of causal factors. For the period 1927–29 the Red Army's political organs classified 51 cases of suicide (out of 1,395 total cases) under the category 'the inattention of superiors' and an additional 33 per cent under the motive 'the inattention and oppression of others.' Both of these categories in turn fell under the broad heading that attributed the suicide to the 'fault of those around [the suicide]' (*vina okruzhaiushikh*). A common theme of suicides placed under this rubric was the failure of others to notice the suicide's personal troubles and to take appropriate action. In each instance, investigators concluded that the suicide resulted from a dangerous combination: a callous officer or Red Army man together with an 'extremely susceptible' (*ostro vospriimchivyi*) individual. For example, the higher authorities had ignored the deceased's entreaties for medical, material, or spiritual assistance, or they had taken disciplinary measures against the individual without being sensitive to how these actions might affect a mentally and emotionally vulnerable individual.[54] This lack of mutual concern and attentiveness among the troops could be expressed statistically in a variety of formulations. Among them were the following: 'due to a bureaucratic and inattentive approach to individual comrades,' 'the inattentiveness of commanders to their subordinates,' and 'abnormal relations among comrades.'[55]

To overcome these breakdowns within the collective, the Red Army's political organization called for heightened sensitivity towards the needs and concerns of the individual. The report on the suicide of Evgenii Funt, for example, recommended that the party's organs in the Volga Military District take steps to know 'the personal life [*lichnaia zhizn'*] and everyday living conditions of each party member ... So that through the constant and daily observations of changes we have a full opportunity to prevent unethical and denigrating acts of the party member and, at the same time, avert accidents like this one.'[56] Similarly, the special commission organized in the Western Military District concluded from its analysis of suicides: 'There exists a need for an individual approach [*individual'nyi podkhod*] on the part of officers towards those under their command, the exposure by them of their subordinate's subjective particularities (this is especially expected from non-commissioned officers), familiarity with the concerns of his family and service life, and an accounting of all these data when deciding any sort of questions regarding the individual.'[57] According to K. Podsotskii, first secretary of the Political Administration, the rationale behind such calls for increased 'attention to the life of the party member' was to prevent 'illnesses' before they happened, so that there would be less need for 'curative' measures, such as the post factum administration of disciplinary or exclusionary measures.[58]

As in the case of 'collective opinion,' the therapeutic logic underlying these and other prescriptions was based on the conception of the self as a collective entity. Such an understanding made mutual surveillance – the continuous observation by and of others – an essential component of the Bolsheviks' strategy for preventing acts of violence against the self. Monitoring and promoting the well-being of the individual effectively became a necessary precondition for creating a healthy collective, which in turn exercised a positive influence on its constituent members. For example, the political activist Moseichuk hoped that the party cells would take the following lesson from studying the suicide in 1929 of comrade Ochkovskii: 'It is necessary to decisively liquidate those cases where a party candidate remains for months isolated from the party environment and outside the party's influence.'[59] More broadly, political reports on suicide in the party and the military routinely recommended that measures be taken to 'create genuine party and comradely relations in the cells towards every party member.' As part of this effort, the cells were to study 'individually [*v otdel'nosti*] every commander, political worker, and Red Army man with the purpose of getting familiar with his life and his feelings [*perezhivaniia*], so that help might be given to any comrade when it is needed.'[60]

These approaches to suicide, which recognized the individual as a distinct but by no means autonomous entity, further established in practice the reciprocal relationship between the part and the whole. In fact, the therapeutic logic behind Bolshevik social practices suggested that greater integration would actually facilitate the process of mutual surveillance. Rather than conceal their 'sufferings' from others out of fear of ridicule or an unsympathetic response, individuals would instead voluntarily come forward to share their personal concerns and problems. In other words, potential suicides would reveal themselves to others *before* they did so by taking their lives. They would recognize their own duty as members of the collective to seek treatment or help before they could 'infect' others.[61] The socially integrated – and thus socially responsible – individual was by definition someone who carried out mutual surveillance because he or she understood the need to see and be seen.

Conclusions: Suicide and the Collective Self

The meaning of suicide, murder, and other forms of violence is based on historically and culturally specific assumptions about the self. Where the individual is conceived as an autonomous being, murder can be thought to reflect love of the self, while suicide can suggest a desire to destroy it. By comparison, the Bolsheviks' understanding of the individual as a social entity made suicide appear the result of an excessive love and concern for one's self. This is not to suggest that the individual mattered less in Soviet Russia; rather, it mattered differently within the context of a regime that encouraged its members to think about themselves as collective, rather than autonomous, beings. Suicide therefore provides a fitting object for investigating how Bolshevik conceptions of the individual helped to define the overlapping spheres of governmental action, personal development, and public participation which together formed the Soviet polity.

Bolshevik responses to suicide ultimately helped to create a society with enormous powers to promote itself and to defend itself from perceived threats. These involved the creation of 'healthy' individuals and the development of a continuous diagnostic regime that would work through the individual. As suggested above, the two processes were intertwined. Ritualized discussions of suicide encouraged the formation of a desired Soviet subject by isolating the transgressors and by communicating a system of values through their objectification. The creation of the collectivist person in turn deepened the possibilities for mutual surveillance and for the gathering of information so vital to the maintenance of society's well-being. Either way, the power of society ran through its individual members.

Ironically, the need to establish some form of control over the individual only increased as the Soviet regime got closer to its goal of creating a holistic society. Bolshevik responses to suicides suggest that one consequence of thinking in terms of the social organism is the realization that the defective or offending elements can come from within. This awareness deepened the anxiety associated with the fear of corruption and furthered the trend towards pathologizing individuals who behaved in ways deemed threatening to the collective. As Martyn Liadov proclaimed in his discussion of the new everyday life, 'It will hurt me to violate these [common] interests, and in the future society they will look upon the person who has violated these interests as a sick person who needs to be cured.'[62] Accordingly, when the individual transgressed society, he or she also transgressed him/herself, since the individual's interests and those of society were the same. Self-defence of the group could therefore be rationalized in terms of individual self-protection.

The implications are important for our understanding of the early Soviet regime. Although this article has focused on the Bolshevik Party's response to acts of violence against the self, the ideas and practices developed within the party had a broader significance for the rest of the population. As the Bolsheviks increasingly exercised a monopoly on power during the 1920s, they aspired to political and cultural hegemony throughout the USSR. Many of their practices associated with the problem of party 'illnesses' such as suicide, including the ritualistic isolation and exclusion of 'unhealthy' elements, later found expression in the physical suppression of 'alien' social groups and the violent terror of the 1930s. Equally important, the party set the key parameters, and thus the possibilities, for how individuals could think of themselves and their place in the new socialist society. Consistent with Bolshevik notions of the organic society, the Soviet citizen of the 1930s was expected to display loyalty through particular forms of public activism, including the identification and reporting of individuals who threatened the social order.[63]

We therefore should not read the information on suicide and violence as mere summaries of reality, but instead interpret them within the larger framework of the revolutionary effort to achieve the dream of collective harmony. Suicide statistics and other social data were, in this respect, part of an effort to measure the assimilation of new values, to identify and eradicate remaining pockets of 'illness,' and to generally know how far the Soviets remained from achieving the socialist utopia. After all, 'illnesses' or bourgeois 'vestiges' such as suicide were supposed to disappear once the new society was created. Rates of suicide and other forms of violence may not provide access to the 'true' intentions of individual actors, but they do permit the study of how the Bolsheviks interpreted these actions as markers of social well-being and how they developed particular policies on the basis of such understanding.

Interestingly, suicide temporarily 'disappeared' in Soviet Russia. Beginning in the early 1930s, the open publication of suicide statistics ceased, and various state-sponsored studies of suicide were brought to a close.[64] To be sure, the Bolshevik Party and the Red Army, as well as other government institutions, continued to investigate acts of suicide; however, these were mostly secretive affairs. Suicide was, as a result, no longer a visible problem troubling the Soviet population. Like other forms of deviance, it could have no place within the social organism that came into existence through the programs of rapid industrialization and collectivization. This disappearance of suicide from the public realm represented the realization of the Bolsheviks' dream – a society where their ideology held sway and where bourgeois or liberal individualism no longer existed. The actions of any person who still ran counter to such tendencies could only be a 'social anomaly' (*sotsial'naia anomaliia*), a concept that separated the deviant part from the healthy whole.[65]

So who, given the Bolsheviks' understanding of the individual and the collective, was the victim of violence against the self in early Soviet Russia? Can we even think in these terms? In the end, the nature of the victim is contingent upon the definitions. In our society we tend to regard a suicide as the loss of a unique individual who possesses an intrinsic value. It remains an act of aggression turned inwards. Bolshevik discourse, with its blurring of boundaries between the individual and society, framed the problem of loss differently. Suicide was seen as an act of violence directed towards another as much as towards the self. Efforts to prevent suicide in the Bolshevik Party may have focused on the individual, but they were conceived in terms of the individual as a threat to society and thus to him/herself. It is tempting, therefore, to suggest that there could be no suicide in early Bolshevik Russia, since it resulted in multiple victims – the individual and the social body to which he or she belonged.

NOTES

The author would like to acknowledge the valuable suggestions of those who commented on earlier versions of this chapter, including the anonymous readers, the participants of the Maryland Workshop on New Approaches to Russian and Soviet History in May 2002, David Hoffmann, Michael David-Fox, and Barbara Riess. Research was made possible by the International Research and Exchanges Board (IREX), the American Council of Teachers of Russian (ACTR), and the Allegheny College Faculty Support Committee.

1 For an example of the Bolsheviks' categorization, including elements more specific to their revolutionary project, see 'Statisticheskii ezhegodnik. Politiko-moral'noe sostoianie RKKA. (Sostoianie distsipliny, samoubiistva, chrezvychainye proisshestviia). 1929/30 god.,' Rossiiskii gosudarstvennyi voennyi arkhiv (hereafter RGVA) f. 54, op. 4, d. 69, l. 32ob.

2 The significance of social science in Russia is explored more broadly in Michael David-Fox, *Revolution of the Mind: Higher Learning among the Bolsheviks, 1918–1929* (Ithaca: Cornell University Press, 1997); and Alexander Vucinich, *Social Thought in Tsarist Russia: The Quest for a General Science of Society* (Chicago: University of Chicago Press, 1976).

3 Igal Halfin raises a similar point in his discussion of Bolshevik class policies, arguing that the Bolsheviks' use of such categories as 'proletariat' cannot be comprehended fully unless it is examined within the broader framework of Marxist eschatology. See Halfin, *From Darkness to Light: Class, Consciousness, and Salvation in Revolutionary Russia* (Pittsburgh: University of Pittsburgh Press, 2000), 101.

4 Irina Paperno, *Suicide as a Cultural Institution in Dostoevsky's Russia* (Ithaca: Cornell University Press, 1997); Michael MacDonald and Terrence R. Murphy, *Sleepless Souls: Suicide in Early Modern England* (Oxford: Clarendon Press, 1993); and Howard I. Kushner, *American Suicide: A Psychocultural Exploration* (New Brunswick: Rutgers University Press, 1991).

5 Paperno, *Suicide as a Cultural Institution*, esp. 1–17; Alexander Murray, *Suicide in the Middle Ages*, vol. I, *The Violent against Themselves* (Oxford: Oxford University Press, 1998); and A. Alvarez, *The Savage God: A Study of Suicide* (New York: W.W. Norton & Co., 1990), 63–93.

6 This emphasis on 'civilization' also shaped the meanings given to different types of violence, such as suicide and murder. Moral statisticians and

others suggested that suicide was a 'higher' form of violence, citing statistics which indicated that rates of suicide and murder rose and fell in inverse proportion. Even today, researchers tend to view suicide and murder as two distinct forms of violence, with suicide being aggression turned inwards, while murder is aggression turned outwards against another human being. They claim that members of the upper classes tend to prefer suicide, while the lower classes tend to prefer murder, as an outlet for their aggression. A fine summary and critique of these views and their origins can be found in N. Prabha Unnithan et al., *The Currents of Lethal Violence: An Integrated Model of Suicide and Homicide* (Albany: State University of New York Press, 1994), esp. 7–34.

7 By 'society' I mean an aggregate of the population that is said to display certain general regularities transcending its individual parts.

8 Ian Hacking, *The Taming of Chance* (Cambridge: Cambridge University Press, 1990), chap. 20; and Theodore M. Porter, *The Rise of Statistical Thinking, 1820–1900* (Princeton: Princeton University Press, 1986), chap. 2.

9 I develop this argument in Kenneth M. Pinnow, 'Making Suicide Soviet: Medicine, Moral Statistics, and the Politics of Social Science in Bolshevik Russia, 1920–1930' (PhD diss., Columbia University, 1998); and Pinnow, 'Cutting and Counting: Forensic Medicine as a Science of Society in Bolshevik Russia, 1920–29,' in *Russian Modernity: Politics, Knowledge, Practices*, ed. David L. Hoffmann and Yanni Kotsonis (London: Macmillan Press, 2000), 115–37.

10 Susan K. Morrissey, 'Suicide and Civilization in Late Imperial Russia,' *Jahrbücher für Geschichte Osteuropas* 43: 2 (1995), 201–17; Paperno, *Suicide as a Cultural Institution*, passim.

11 Calling for the establishment of government statistical bureaux throughout Russia, the pre-revolutionary physician Grigorii Izrailevich Gordon lamented, 'The vast majority [of suicides], especially within the villages and small cities, completely escape notice because in our country we do not yet see suicides as important social phenomena demanding the most serious attention.' See Gordon, 'Samoubiistva v Rossii,' *Bodroe slovo*, no. 15 (August 1909), 72.

12 Halfin, *From Darkness to Light*, 287–8; Jochen Hellbeck, 'Self-Realization in the Stalinist System: Two Diaries of the 1930s,' in *Russian Modernity*, ed. Hoffmann and Kotsonis, 229; and Oleg Kharkhordin, *The Collective and the Individual in Russia: A Study of Practices* (Berkeley: University of California Press, 1999), 199–201.

13 Kharkhordin, *The Collective and the Individual in Russia*, passim.

14 Peter Holquist, 'What's So Revolutionary about the Russian Revolution?

State Practices and the New-Style Politics, 1914–21,' in *Russian Modernity*, ed. Hoffmann and Kotsonis, 87–111; and David L. Hoffmann, 'European Modernity and Soviet Socialism,' in *Russian Modernity*, ed. Hoffmann and Kotsonis, 245–60.

15 G. Gordon, 'Samoubiitsy i ikh pis'ma,' *Novyi zhurnal dlia vsekh*, no. 28 (February 1911), 107.

16 On the significance of organismic metaphors within Bolshevik thought, see Eric Naiman, *Sex in Public: The Incarnation of Early Soviet Ideology* (Princeton: Princeton University Press, 1997); and Eric van Ree, 'Stalin's Organic Theory of the Party,' *Russian Review* 52: 1 (January 1993), 43–57.

17 Martyn Nikolaevich Liadov, *Voprosy byta (Doklad na sobranii iacheiki sverdlovskogo kommun. Un-ta)* (Moscow, 1925), 21–2.

18 Ibid., 32. The context of Liadov's comments was a marked increase in suicides among party members in 1924–5, a fact that served as a catalyst for several studies of suicides in the organization. See V.S. Tiazhel'nikova, 'Samoubiistva kommunistov v 1920–e gody,' *Otechestvennaia istoriia* 6 (1998), 158–73.

19 Liadov, *Voprosy byta*, 20. More broadly, Marxist eschatological discourse emphasized the belief that the proletariat was the only social class untainted by the ownership of private property and thus from a view of the world which emphasized the 'I' over the 'we.' See Halfin, *From Darkness to Light*, 96–104.

20 'O samoubiistve. Nasha anketa,' *Vecherniaia moskva*, no. 5 (7 January 1926), 2.

21 P. Tsel'min, 'O samoubiistvakh,' *Sputnik politrabotnika*, no. 13 (31 March 1926), 22.

22 The link between suicide and desertion was first established in party discourse following the introduction of the New Economic Policy in 1921, when suicide and resignation were two of the most visible responses among disenchanted party members. For an example of this linkage see Em. Iaroslavskii, 'Nuzhno surovo osudit' samoubiistva,' *Pravda*, 9 October 1924, 4.

23 'Vypiska iz protokola obshchego sobraniia chlenov i kandidatov kollektiva RKP(b) 7–go polka sviazi ot 5/11–1924 g.,' RGVA f. 9, op. 28, d. 781, l. 31. In this respect, the suicide was the opposite of the new regime's championed values of inner strength, will power, and unflagging optimism. For a discussion of these traits and their encapsulation in party discourse, see Katerina Clark, *The Soviet Novel: History as Ritual*, 3rd ed. (Bloomington: Indiana University Press, 2000), 46–89.

24 Suicide therefore transgressed the ideal of selflessness that animated the

revolutionary intelligentsia in Tsarist Russia and continued to be upheld by the more radical elements of the Bolshevik Party. At least one 1924 gathering of the party emphasized that the Bolsheviks differed from other socialist parties because they made no distinction between private (*lichnyi*) and public (*obshchestvennyi*) life. See 'O partetike. Proekt predlozhenii preziduma TsKK II plenumu TsKK RKP(b),' in *Partiinaia etika. Dokumenty i materialy diskusii 20-kh godov* (Moscow: Izdatel'stvo politicheskoi literatury, 1989), 152–3.

25 Tsel'min, 'O samoubiistvakh,' 22.

26 My thanks to Claudio Ingerflom for suggesting the example of Lenin and his body. See Claudio Sergio Ingerflom and Tamara Kondratieva, 'Pourquoi la Russie s'agite-t-elle autour du corps de Lénine?' in *La mort du roi: Autour de François Mitterand: Essai d'ethnographic politique comparée*, ed. Jacques Julliard (Paris: Éditions Gallimard, 1999), 264–5.

27 Vladimir Ivanovich Velichkin, 'Pravo na smert,'' *Sovremennyi vrach*, no. 17–18 (1930), 765–66. Velichkin was responding to the discussion by Maksim Gor'kii (Maxim Gorky) of the poet Vladimir Maiakovskii's 1930 suicide, in which the great writer suggested that suicide might be justified or excused in some instances (such as a terminal illness that robbed the individual of his ability to be a productive member of society). For Gor'kii's comments, see his 'O solitare,' *Nashi dostizheniia*, no. 6 (June 1930), 5–6.

28 I have chosen here to translate *obshchestvennoe mnenie* as 'collective opinion' rather than use the more literal and common translation 'public opinion.' 'Collective opinion' better conveys the distinguishing aspects of *obshchestvennoe mnenie* under the Soviets. In particular, it captures the idea of widely held views and beliefs that have been actively shaped and then consciously internalized by the members. This concept contrasts with the pre-revolutionary notion of 'public opinion' as a commonality of viewpoints that developed naturally among members of educated society (*obshchestvo*) through the free and rational exchange of ideas. On the distinctive characteristics of Soviet 'collective opinion,' see Pinnow, 'Making Suicide Soviet,' 66–7; and Kharkhordin, *The Collective and the Individual*, 114–15. My particular thanks to Michael David-Fox and Peter Holquist for their helpful comments and suggestions regarding the thorny issues of translation and meaning.

29 During the 1920s the party regularly instructed its local organs to organize 'collective opinion' around all occurrences of suicide. For example, Gaitskhoki, a political instructor who was charged with investigating a number of incidents within the Leningrad Komsomol organization, con-

sidered the process of constructing a single, collective voice essential to controlling the problem of suicide. Among his primary suggestions for the 'eradication' of suicide was the following: 'To foster around every case of suicide a collective opinion of the organization's members condemning this act, pronouncing it at a meeting of the party cells and collectives, and widely illuminating it in wall newspapers.' See 'V sekretariat leningradskogo gubkoma VLKSM,' Tsentral'nyi gosudarstvennyi arkhiv istoriko-politicheskikh dokumentov sankt-peterburga (hereafter TsGAIPD [SPb]) f. 601, op. 1, d. 735, l. 2. Broader discussions of party ethics also emphasized the importance of a clear and firm party 'opinion,' which would help to guide members and keep them from succumbing to various immoral temptations. See, for example, 'O partetike,' in *Partiinaia etika*, 157.

30 This interpretation follows Oleg Kharkhordin's distinction between 'individuality' and 'individuation,' with the latter signifying the process of separating the individual from others in order to make him/her an object of study. See Kharkhordin, *The Collective and the Individual*, 164.

31 Iaroslavskii, 'Nuzhno surovo osudit' samoubiistva,' 4. Iaroslavskii may have emphasized the 'individual' character of suicide in order to establish a boundary between the suicide and the rest of the organization, which he declared to be 'healthy.' Accordingly, he concluded that suicides had nothing to do with *partiinost'*, or the state of the party organization.

32 For example, one report concluded, 'In the future there must be deeper and more attentive study of the causes and motives of every case of suicide.' See 'O samoubiistvakh sredi chlenov RKP(b) v partorganizatsii krasnoi armii i flota,' RGVA f. 9, op. 28, d. 736, l. 5.

33 Pinnow, 'Making Suicide Soviet,' chap. 5.

34 Here too comparisons between such gestures and religious responses to suicide are unavoidable. As an act of ritual excommunication, for example, the refusal to escort the body or to provide it the usual honours echoed the practice of many churches, including the Orthodox Church, to forbid internment of the suicide in hallowed ground. A direct parallel here was the party leadership's decision regarding the civil war hero Evgeniia Bosh following her suicide in 1925. Victor Serge claimed that Bosh's death provoked intense debate among the leadership over how to handle her burial. Although the 'more rigorous comrades' claimed that suicide was often justified in the case of illness, many considered Bosh's suicide an act demonstrating a lack of discipline and viewed the means of death as proof of her oppositionist political leanings. In a decision

reminiscent of older church sanctions against suicide, party leaders
denied her an official funeral and refused to inter her ashes in the wall of
the Kremlin: she was banished from the sacred burial place of the Revolution's heroes. See Serge, *Memoirs of a Revolutionary, 1901–1941* (London:
Oxford University Press, 1963), 194.

35 This is not to suggest, however, that a single 'Soviet line' on suicide was
ever achieved. Indeed, the self-professed need to cultivate a specific 'line'
of opinion among the party cadres was itself a recognition that multiple
definitions and attitudes existed within the organization. See, for
example, the questioning of the refusal to grant Evgenii Funt full burial
honours. Apparently, some party members noted that such distinction
had been accorded to Lev Trotsky's secretary, Glazman, who was also a
suicide. See 'Vypiska iz vnesrochnogo doneseniia No. 5 Politupravleniia
Privo ot 22/XI-1924 g.,' RGVA f. 9, op. 28, d. 781, l. 55. Nevertheless, the
dispute surrounding the suicide in 1927 of the oppositionist Adol'f
Abramovich Ioffe demonstrates that arguments about the meaning of
suicide occurred within a common conceptual framework centred on the
dichotomies of pessimism/optimism, strength/weakness, and
health/degeneration. Supporters of Ioffe argued that his suicide was an
act of selflessness and a 'death in the name of life and struggle,' whereas
his adversaries labelled it the result of pessimism and ideological degeneration. See, for example, Em. Iaroslavskii, 'Filosofiia upadochnichestva,'
Bol'shevik, no. 23–4 (31 December 1927), 135–44.

36 'Protokol No. 13 ekstrennogo zakrytogo zasedaniia politsoveshchaniia
32-i str. divizii sostoiavshegosia 8 sentiabria 1924 g.,' RGVA f. 9, op. 28, d.
781, l. 50.

37 On the prophylactic character of these discussions, see 'Proekt rezoliutsii
TsVPS o samoubiistvakh,' RGVA f. 9, op. 28, d. 1175, l. 42; 'Boleznennye
iavleniia v organizatsii (informatsionnyi obzor),' Rossiiskii gosudarstvennyi arkhiv sotsial'noi i politicheskoi istorii (hereafter RGASPI) f. 17, op.
85, d. 66, l. 66ob; and M. Dubrovskii and A. Lipkin, 'O samoubiistvakh,'
Revoliutsiia i kul'tura, no. 5 (15 March 1929), 33.

38 'Protokol No. 13 ekstrennogo zakrytogo zasedaniia politsoveshchaniia,'
ll. 50–2.

39 Nevertheless, the political meeting made an effort to learn from Funt's
suicide. It called for further investigation into the 'difficult material conditions' of the command-political staff, suggested the organization of a campaign against suicide and other immoral actions, and resolved that further
attention be paid to this case 'as an example of insufficient party steadfast-
ness and tempering existing among RKP(b) members' (ibid., l. 52).

40 'Zakliuchenie. Voenkom otdela artsnabzheniia R.K.K.A.,' RGVA f. 9, op. 28, d. 712, l. 103.

41 'Protokol No. 2 Obshchego partsobraniia iacheiki R.K.P. 2-i roty T.O.Sh.,' RGVA f. 9, op. 17, d. 186, l. 24; and 'Protokol No. 6 Obshchego zakrytogo partsobraniia 4–i Tashkentskogo Ob'edinennoi imeni tov. Lenina Komandnoi Shkoly,' RGVA f. 9, op. 17, d. 186, l. 25ob.

42 Ibid., ll. 25ob–26.

43 'Obzor samoubiistv sredi chlenov i kandidatov partii v armeiskikh par-torganizatsiiakh,' RGVA f. 9, op. 28, d. 73, l. 2ob; my emphasis.

44 The same report, for example, included an instance where timely inter-vention – a combination of material assistance, medical treatment, and 'comradely moral support' – prevented the joint suicide of a party member and his wife. (ibid., l. 2ob).

45 Tsel'min, 'O samoubiistvakh,' 20. The suicide's lack of complete 'diges-tion' by the factory workplace is also cited in the study of the Leningrad Komsomol organization. See 'V sekretariat leningradskogo gubkoma VLKSM,' l. 1.

46 Dubrovskii and Lipkin, 'O samoubiistvakh,' 34.

47 Iaroslavskii and other commentators cited isolation from the party and the working masses as a primary cause of suicides. See Iaroslavskii, 'Nuzhno surovo osudit' samoubiistva,' 4; and Dubrovskii and Lipkin, 'O samoubiistvakh,' 35–6. The comrades of A. Karasev came to a similar conclusion about his suicide. As a result of Karasev's isolation from 'social life,' which meant that he did not partake in social or political work, he could only see the 'negative side' of things through the 'prism' of his personal life. See 'Boleznennye iavleniia v organizatsii (informat-sionnyi obzor),' l. 67.

48 Perhaps the best example of this thinking is 'Eseninism' (*eseninshchina*), a wastebasket diagnosis that encompassed a wide variety of 'morbid' con-ditions and behaviours, including apathy, disenchantment with the prospects of the Revolution, uncontrolled individualism, decadence, ide-ological degeneration (*upadochnichestvo*), and a more general sense of alienation. Party leaders thought that Eseninism could quite literally 'infect' an individual. For a flavour of its meaning and uses, see *Upadochnoe nastroenie sredi molodezhi: Eseninshchina* (Moscow-Leningrad, 1927); G. Pokrovskii, *Esenin – Eseninshchina – religiia* (Moscow, 1929); and I. Bobryshev, *Melkoburzhuaznye vliianiia sredi molodezhi* (Moscow-Leningrad, 1928), 98.

49 'V sekretariat leningradskogo gubkoma VLKSM,' l. 1; Dubrovskii and Lipkin, 'O samoubiistvakh,' 33.

50 'Informatsionnaia svodka Polit. Upravleniia RKKA. No. 336 ot iiunia
    mesiatsa 12 dnia 1926 goda,' RGASPI f. 17, op. 85, d. 127, ll. 192–3. On the
    need for the party to have its own counter-influence (*kontr-vliianie*), see
    Redaktsiia, 'Nashe zakliuchenie,' *Voennyi vestnik*, no. 35 (22 September
    1928), 53–6.
51 On soldiers concealing their personal experiences from others, see
    'Samoubiistva v chastiakh M.V.O. (Obzor za 1923 i 24 g.g. po dannym
    Prokuratory MVO),' RGVA f. 9, op. 28, d. 739, ll. 49ob–50. See also the
    mention of suicides in S. Nevskii, 'Litso, kotoroe skryto,' *Voennyi vestnik*,
    no. 14 (21 May 1927), 39–40.
52 'Obzor direktiva o samoubiistvakh v chastiakh Turkfronta za vremia
    avgust-dekabr' 1924 g.,' RGVA f. 9, op. 28, d. 781, l. 84. My thanks to Eliot
    Borenstein for his suggestions on this translation.
53 'Samoubiistva v chastiakh M.V.O. (Obzor za 1923 i 24 g.g. po dannym
    Prokuratory MVO),' RGVA f. 9, op. 28, d. 739, l. 49. A report on suicides
    in the military party apparatus also noted the lack of critical attention by
    some party organs to the behaviour of individual soldiers in their units.
    It stated, 'There are also instances when a party member disintegrates
    [*razlagaetsia*] before the eyes of the entire party organization, but the latter
    doesn't take any sort of preventative measures.' These were contrasted to
    those suicides committed by individuals who displayed a disciplined
    and active public face before they unexpectedly took their own lives. See
    'Obzor samoubiistv sredi chlenov i kandidatov partii v armeiskikh par-
    torganizatsiiakh,' l. 3.
54 'Statisticheskii ezhegodnik za 1928/29 god. Politiko-moral'noe sostoianie
    RKKA.,' RGVA f. 54, op. 4, d. 64, ll. 44ob, 45ob; and 'Statisticheskii ezhe-
    godnik. Politiko-moral'noe sostoianie RKKA ... 1929/30 god,' ll. 32, 33.
55 'Obzor samoubiistv sredi chlenov i kandidatov partii v armeiskikh par-
    torganizatsiiakh,' ll. 1, 3ob; 'Samoubiistva v RKKA za 1926/27 god.,'
    RGVA f. 9, op. 28, d. 73, l. 13ob; and 'Samoubiistva M.V.O. za 1923 i 1924
    goda,' RGVA f. 9, op. 28, d. 739, l. 4.
56 Reprint of a 24 September 1924 letter from Tret'iakov, head of the 32nd
    Division's political department, to the 'Military Commander and Execu-
    tive Secretary of the RKP(b) cells of all units,' RGVA f. 9, op. 28, d. 781, l.
    48.
57 'Samoubiistva v voiskakh Zapadnogo Voennogo Okruga,' RGVA f. 9, op.
    28, d. 781, l. 68ob.
58 K. Podsotskii, 'Vnimanie k zhizni partiitsa,' *Voennyi vestnik*, no. 14 (9
    April 1927), 40–1. Podsotskii was a participant in the political leader-
    ship's discussions of suicide inside the Red Army. He was present, for

example, at the March 1926 gathering of the Central Political Meeting, which was devoted to the topic of suicide. See 'Protokol No. 3: Zasedaniia tsentral'nogo politsoveshchaniia 24 marta 1926 g.,' RGVA f. 9, op. 28, d. 1175, l. 50.

59 Moseichuk, 'O nekotorykh momentakh prakticheskoi raboty v sviazi s chistkoi partii,' *Voennyi vestnik*, no. 19 (21 May 1929), 34–6. Specifically, Moseichuk criticized the local cell for 'not taking an interest in how Ochkovskii worked and lived over the course of months, so that not a single measure was taken to protect him from the rot of his everyday life [*bytovoe zagnivanie*].'

60 'O samoubiistvakh sredi chlenov RKP(b) v partorganizatsii krasnoi armii i flota,' l. 4ob; and 'Obzor "Samoubiistva v chastiakh UVO v period ianvar"-iiun' 1924 g.,' RGVA f. 9, op. 28, d. 738, l. 39ob. These measures were usually combined with calls to 'pull' into social work individuals 'who display a propensity towards individualism.' See, for example, 'Samoubiistvakh v voiskakh Zapadnogo Voennogo Okruga. Doklad Komissii iz predstavitelei V/Prokuratury ZO, Voenno-Politicheskogo Upravleniia i Voenno-Sanitarnogo Upravleniia,' RGVA f. 9, op. 28, 781, ll. 68–68ob.

61 On the desire for Red Army men to share their personal experiences with officers, see 'Samoubiistva v chastiakh M.V.O.,' l. 51.

62 Liadov, *Voprosy byta*, 23. At least one early commentator recognized the danger of such thinking for the autonomous being. Evgenii Zamiatin's dystopian novel *We* (1920) satirizes the total merger of the part and the whole in the nightmarish vision of the One State. In the end, the complete union of the two is only possible through an act of therapeutic violence carried out against the individual – the so-called great operation, which removes the person's imagination.

63 For more on the important relationship between conceptions of 'society' and expectations of public activism, see Michael David-Fox, 'From Illusory "Society" to Intellectual "Public" Works: VOKS, International Travel and Party-Intelligentsia Relations in the Interwar Period,' *Contemporary European History* 2: 1 (2002), 7–32; and David-Fox, Review of Irina Nikolaevna Il'ina, *Obshchestvennye organizatsii Rossii v 1920–e gody*, in *Kritika* 3: 1 (Winter 2002), 173–81.

64 Among the programs terminated were the special studies carried out by the Department of Moral Statistics in the Central Statistical Bureau (TsSU) and by the Department of Forensic-Medical Expertise in the People's Commissariat of Public Health (Narkomzdrav). Suicides, however, continued to be counted by government statisticians as a form

of unpublished demographic data during the 1930s. See 'Svedeniia ob umershikh po polu, vozrastu i prichinam za 1937 g.,' Rossiiskii gosudarstvennyi arkhiv ekonomiki (RGAE) f. 1562, op. 20, d. 93. For later Soviet attitudes towards suicide, see Martin A. Miller and Ylana N. Miller, 'Suicide and Suicidology in the Soviet Union,' *Suicide and Life-Threatening Behavior* 18: 4 (Winter 1988), 303–21.

65 This understanding found concrete expression in Soviet psychological theories during the 1930s. According to Raymond A. Bauer, environmental theories of human behaviour, which dominated in the 1920s, were increasingly displaced by explanations that focused on personal responsibility. Psychologists and others could therefore treat the deviant individual as someone unreflective of the dominant social order. See Bauer, *The New Man in Soviet Psychology* (Cambridge: Harvard University Press, 1952).

10 Race and the Intellectualizing of Suicide in the American Human Sciences, circa 1950–1975

ANDREW M. FEARNLEY

Among both human scientists and the American public at large, the subject of suicide was much discussed in the decades of the immediate postwar era. According to one estimate, articles appearing in the professional literature rose from fewer than twenty per year in the 1940s to almost ninety by the mid-1950s. Figures for causes of death regularly featured in the nation's leading journals of opinion, and physicians and mental health officials, in keeping with the country's therapeutic ethos, frequently wrote didactic pieces alerting people to the ways they could identify suicidal tendencies in relatives and neighbours. In short, suicide became a topic of some considerable cultural authority: depicted in film and novel, spoken about before congressional committees, and the inspiration for a series of campaigns by law-enforcement agencies and religious groups. But exactly how was it intellectualized in this period? Put simply, how did scholars and researchers write about suicide? What did their empirical studies look like? Why were certain research methods more popular than others for exploring this most fascinating topic? By looking at the process by which suicide became a subject of systematic and sustained scrutiny for the United States' burgeoning human sciences, this chapter seeks to engage those questions.[1]

Histories of suicide have commonly been written from the perspectives of social and cultural history. Famously, one author wrote that the 'import of the history of suicide lies in what it reveals about the nature of clinical and social change.'[2] Nevertheless, the view abounds that most histories of suicide are written as works of intellectual history. Yet such assessments are misplaced if by that term we mean an understanding of how the subject has been formally interrogated, rationalized, and understood. Past accounts that people commonly identify as

providing intellectual histories of the subject are little more than considerations of how men traditionally regarded as intellectuals – David
Hume and J.J. Rousseau – thought about the topic. But for these men,
suicide was always a moral issue, debated as a problem in meta-
physics. If we perceive intellectual history to mean the sociology of
knowledge, then we have a very shallow understanding of how
suicide was intellectualized in previous historical contexts. With only
a few exceptions, we know little about the tools, types of empirical
research, or interpretive theories with which those interested in the
subject gathered, dissected, and explained the phenomenon. Focusing
on these types of conceptual apparatus, this chapter seeks to demonstrate how an interest in the interpretive methods used by researchers
and the models of empirical data from which they launched their
claims can reveal much about the processes of knowledge production
and the state of scientific inquiry in a particular context.[3]

Raising questions about research methods of course leads us to
ponder both technical and epistemological dimensions of scholarship,
as well as the relationship between the two. Contemporaries wrote
much and often about these subjects, and peevish rivalries frequently
broke out between disciplines over the validity of their methods. Psychoanalysts attacked the generalizing, statistically based approaches
of sociologists; sociologists questioned the validity of conclusions psychiatrists drew from their single-figure samples; the biologically oriented declared that too much importance was given to social factors;
and so forth. And the stench of these surface tensions has been taken
by some as proof of a lack of interdisciplinary cooperation with regard
to the subject. But if we shift our attention away from scholars' rhetoric and towards their basic approaches to research instead, it is clear
that interaction also took place between disciplines. Methods, for the
most part, were shared by scholars regardless of their disciplinary
background.[4] According to the historian of science Theodore Porter,
for example, methods such as statistics 'provided a degree of unity for
social science, even if they assumed distinctive forms within the
various disciplines and subdisciplines.'[5] When the scholarship is cast
in this light, it becomes clear that genuine cooperation was as much
the tone as was division. As one leading sociologist of suicide admitted in 1962, 'the study of suicide is not the exclusive property of any
particular field.'[6]

Uncharacteristic of the period's broader trends within the American
human sciences at large was the lack of attention those who studied

suicide gave to the collection of data. Hardly any new empirical samples about suicide were collected between the 1950s and the mid-1970s, researchers instead preferring to use data sets obtained from police bureaux or health departments.[7] Trends in writing about suicide during these decades did differ from previous eras, however. Findings generally appeared along two, largely opposed axes. Firstly, suicide became an area of study in its own right, and work was grouped under the heading 'suicidology.' Within a few years suicidology was a thriving area of scholarship, with its own literature, professional organizations, fellowships, and, in a few instances, assumed institutionalized form. In 1968 the American Association of Suicidology was formed. At the same time, academic periodicals on the topic appeared: the American Psychiatric Association launched the *Bulletin of Suicidology* (1967); a general journal about death, mourning, and suicide – *Omega* (1970) – followed three years later; and the long-lasting *Suicide and Life-Threatening Behavior* (1971) began publication. But concurrent with these trends were those that moved in the opposite direction, making the subject less specialized and placing it within a broader literature about social dysfunction. Alongside habits such as drug use and alcoholism, suicide became just another index for measuring social breakdown. A 1965 article in the *Archives of General Psychiatry*, for instance, had three psychiatrists consider the connection between being raised in a 'broken home' and later committing suicide.[8] Both these trends had implications for the way the topic was understood and debated.[9] One of the most striking ramifications was the effect these changes had on the way race was configured within such conversations.

For centuries, racialized assumptions had underpinned understandings of which people killed themselves. Throughout the nineteenth century, suicide had regularly served as one of the best-known scales for measuring supposed evolutionary hierarchies, commonly invoked as an indicator of the primitive and inferior capacities of lower races. Seldom did non-white people take their own lives, it was said. Beginning in the postwar period, these assumptions changed, and dramatically so, replaced seemingly overnight by the view that suicide was as much a problem among non-white groups as it was for white people. Such views represented a seismic shift in thinking, the most popular work on the subject boldly declaring that suicide among New York City's adolescent population showed rates among black youths to be double those of their white counterparts.[10] Yet if we consider what suicidologists wrote about how and why black people committed suicide, rather than just the rates at which they did so, the hold of older patterns of thinking can be seen. Agency, initiative, and internalization were all qualities that continued to be denied in the general depiction of black people's suicides – suicides that were instead considered violent, rash, and uncontrollable.[11] To explain precisely how these changes took place and how the study of suicide was reshaped in these decades, we must focus less on the insights of any particular author or the emergence of new data and more on the modified ways in which the subject itself was conceptualized.[12]

Changing Conceptions of Race and Suicide

What was the relationship between ideas of race and understandings of suicide in the United States between roughly 1865 and 1945? As long as people had been thinking in terms of race, they had been arguing that people of 'Negroid' ancestry rarely suffered bouts of depression and seldom took their own lives. Such opinions were widely held, stated with unwavering certainty not just by American commentators but by those writing in parts of the British Empire too, and they served as a little-noticed axiom in raciological thought. Like the claims made in earlier periods from the fields of craniology and comparative anatomy, suicide was a crucial topic within which ideas of race were produced.

In the post-bellum period, with slavery no longer demarcating the boundaries of racial separation, greater attention began to be called to alleged physical and behavioural differences between groups. Adding to the burgeoning literature that sprang up around claims of freedmen's proclivity towards drunkness, their tendency to be sloven and lazy, and their rampant sexuality, their failure to commit suicide was noted. Importantly, such opinions enjoyed a popular currency, recited in works of fiction and journals of opinion. Philip Bruce's *The Plantation Negro as Freedman* (1889), was typical in its conviction 'that the blacks rarely commit suicide,' a statement the author explained was justified if one had 'a full knowledge of the character of the race.' Pointing to the Negro's impulsive and ebullient nature, his 'inability to retain any one thought long enough to influence his conduct permanently,' Bruce, like many writing about the subject, supported his claims on the basis of a presumed privileged position of observation and on racial lore. More scientific treaties on the subject made the same point. The statistician and prominent racial theorist Frederick Hoffman wrote in 1896, 'Nowhere is there shown a specific tendency

towards self destruction [in the Negro].' Before the Massachusetts Historical Society, G. Stanley Hall, president of Clark University and one
of the country's leading psychologists at the time, told his audience
that Negroes 'are naturally cheerful, and so very rarely suffer from
melancholia or commit suicide.' The Swedish economist Gunnar
Myrdal, writing in his landmark work *An American Dilemma* (1944),
felt such trends worthy of mention too.[13]

Among alienists and their twentieth-century successors, psychiatrists, such opinions continued to be upheld, at least until the mid-
1950s. At the eighty-fifth annual meeting of the American Psychiatric
Association in 1929, Eugene Horger read a paper in which he told colleagues that suicide was rarely seen in the Negro. 'He does not worry
as much as the white man,' Horger claimed. Nolan D.C. Lewis, a man
sitting alongside Horger the day he read his paper and by mid-century
one of the most distinguished psychiatrists in the United States,
penned a number of articles and book chapters dealing explicitly with
the subject. In one from 1933 Lewis effectively endorsed Horger's
observations, stating that where Negroes had been found to take their
own lives, they had not been of pure Negro ancestry. An 'admixture of
white blood' had been found in them, Lewis explained. Prominent suicides of black people, like that in 1916 of Ota Benga, the Congolese
man exhibited in the Bronx zoo, were batted away with evolutionary
explanations. Benga was 'a savage who [had] vainly tried to leap from
savagery to civilization, over the intermediate stage of barbarism,' one
commentator claimed.[14]

Beginning in the postwar era and helped by the massive expansion
of the American university system, the study of suicide became more
structured, routine, and sophisticated. Gradually, previously held
axioms loosened. Though imperceptible at first, changes in the way
scholars approached the subject had by the late-1960s flipped the view
that it was just white people who committed suicide to a recognition
that non-white groups did so too, and in some cases at higher rates
than white people. By far the most recognized work on the subject was
one written by a New York psychoanalyst named Herbert Hendin.
Titled *Black Suicide* (1969), the work marked the culmination of trends
that had been vaguely perceptible across the human sciences for a
number of years. Reviewed in the pages of the *New York Times* three
months before its September publication and discussed by the distinguished novelist John Updike in the *Atlantic* a year later, the book had
an impact that cannot be doubted.[15]

Hendin's work, aimed at the general reader, popularized arguments that had already begun to win favour within academic settings. 'Most people,' it began, 'are surprised to learn that among young urban Negroes suicide is a serious problem.' But Hendin went further. 'Among blacks of both sexes between the ages of 20 and 35,' he wrote in an academic article that appeared concurrently with his book, 'suicide is decidedly more of a problem than it is in the white population of the same age.'[16] Importantly, Hendin argued that the suicides by black people were expressions of frustration and rage-like symptoms at their position in American society. Black children were raised in families deformed by racialized employment patterns that emasculated black men and turned black women into overbearing superwomen.[17] For all the work's iconoclasm and hype, few who picked up a copy of *Black Suicide* while browsing their bookstore's shelves would have been unfamiliar with the register in which Hendin was writing. Parallels with Abram Kardiner and Lionel Oversay's work *Mark of Oppression* (1951), and Price Cobbs and William Grier's *Black Rage* (1969), a work published just a few months earlier, were unmistakeable. Yet the claims Hendin made were significant and formed part of a larger transformation in the way race was thought to affect suicide.[18]

As much as *Black Suicide* was a work based on a specific set of arguments, it was also a study intent on promoting the merits of the psychoanalytic approach. Free associations and interrogation of dreams were at the core of the study. Hendin, like many of his colleagues, hoped to demonstrate the rewards derived from such methods. Following in the style of his better-known colleague Abram Kardiner, Hendin remained testy about other approaches to the subject. He bemoaned, for example, what he identified as sociologists' tendencies to write work that he said was like 'Hamlet with Hamlet removed.'[19] Statistical methods and generalizing theories were what analysts most took exception to, emphasizing the inability of such approaches to get at 'the human consequences of the ghetto.'[20] These portrayals of the social-science disciplines were little more than bluster, though. Whether they realized it or not, in practice psychiatrists showed little hesitancy in using the methods they criticized in others. Indeed, perhaps the greatest irony of *Black Suicide* was that, although it was principally constructed around particular encounters and discussions with analysands, it owed its overarching success and longevity to the use it made of statistical data.

For most human scientists working in the postwar era, numerical data provided an important dimension to research about suicide. This is not to say that American mental health officials placed an emphasis on statistics that was lacking in previous generations' studies. Indeed, even a cursory glance at the extensive surveys conducted by the likes of Louis Dublin or Frederick Hoffman would repudiate such arguments. Rather, what distinguished their work was the particular way in which statistical methods were absorbed and the ramifications this approach had for the types of arguments and interpretations they could make. In striking contrast to an earlier generation of writers whose interest in statistical data focused on the aggregate and the mean, an approach that recorded data just as Adolphe Quételet did with his *homme moyen*, in the immediate post war era, American human scientists turned their attention to much narrower statistical groups. Encouraged by Cold War scientism and the rise of the 'variable' as the key unit of data among the social-science community, regressive analysis became the most common method for modelling the relationship between figures. But use of such models did not just point to a shift in method; it also brought about new ways of describing the reality investigated, in turn having implications for the way people thought and spoke about certain subjects. This was certainly true of academic conversations about suicide.[21]

For Hendin and others who thought about how they might investigate the incidence of suicide among various groups, multivariate analysis – in spite of the anxiety they expressed towards statistics – proved a common tool of research. As Hendin was candid enough to point out, *Black Suicide* actually began as a 'statistical study of suicide in New York City that I completed in 1967.'[22] Working with the extensive records kept by the city's department of health, Hendin was able to establish a rough outline of the rates at which the various races were shown to take their own lives. His single greatest contribution to this body of research, however, was the way he applied the period's most fashionable statistical methods to the dissection of an older data set, thereby introducing 'age' as a variable. As the then-young black psychiatrist James Comer explained a few years later, before Hendin arranged the data according to age groups, 'the extremely high rate of suicide among older Whites [had] distort[ed] the average and [had been] one of the factors that ... led to the mistaken notion that suicide [was] much less a problem among Blacks.'[23] Hendin's work did not supply new data but, rather, a new way of viewing those data.

Not only did these methods produce startling new conclusions, as was the case with Hendin's claims; equally important was the effect they had in producing new groups of observation. Regressive analysis meant that rather than speaking about the suicidal tendencies of broad, general groups – 'Negroes,' 'men,' or much less frequently 'Negro men' – human scientists began systematically measuring the impact of other factors, such as age, class, and income. Rather than speak of the incidence and type of suicide committed by 'white men' or 'black women,' then, the introduction of other variables, the addition of another layer of detail, led researchers to begin speaking of new constituencies, such as 'young black men' or, even more specifically, 'black men between the ages of twenty and thirty five.' The change this new focus wrought upon the terms of debate can be heard in the measured and calculated language that Hendin employed in his study. In the way he articulated his principal claim – that suicide was 'twice as common' – and the precise way he qualified that statement – 'among Negro men aged 20 to 35' – Hendin's work captures quite well the changes in tone, direction, and judgment that human scientists made because of the different research methods they used.

Attention to the incidence of suicide among adolescents was a trend that extended beyond Hendin's own research priorities, however. Publication of a work by a Berkeley psychologist titled *Suicide among the Young* [1969] hinted at the fact age was becoming a significant area of inquiry, applied to all aspects of suicide.[24] Still, it was no coincidence that this turn to adolescent suicide ran concomitantly with the acceptance that non-white people also killed themselves. The associations this view carried became clear in the studies that appeared on suicide and age.

Although some research was done on suicide among white adolescents, this never amounted to a critical body of work. Most studies simply started from the premise that adolescent suicide was a defining characteristic of non-white groups, and surveys were designed accordingly. A paper written in the mid-1980s narrated these distinctions best when it stated that 'Indian suicides are disproportionately young which is a pattern quite different from that of the general U.S. population, but somewhat similar to that of other non-Whites.'[25] Pages of contemporary suicide journals and mainstream newspapers continue to refer to suicide among non-white peoples as a problem of 'youth.' A major initiative launched by the National Institute of Mental Health to reduce health disparities, for example, listed one of its core aims as being 'to decrease the incidence and disproportionate burden of depressive disorders and suicide within minority populations at increased risk (e.g., Native American and Alaska Natives and African

American males aged 15–19).' Such characterizations chime with the sense that these suicides were caused principally by behaviour that was reckless, violent, and an expression of social disenchantment.[26]

Reviewers of *Black Suicide*, writing in both specialist and mainstream publications, were quick to elaborate on Hendin's point about how suicide differed between black and white Americans. And the general characterizations of suicide that they offered – as something associated with youth, carried out impulsively, the result of rage and frustration – served, not as indices of black people's cultural and intellectual advancement, but as markers of their dysfunction. The esteemed novelist John Updike, reviewing two of Hendin's works for the *Atlantic*, wrote in 1971 that 'in the black ghettos of America, suicide is one face of a rage that, though ultimately caused by the Negro's frustrating position in the society, originates for almost every individual in maternal rejection.' A review in the flagship *American Journal of Psychiatry* the previous year also identified Hendin's depiction of suicide in black people as being 'conscious hostility erupting in episodic violence.' Such behaviour, this reviewer noticed, 'is markedly different from the Freud and Abraham formulation of suicide associated with depression: dependent ambivalence, guilt, oral incorporation fantasies, and inwardly turned hostility.' [27] In the collective view, then, suicide continued to be used as a subject for denying the capacity of non-white people to act rationally and according to their own intentions. This trait pervaded the field and provides one example of the very particular way in which experts 'effectively diminish[ed] individual responsibility for the decision to die.'[28]

Culture and the Study of Behaviour

Though they were subject to ever more serious challenges from a resurgent biologism, social and environmental explanations of human behaviour remained regnant within the American human sciences until at least the mid-1970s. While the advent of antidepressants and antipsychotic medications had from the mid-1950s encouraged a growing interest and faith in what was becoming known as 'biological psychiatry,' it was the category of culture that received the most extensive support from those interested in the subject of suicide in these decades.[29]

Culture entered the clinic as both a field in its own right, via people such as Marvin Opler, the cultural anthropologist interested in mental health, and as a perspective widely applied across the human sciences.

While anthropologists and social psychiatrists undertook large-scale surveys, comparing the rate and form of suicide in different parts of the world, culture was also integrated into existing conceptual apparatus. Family therapists such as Nathan Ackerman and psychoanalysts such as Abram Kardiner thus began to think about how social institutions such as the family were shaped by cultural patterns, and how in turn those units affected the formation of personality.[30] As a student of Ackerman and a colleague of Kardiner, Hendin not surprisingly became one of the leading advocates for cultural explanations of suicide. Given the use to which the language of culture was put in discussions about race and ethnicity, it was also no coincidence that much of his work focused on these issues.

As he repeated throughout *Black Suicide* and his earlier study, *Suicide in Scandinavia* (1965), Hendin wanted his colleagues to understand that 'culture influences character.' The way he thought it did so was instructive. Like most analysts writing in this period, Hendin appropriated culture psychodynamically. That is, he directed his interest towards the effect different cultural patterns had on concepts such as ego development, the Oedipal complex, and self-image.[31] In the case of black people, the argument came about that they committed suicide out of frustration and rage, which they developed because of the way society had deformed their families, creating matriarchal homes from which children gained little emotional nourishment and which proved a source of endless turmoil.

Drawing on anthropological studies usually long past their 'sell-by' date, a good deal of the work on suicide that took a cultural perspective was notable for its reductionism. The period's emphasis on cultural particularism – the view that groups have their own discrete values – informed most writing during these decades and fostered a tendency to indulge in simplistic dichotomies. A former student of Marvin Wolfgang's wrote that 'the dramatic contrast of suicide-homicide rates for whites and Negroes may indicate that we are dealing with two separate cultural systems.'[32] Stock portraits of cultures suffused the literature. A 1975 epidemiological survey, funded by the National Institute of Mental Health, used participant responses to show that Japanese Americans and Mexican Americans belonged to 'collectivistic cultures,' 'orientated strongly towards preserving in-group solidarity,' whereas Black and Caucasian Americans 'appear[ed] more individualistic in their orientations.'[33] Family patterns were the most obvious markers of supposed cultural difference between groups. Minority families were frequently shown to be organized by a power asymmetry between parents, a detail usually represented by absentee fathers and overbearing mothers. This was certainly thought to be characteristic of both Jewish and Negro families.[34] For analysts such as Hendin and Ackerman, the interest lay in exploring the possible links between how different patterns of family life affected childhood psychological development, and how in turn these patterns either increased or lessened the likelihood of suicidal ideation in later life. Others within the human sciences used culture differently, often thinking more about how various groups interacted with each other, and how those cultures damaged by such exchanges might encourage suicidal tendencies in their members.

How might the processes of integration and acculturation affect patterns of suicidal ideation? At a time when integration discourse was prominent in American social thought and when a number of groups were making loud claims for full legal and social inclusion, interaction between cultures was an issue that greatly interested those who wrote about suicide. Were matriarchal families, for example, causative of higher rates of suicide because they were anomalous in a patriarchal society? Not all commentators thought this was so, some arguing that differences between cultures did not necessarily make them incompatible and thus might not necessarily be causative of suicidal ideation. As Daniel Patrick Moynihan wrote in his infamous 1965 report *The Negro Family: A Case for National Action*, 'it is clearly a disadvantage for a minority group to be operating on one principle, while the great majority of the population ... is operating on another.'[35] Overwhelmingly, however, the process of acculturation was found to be a turbulent one, perhaps even causative of suicide. Work on Native Americans frequently pointed out that the highest rates of suicide were found on those reservations closest to the country's industrialized cities.[36] Usually such arguments insisted that it was second-generation adolescents who felt the transition most acutely. '[T]he younger Indian is caught in the cross-cultural conflict,' public health officials typically wrote.[37] Others claimed differently. Among migrants from China, the reverse seemed to be true, such that cultural dissonance was thought to afflict an older generation. Peter Bourne, an assistant professor in Emory University's Department of Psychiatry, read a paper before the American Psychiatric Association in 1973 in which he argued that the falling rate at which Chinese people in San Francisco took their own lives was linked to a reduction in 'older isolated men living alone in boarding houses.' Such men, Bourne said, committed suicide because of their 'disrupted lives and ... fail[ure] to become integrated into society.'[38] It was revealing of the extent to which cultural explanations had infiltrated the human sciences that a psychiatrist would show no hesitation in offering such assessments before a distinguished gathering of his peers.

If they were unable to agree which age groups were most at risk of suicidal ideation because of acculturative stress, scholars were unanimous in depicting such problems as those of masculinity. 'The role of the contemporary Papago man is poorly defined,' one researcher noted, 'largely as a result of acculturation and its concomitant erosion of role definition.' Modern society undermined traditional values and practices: 'Anglo priests and ministers have usurped the role of spiritual leader, government physicians have replaced the medicine man in the society's healer role ... All these roles and related functions once belonged to the Papago man.'[39] Instructively, no investigation was conducted at this time into how suicide patterns of white people might also be affected as a result of living in a culturally changing society. Instead, the process of acculturation was only ever cited as a causative factor in minority groups' suicides, as their cultural patterns crumbled. Shot through with an underlying presumption that acculturation referred to the interaction between simple, traditional cultures of non-white peoples, on the one hand, and the advanced, industralized culture of modern society, on the other, such interpretations often reinvoked the civilizationalist rhetoric of previous eras.

In the way they were incorporated into explanations of suicide, cultural methods were revealing of an interaction between sociological and psychodynamic perspectives. Contemporaries often called attention to such hybridity without realizing it. In 1973 James Comer, now a psychiatrist at Yale University, claimed that 'it is very likely that the life style and/or culture of a group makes it relatively vulnerable to suicide ... It is equally likely that the way a child is reared and his or her experiences do the same.'[40] Furthermore, by taking the family as a unit on which culture had an effect, analysts effectively treated it as sociologists might approach other institutions – as a part of the social structure. This slippage of methods across disciplines was proof that much of the work done on suicide in this period was united by a common technical element.

References to culture also figured in those studies that plotted a connection between frustration and rage, on the one hand, and the aetiology of suicide, on the other. Unlike previous interpretations that had generally positioned suicide in an inverse relationship to homicide, tracing its causation through factors such as depression, suicide in the postwar decades was increasingly regarded as a violent form of behaviour, caused by such things as one's annoyance with society. Such contentions demanded a mode of analysis that looked at how particular groups interacted with social institutions and the attitudes they formed as a consequence. In short, it required a mode of explanation that was informed by an understanding of culture.

Traditional studies on suicide had been underpinned by an implicit sense that the rate at which members of a particular group took their own lives was inverse to the rate at which such people committed homicide. 'Where the suicide rate is low, the incidence of aggressive acts against other people or objects is usually high,' one psychiatrist explained in 1967.[41] Given the high rate at which it was alleged black Americans committed homicide, the logical weight of such theories had encouraged the view of their supposedly low rates of suicide in the pre-1945 era. By the 1960s, however, even though homicide rates among blacks were still thought to outstrip those of white people, the suicide rates of black people were also deemed to be high. What might have seemed like a contradictory situation to an older generation of scholars – high rates of *both* suicide and homicide – was reconciled only by the fact these suicides were now regarded as expressions of frustration, described in exactly the same terms as violent acts like homicide. This perspective has remained in place subsequently, as testified by a government report from 1989 in which one psychiatrist noted that 'self-hatred and intense rage characterized ... suicide attempters, particularly the black males.'[42]

Interest in analysing the relationship between suicide and homicide was of lessening importance in these years, as researchers instead began to resort to broader cultural explanations. Frequently it was insisted that phenomena such as suicide and homicide were actually inseparable events, both the products of the culture in which a particular group was immersed. Hendin thus wrote that 'underlying suicide as well as homicide is the central common factor of the attempt by the young black population to deal with its rage and violence.' He would remain unwavering in these observations, making exactly the same point fifteen years later.[43] Indian Health Service specialists writing in these years offered similar observations about the comparable rates at which young Native Americans committed both homicide and suicide. One article from 1970 made its point on this subject diagrammatically, pointing to the similar trajectory at which Native Americans took their own lives and that for other members of society. Intellectual curiosity inspired further research to extend this point further. How might other manifestations of maladjustment – alcoholism, family breakdown, drug addiction, other mental disorders – be related to the incidence and causation of suicide? Hendin's scepticism that there was anything essential about individual phenomena such as suicide among black people was typical of the perspective that emerged: 'Whether the individual acts on homicidal impulses, tries to drown them in alcohol, "cools" them by emotional detachment, controls them through religious faith, projects them as hallucinations or turns all feelings inward in suicide, the picture that emerges of young black adults struggling with conscious murderous impulses is a far different picture than emerges from most studies of white suicide.'[44]

Connections between violence and suicide were thus part of a broader set of transformations concerned with the causation of suicide in this period. While the aggression concept grabbed headlines and helped to make suicide a distinctive and much-spoken-about topic of the day, other trends worked to absorb it within a broader literature about social dysfunction and maladjustment. Written predominantly by and for American mental health professionals, this literature attempted to view suicide less as a discrete phenomenon than as just one type of dysfunctional behaviour. 'As tragic and as final as suicide and homicide are, they are but symptoms of deeper problems,' an article about Native Americans pointed out; 'other symptoms of maladjustment among Indians are excessive use of alcohol, broken homes, neglect of children, juvenile delinquency, truancy, and school dropouts.'[45] Ronald Maris, the Dartmouth professor of sociology, commented around the same time that a study of the subject ought to be done with one eye on 'related social problems such as drug addiction, alcoholism, homicide, assault, accidents, mental illness, martial discord, work problems and prostitution.'[46] Hendin put the point most succinctly, writing about how 'people in difficulty are apt to express the difficulty in more than one way.'[47] Applied almost exclusively to non-white peoples, though, these characterizations only helped to create an image of deformity among such groups, all the while stripping their suicide of its most distinctive attributes.

Changes in the terms commonly used to describe study of this subject signal the types of shifts that took place in these decades with regard to thinking about the causation of suicide. Increasingly, authors refrained from describing their work as being just about suicide. By the early 1970s, the preferred term was in fact 'self-destructive' or 'life-threatening' behaviours, terminology that hinted at the more capacious view taken of causation.[48]

Concepts, Methods, and Empirical Research

If Hendin revised and rejected the homicide/suicide paradigm, the attention he gave it is noteworthy, at least revealing of the hold such formulations continued to have over the study of the subject. His suggesting that suicide and homicide ought not to be seen as inversely related but as two discrete symptoms of a particularly violent culture was also typical of an emerging strain within the study of suicide. Erwin Stengal, a psychiatrist and vice-president of the International Association for Suicide Prevention, cautioned colleagues at a 1967 symposium in Washington, DC, that, 'as students of human behavior, we cannot view suicide in isolation but as only one of the manifestations of aggressive tendencies.'[49] Aggression was becoming a guiding motif of the field, particularly when applied to the suicides of non-white peoples. Placing an emphasis on violence and on social dysfunction, these new ways of thinking about suicide immediately piqued the interest of criminologists. And they too directed their work towards exploring the relationship between these two types of death.

In what was arguably the most successful reformulation of the homicide/suicide paradigm, Marvin Wolfgang, a psychoanalytically oriented sociologist and future world-renowned criminologist, argued in a series of papers in the late 1950s that occasionally behaviour was mistakenly recorded as homicidal when in fact it was suicidal. Working from data sets obtained from the Philadelphia police department's Homicide Squad, Wolfgang composed two research papers, the first looking at 'homicide-suicide'; the second, a year later, at 'victim-precipitated homicide.' The topic of this later paper referred to those instances when people committed suicide by goading another person into killing them. In short, the person was not the agent of their own suicide. Wolfgang's model was a direct, though little recognized, antecedent of what ultimately would become known as suicide-by-cop. In the way he discussed such behaviour as suicidal, he revealed the field's abiding interest in seeing it as an expression of aggression.

Victim-precipitated homicide, Wolfgang argued, was more common among black Americans than among any other group: 'a significantly higher proportion of Negroes (79 per cent) than of whites (21 per cent) commit suicide by becoming willing victims of homicide.' Explaining these trends, he wrote that Negroes were less likely to commit conventional, or 'ordinary,' suicide because such behaviour was 'outside [their] frame of reference as a means of solving problems or alleviating tension.' Furthermore, suicide was also thought not to be a masculine form of behaviour for people of colour, Wolfgang argued. In a subculture that emphasized 'external, overt, other-oriented aggression,' conventional methods of suicide went against the grain of life. Victim-precipitated homicide instead chimed with black cultural patterns: 'The victim-precipitated homicide victim may give up the struggle and willingly submit to the retaliation, but he has destroyed himself by engaging in an active fight.'[50] In devising a way of thinking about suicide that purported to show the existence of suicidal tendencies among black people, Wolfgang's work was revealing of the nascent tendencies within the field, trends that Hendin's later work would confirm. Increasingly, scholars were coming round to the idea that black people did commit suicide. But there was little change in the characterizations they made about what motivated these suicides, which stripped that term of almost everything it signified when they were speaking about white people, most notably the subject's agency.

Judging black people's suicides to be the result of social pressures rather than conscious will was another way in which academics' studies in this period uncoupled agency from the act. Ronald Maris told readers of his *Social Forces in Urban Suicide* (1969) that such behaviour 'does not seem to be a product of excessive individuation but rather of a malfunctioning of social interaction.'[51] It was an image that associated suicide not with middle-class urbanity but with a breakdown in the fabric of the black community, perhaps a suggestion of incompatibility between so-called black and white cultures.

In the decades following the Second World War, research across the human sciences was dominated by two trends. The first was the concern researchers showed towards issues prominent in the public eye. People did not wish just to think about suicide but also to act to prevent it, and accordingly, many of these scholars were at the forefront of efforts to establish suicide-prevention bureaux. The second, somewhat related trend was the tendency of researchers to assess older theories in light of contemporary problems, testing, revising, and synthesizing those theories in relation to new empirical findings. And in this sense, no scholar's work was invoked more frequently than that of the French sociologist Émile Durkheim.

The neglect shown Durkheim's work before 1945 has been taken by some scholars as indicative of the rigid divisions that existed between American academic disciplines. Karl Menninger's failure to reference the French sociologist's work in his influential study *Man against Himself* (1938), and psychoanalysts' preoccupation with other modes of explanation have thus been said to illustrate biological scientists' refusal to accept sociological explanations. Yet it would have been only the most abstruse sociologist who cited Durkheim's work before the postwar era; the vast majority of American sociologists remained ignorant of his research too.[52] Only in the late 1950s did Durkheim begin to enjoy something of a renaissance in the way he was both used and appraised. The centenary of his birth in 1958 was marked by a host of conferences and graduate seminars reporting favourable verdicts of his work. More relevant for those interested in the subject of suicide was the appearance of the first English translation of his work *Le suicide* in 1951. Instantly embraced by social scientists and well-liked because it chimed with the period's 'interests in comparative method and in techniques of multivariate analysis,' *Suicide* had a serious influence on the investigation of this subject in the postwar United States. Twenty-five years after the first English translation of the work was released, an entire study devoted to the book appeared. The title of this book was instructive: *Durkheim's Suicide: A Classic Analyzed.*[53] By the mid-1960s 'it was normal to treat Durkheim as a key figure,' one scholar reminds us, speaking about him alongside figures such as Karl Marx and Max Weber.[54] By the late 1960s such praise of his methods was as likely to be made by physicians and psychiatrists as it was by those working in the American social sciences.[55]

The popularity of Durkheim's theories on suicide was in part a consequence of the attention they were given by some of the period's leading intellectuals. Robert Merton at Columbia University was one of his most significant boosters. In an article he wrote in 1938 about 'anomie,' Merton gave new life to Durkheim's work, providing a way of thinking about his theories that related them to contemporary problems. Anomie, according to Merton, was the disjuncture that often existed between socially held ideas and social reality. As Gunnar Myrdal's *An American Dilemma* had made clear, this was an observation that described the United States' treatment of race especially well. For those who had experienced the worst excess of American racism and the daily celebration of the country's lofty ideals, might such moral hypocrisy not be causative of suicide, scholars wondered in these decades. Indicative of the racialized nature of research in these years was the fact that no one thought to investigate the effect this moral dilemma might have upon rates of suicide among white people.[56]

One of the best known of Durkheim's models for explaining suicide was his so-called theory of status integration. As with acculturation approaches, it was a theory well suited to the concerns of postwar American society. Status-integration theory was concerned principally with how social regulation and social stability affected the incidence of suicide. What is interesting about the theory is the widespread acceptance it won across various disciplines. When the sociologist Jack Gibbs was asked at a symposium in 1967 to explain the low rate of suicide among blacks, he answered with reference to the theory. Lower rates among blacks, Gibbs told his audience, 'is entirely consistent with the notion that status integration varies inversely with the suicide rate. Negroes in the United States have much higher occupational integration than do whites; that is, they are concentrated in particular occupations more than are the whites.'[57] Gibbs's comments were hardly surprising, given that he had just co-written a work drawing extensively on the theory. What his remarks do indicate, however, is the general acceptance they had among an audience of psychiatrists.

Revealing of the methodological exchanges that underpinned the study of suicide in these years was the degree to which those trained within the biological sciences would proudly display their use of sociological concepts. One Berkeley behavioural scientist drew on Merton's theory of anomie when he wrote that 'in a period of rapid, forced and unequal change, expectations or hopes are created far more rapidly than they are fulfilled, and feelings of frustration and despair are thus intensified.'[58] His use of sociological theories was by no means an isolated case among those with medical training. When asked about the low rates of suicide among blacks, Erwin Stengal answered that such trends were 'possibly because of the closer social cohesion of minority groups and their lower social status.'[59] That neither of these authors acknowledged or probably understood the intellectual genealogy of their observations does not diminish the fact they were making use of ways of thinking formed within social science. Intellectual traditions, as Jennifer Platt and a number of other scholars have argued, take shape as bricolage, pieced together from a number of ideas. While rivalries and one-upmanship may have seethed publicly between disciplines, in most cases methods and empirical studies were surprisingly similar.

In *Suicide*, for all the various permutations he was thought to have given the subject, contemporaries believed Durkheim's principal concern to be in exploring the cohesiveness of societal arrangement. The four types of suicide that he identified were all examples of how individuals were affected by social structures. And the general picture that emerged was that too little or too much social regulation of a person's life was likely to encourage suicidal ideation. In a period when anxieties about generational, sexual, and racial divisions were feverishly discussed, theories that explored the impact of social cohesion on rates of suicide were naturally attractive. One of the ways in which this was done was to look at attitudinal divisions among people, trying to understand how the embrace of a certain viewpoint might lead to a sense of connection with other people. Alton Kirk, a sociologist at Michigan State University, wrote a prize-winning paper in the late 1970s in which he insisted that black consciousness strongly correlated to lower rates of suicide. Those who did experience suicidal ideation had expressed 'doubts about their personal identities and great uncertainty about their identity as members of the black race,' Kirk wrote, 'they felt isolated and of not being full, participating members in society as a whole and in the black race.'[60] This mixture of the psychological and the sociological was typical of studies done in this period along such lines. It was revealing both of the way structural-functional concepts were described in accordance with the field of behaviourism and of the way methods were used in a pick-and-mix fashion. In more recent times, research on suicide has continued to look at other issues in a similar way, investigating, for instance, how heightened rates of religiosity might correlate with low rates of suicide.[61]

Studies of suicide in this period were buffeted by the period's political tensions and, in particular, the problem of the United States' racial heritage. One of the dominant axioms of social-science research in these years was the view that segregation and discrimination had caused untold damage to the black psyche. It was a contention cited in the *Brown* decision of May 1954, Senator Moynihan's 1965 report, and almost every social-science textbook of the period. Those interested in the subject of suicide were equally moved to consider the validity of such arguments. In the early 1970s a young sociologist called Warren Breed dealt directly with this topic, taking Durkheim's little-remembered theory of fatalistic suicide as his prompt for considering whether societal oppression was causative of suicidal ideation among black people. Fatalistic suicide was a Durkheimian term, and as Breed told his readers, it referred to a type of suicide thought to 'deriv[e] from excessive regulation.' It was, then, a behaviour most likely to be observed in 'persons with futures pitilessly blocked and passions violently choked by oppressive discipline.'[62] Working from medical records obtained from the New Orleans health board, Breed went on to argue that involvement with the police was common among the cases of black suicides and thus might be an expression of the social control of such groups.

Conclusion: New Methods, Changed Debates, Old Characterizations

In the years between roughly 1950 and 1975, a series of intellectual and institutional transformations within the American academy transformed suicide from a marginal topic into a subject in its own right, written about in dedicated journals from papers given at conferences convened for scholars who might refer to themselves as 'suicidologists.' There was no doubting the scale of these changes. General intellectual currents had a similarly effervescent effect on how people thought about suicide and how they went about researching it. It is worth recounting here the changed intellectual contours of the period.

Firstly, it needs to be noted that suicide, as well as becoming an area of research in its own right, was also written about within a broader social-science literature on social dysfunction. These latter currents were in part responsible for altering what had previously been blandly termed the study of 'suicide' into a bundle of topics known as the study of 'life-threatening behaviours.' But secondly, the shift in nomenclature also gestured at the more capacious way in which the causality of suicide – indeed, what was considered to constitute suicidal *behaviour* – was described. Thus a 1970 conference organized by Kenneth Clark's Metropolitan Applied Research Center cited 'underachievement' as one of the many types of 'Self Destructive Patterns in the Black Community.' More recently, one prominent psychiatrist would refer to 'slow forms of suicide.'[63] By the late 1960s, in contrast to earlier decades, killing oneself was no longer necessarily regarded as simply the result of one's sophisticated surroundings or the pressures of modernity. For now the converse was also true, such that from this period onwards, suicide was thought of as the ultimate expense paid by those living in isolated, poverty-stricken, precarious, and violent surroundings. Overwhelmingly, this second type of characterization has been applied to non-white groups. As one columnist scribbled in 1978, 'Black men who committed suicides include dejected lower-class Black men burdened by a feeling of worthlessness and middle-class men frustrated because they were not moving up as fast as they had thought they should.'[64]

The scale of the shift from the pre-1945 belief that black people did not commit suicide to a postwar view that they do kill themselves cannot be overplayed. The incidence and patterns of suicide among races were what really occupied those studying the subject in these decades. Yet to understand the direction and degree of change in how suicide was conceptualized in these years, it is better if we focus on the characterizations scholars offered of particular races' behaviour, for exactly what non-white people's suicides were believed to signify changed surprisingly little. The different characterization offered of black people's suicides continued the practice of describing their actions in the same way as an earlier generation of anthropologists had explained the suicides of Africans – as ritualistic or signs of weakness. The suggestion that black people committed suicide principally out of frustration and rage, rather than introspection and depression, was a particularly obvious use of the long-standing associations of blackness and violence.

NOTES

1 Richard Seiden provides an estimate of the number of articles published on the subject in *Suicide among the Young: A Review of Literature, 1900–1967* (Washington, DC: US Government Printing Office, 1969), 1. Articles about various aspects of suicide appeared yearly in the pages of the *New York Times*. See 'Psychiatrist Says Potential Suicides Can Be Recognized,' *New York Times*, 10 September 1967, 63; Jane E. Brody, 'Spotting Suicidal Patients,' *New York Times*, 5 February 1967, D5. On the American therapeutic ethos, see Ellen Herman, *The Romance of American Psychology: Political Culture in the Age of Expert* (Berkeley: University of California Press, 1995).

2 Michael MacDonald and Terence R. Murphy, *Sleepless Souls: Suicide in Early Modern England* (Oxford: Clarendon Press, 1990), 338. See also Michael MacDonald, 'The Medicalization of Suicide in England: Laymen, Physicians, and Cultural Change, 1500–1870,' *Milbank* Q 67 1, Supplement 1 (1989), 69–91.

3 For the claim that the intellectual history of suicide has already been written, see Jeffrey R. Watt, ed., *From Sin to Insanity: Suicide in Early Modern Europe* (Ithaca: Cornell University Press, 2004). See esp. Jeffrey Merrick, 'Chapter 9: Suicide in Paris, 1775.'

4 Howard Kushner has argued that interdisciplinary research on the subject of suicide was not possible because of the rigid boundaries

between academic disciplines. See Kushner, 'American Psychiatry and the Cause of Suicide, 1844–1917,' *Bull. Hist. Med.* 60 1 (Spring 1986), 36–57; and his *Self-Destruction in the Promised Land: A Psychocultural Biology of American Suicide* (New Brunswick: Rutgers University, 1989). My argument does not directly challenge Kushner's insomuch as I am arguing less for the rise of a unified theory of suicide within the American human sciences as for a sharing of methods among disciplines.

5 Theodore M. Porter, 'Statistics and Statistical Methods,' in *The Cambridge History of Science*, vol. 7, *The Modern Social Sciences* (Cambridge: Cambridge University Press, 2003), 50.

6 Jack Gibbs, 'Suicide,' in *Contemporary Social Problems*, ed. Robert K. Merton, and Robert A. Nisbet (1961; 2nd ed., New York: Harcourt, 1966), 288.

7 See, for example, Marvin Wolfgang's studies 'An Analysis of Homicide-Suicide,' *J. Clin. Exp. Psychopath.* 19 3 (September 1958), 208–18, and 'Suicide by Means of Victim-Precipitated Homicide,' *J. Clin. Exp. Psychopath.* 20 4 (December 1959), 335–51; as well as J.A. Ward, 'A Suicide Epidemic on an Indian Reserve,' *Can. Psychiatri. Assoc. J.* 22 8 (December 1977), 423–6; and Richard Kalish, 'Suicide: An Ethnic Comparison in Hawaii,' *Bull. Suicidol.* 2 4 (December 1968), 37–43.

8 Thoedore L. Dorpat, Joan Jackson, and Herbert Ripley, 'Broken Homes and Attempted and Completed Suicide,' *Arch. Gen. Psychiatr.* 12 2 (February 1965), 213–16.

9 For contemporaries' responses to the rise of suicidology in the late 1960s and early 1970s, see E. Webster, 'Review: *Race and Suicide in South Africa*, by Fatima Meer,' *Am. J. Sociol.* 84 1 (July 1978), 262–3. Instructively, the first book to take that term as its title appeared in these years; see Edwin Shneidman, *Suicidology: Contemporary Developments* (New York: Grune and Stratton, 1976).

10 Herbert Hendin, *Black Suicide* (New York: Basic Books, 1969).

11 The literary scholar Lisa Lieberman similarly contends that all modern understandings of suicide as described in psychiatric approaches deny the 'liberty, self-determination, free will' of such actions. See her *Leaving You: The Cultural Meaning of Suicide* (Chicago: Ivan R. Dee, 2003). My argument departs from Lieberman's in that I emphasize the racialization of this process.

12 My understanding of change in scientific thought is led by Michel Foucault's emphasis on a 'systematic ensemble' rather than an individual author. See his 'What Is an Author?' in *The Foucault Reader*, ed. Paul Rabinow (New York: Pantheon Books, 1984), 109. See also his *The Order of*

Things: An Archaeology of the Human Sciences (1966; trans., London: Tavistock Publications, 1970).

13 Philip Bruce, *The Plantation Negro as a Freeman: Observations on His Character, Condition, and Prospects in Virginia* (New York: G.P. Putnam's Sons, 1889), 158n57; Frederick Hoffman, *Race Traits and Tendencies of the American Negro* (Publication of the American Economic Association 11 nos.1–3: New York: Macmillan Co., 1896), 1–329, folder 36, box 11, Frederick Hoffman Papers, Manuscripts and Rare Books, Columbia University; G. Stanley Hall, 'A Few Results of Recent Scientific Study of the Negro in America,' *Proceed. Mass. Hist. Soc.* 2nd Series 19 (1905), 99; Gunnar Myrdal, *An American Dilemma: The Negro Problem and Modern Democracy* (Harper & Brothers Publishers: New York, 1944), 979–82.

14 See Eugene L. Horger, 'A Comparative Psychiatric Study of the Whites and Negroes Admitted to the South Carolina State Hospital from 1916 to 1927, Incl.,' [n.d., c.1927], folder 8, box 1, Eugene Leroy Horger Papers, South Caroliniana Library, University of South Carolina; Nolan D.C. Lewis, 'Studies on Suicide: Preliminary Survey of Some Significant Aspects of Suicide,' *Psychoanal. Rev.* 20 3 (July 1933), 246; 'Editorial: Suicide of Ota Benga, the African Pygmy,' *Zoolo. Soc. Bull.* 19 3 (May 1916), 1356.

15 Harold Schmeck, 'Study Shows High Rate of Negro Suicides in City,' *New York Times*, 21 June 1969, 28; John Updike, 'Black Suicide,' *The Atlantic* 227 2 (February 1971), 108–12.

16 Hendin, *Black Suicide*, 3; Herbert Hendin, 'Black Suicide,' *Arch. Gen. Psychiatr.* 21 9 (October 1969), 407–22.

17 Describing family dysfunction as being due to matriarchy was a common theme in this period, applied to particular ethnic and racial groups. See, for example, Nathan Ackerman and Marie Jahoda, *Anti-Semitism and Emotional Disorder* (New York: Harper & Brothers, 1950). Historically, such portraits were made especially about black women. See Michele Wallace, *Black Macho and the Myth of the Superwoman* (1978; New York: Verso, 1996) for a contemporary's reaction to such charges.

18 A general overview of scholarship on race and alleged mental deformity can be found in Daryl Michael Scott, *Contempt and Pity: Social Policy and the Image of the Damaged Black Psyche, 1880–1996* (Chapel Hill: University of North Carolina Press, 1997), esp. chap. 5.

19 Abram Kardiner and Lionel Oversay, *The Mark of Oppression: A Psychosocial Study of the American Negro* (New York: W.W. Norton and Company, 1951), xii.

20 Hendin, *Black Suicide*, 6.

21 Dorothy Ross, 'Changing Contours of the Social Science Disciplines,' in *The Cambridge History of Science*, vol. 7, *The Modern Social Sciences*, ed. Theodore M. Porter, and Dorothy Ross (Cambridge: Cambridge University Press, 2003), 231–2; Kurt Danziger, *Naming the Mind: How Psychology Found Its Language* (London: Sage Publications, 1997), 163–9. For more on the relationship between social thought and statistical knowledge in the postwar United States, see Sarah E. Igo, *The Averaged American: Surveys, Citizens, and the Making of a Mass Public* (Cambridge: Harvard University Press, 2007).

22 Herbert Hendin, 'Racial Oppression and Black Suicide,' *Current* 114 (January 1970), 30.

23 James Comer, 'Black Suicide: A Hidden Crisis,' *Urban Health* 2 4 (August 1973), 41.

24 Seiden, *Suicide among the Young*.

25 Nancy Westlake Van Winkle and Philip A. May, 'Native American Suicide in New Mexico, 1957–1979: A Comparative Study,' *Human Organization* 45 4 (Winter 1986), 302; See also Van Winkle and May, 'An Update on American Indian Suicide in New Mexico, 1980–1987,' *Human Organization* 52 3 (Fall 1993), 309.

26 Details of the NIMH initiative can be found in 'Five-Year Strategic Plan for Reducing Health Disparities,' National Institute of Mental Health (Washington, DC, 16 November 2002), 20. On contemporary human scientists' tendency to describe non-white people's suicide as a youthful, irrational, and violent phenomenon, see Nicolas Ialongo et al., 'Suicidal Behavior among Urban African American Young Adults,' *Suicide Life. Threat. Behav.* 32 3 (Fall 2002), 256–71; Sean Joe and Mark Kaplan, 'Firearm-Related Suicide among Youth African-American Males,' *Psychiatr. Serv.* 53 3 (March 2002), 332–4. Such trends have seeped into popular accounts too. See Rene Sanchez, 'Black Teen Suicide Rates Increases Dramatically,' *Washington Post*, 20 March 1998, A1, A17; Evelyn Nieves, 'Indian Reservation Reeling in Wave of Youth Suicides and Attempts,' *New York Times*, 9 June 2007.

27 Updike, 'Black Suicide,' 109; Charles B. Wilkerson, 'Review of *Black Suicide* by Herbert Hendin,' *Am. J. Psychiatr.* 127 2 (August 1970), 260.

28 Lieberman, *Leaving You*, 7.

29 See A. E. Bennett, 'Biological Psychiatry,' *Am. J. Psychiatr.* 110 4 (October 1953), 244–52. On the syncretic relationship that came about between biological and cultural modes of explaining human behaviour in this period, especially among psychiatrists, see Jonathan Metzl, *Prozac on the Couch: Prescribing Gender in the Era of Wonder Drugs* (Durham: Duke University Press, 2003).

30 The best work on the rise of culture as a clinical category in the postwar period is Debbie Weinstein, 'Culture at Work: Family Therapy and the Culture Concept in Post–World War II America,' *J. Hist. Behav. Sci.* 40 1 (Winter 2004), 23–46.

31 Herbert Hendin, *Suicide in America* (1984; 2nd ed., New York: W.W. Norton & Company, 1995), 115.

32 Michael Lalli and Stanley H. Turner, 'Suicide and Homicide: A Comparative Analysis by Race and Occupational Levels,' *J. Crim. Law. Criminol. Police Sci.* 59 2 (June 1968), 195.

33 David Reynolds, Richard Kalish, and Norman Faberow, 'A Cross-Ethnic Study of Suicide Attitudes and Expectations in the United States,' in *Suicide in Different Cultures*, ed. Norman Faberow (Baltimore: University Park Press, 1975), 42–44.

34 See Weinstein, 'Culture at Work,' 30–2.

35 Daniel Patrick Moynihan, 'The Negro Family: The Case for National Action' [1965], in *The Moynihan Report and the Politics of Controversy*, ed. Lee Rainwater and William L. Yancey (Cambridge: M.I.T. Press, 1967), 29.

36 Ward, 'A Suicide Epidemic on an Indian Reserve,' 423–6. For a more recent example of these arguments, see Van Winkle and May, 'Native American Suicide in New Mexico,' 307.

37 Rex D. Conrad and Marvin W. Kahn, 'An Epidemiological Study of Suicide and Attempted Suicide among the Papago Indians,' *Am. J. Psychiatr.* 131 1 (January 1974), 69.

38 Peter Bourne, 'Suicide Among Chinese in San Francisco,' *Am. J. Public Health* 63 8 (August 1973), 749.

39 Conrad and Kahn, 'An Epidemiological Study,' 71.

40 Comer, 'Black Suicide,' 42.

41 Erwin Stengal, 'National and Cultural Aspects of Suicide and Attempted Suicide,' in *Symposium on Suicide*, ed. Leon Yachelson (Washington, DC: George Washington University School of Medicine, 1967), 44.

42 F.M. Baker, 'Black Youth Suicide: Literature Review with a Focus on Prevention,' in *Report of the Secretary's Task Force on Youth Suicide*, vol. 3 (Washington, DC: US Government Printing Office, 1989), 177.

43 Hendin, *Suicide in America*, 116.

44 Hendin, *Black Suicide*, 45.

45 Michael Ogden, Mozart Spector, and Charles A. Hill, 'Suicide and Homicides among Indians,' *Public Health Rep.* 85 1 (January 1970), 75–80.

46 Ronald Maris, *Social Forces in Urban Suicide* (Homewood, Ill.: Dorsey Press, 1969), ix.

47 Hendin, *Black Suicide*, 46.

48 On more recent discussions of the historical meanings attached to the term 'suicide,' see Morton Silverman, 'The Language of Suicidology,' *Suicide Life Threat. Behav.* 36 5 (October 2006), 519–32.

49 Stengal, 'National and Cultural Aspects of Suicide,' 44.

50 Wolfgang, 'Suicide by Means of Victim-Precipitated Homicide,' 345.

51 Maris, *Social Forces*, 105.

52 Howard Kushner makes much of Menninger's failure to cite Durkheim's work, taking this apparent slight as a mark of a lack of interdisciplinary cooperation in the study of suicide. See Kushner, 'American Psychiatry and the Cause of Suicide,' 56–7. On the shift in the reception given to Durkheim by American intellectuals, see Jennifer Platt, 'The United States Reception of Durkheim's "The Rules of Sociological Method,"' *Sociol. Persp.* 38 1 (Spring 1995), 77–105.

53 Whitney Pope, *Durkheim's Suicide: A Classic Analyzed* (Chicago: University of Chicago Press, 1976).

54 Jennifer Platt, *A History of Sociological Research Methods in America, 1920–1960* (Cambridge: Cambridge University Press, 1996), 68.

55 Ibid., 90.

56 Robert Merton, 'Social Structure and Anomie,' *Am. Sociol. Rev.* 3 5 (October 1938), 672–82.

57 Jack Gibbs, 'Views of Suicide,' in *Symposium on Suicide*, 59.

58 Richard Seiden, 'We're Driving Young Blacks to Suicide,' *Psychology Today*, August 1970, 26.

59 Stengal, 'National and Cultural Aspects of Suicide,' 46.

60 'Feelin' Good: About Young Black Men Who Have Attempted Suicide,' *Sepia* 26 8 (August 1977), 44.

61 Kevin Early, *Religion and Suicide in the African-American Community* (Westport, Conn.: Greenwood Press, 1992).

62 Émile Durkheim, *Suicide* (1951), quoted in Warren Breed, 'The Negro and Fatalistic Suicide,' *Pacific Sociol. Rev.* 13 3 (Summer 1970), 160.

63 Draft letter, Ulrich Haynes, 17 August 1970, folder: Self-Destructive Patterns in the Black Community, 1970, box 342, Kenneth Clark Papers, Library of Congress, Washington, DC; Alvin F. Poussaint and Amy Alexander, *Lay My Burden Down: Suicide and the Mental Health Crisis among African-Americans* (Boston: Beacon Press, 2000), 8.

64 'Fewer Blacks Commit Suicide than Whites in D.C.,' *Jet* 53 22 (16 February 1978), 5.

11 Questioning the Suicide of Resolve: Medico-legal Disputes Regarding 'Overwork Suicide' in Twentieth-Century Japan

JUNKO KITANAKA

> *Suicide* ... the act of intentionally destroying one's own life ... Its existence is looked upon, in Western civilization, as a sign of the presence of maladies in the body politic which, whether remediable or not, deserve careful examination. It is, of course, impossible to compare Western civilization in this respect with, say, Japan, where suicide in certain circumstances is part of a distinct moral creed.
>
> *Encyclopedia Britannica*, 11th ed. (1910–1911)[1]

'Suicide of Resolve' versus 'Overwork Suicide'

Though psychiatry has been institutionally established in Japan since the late nineteenth century, psychiatrists have had little impact on the way Japanese have conceptualized suicide. This may be because Japanese have long normalized suicide, even aestheticizing it at times as a culturally sanctioned act of individual freedom.[2] While they have certainly recognized different degrees of intentionality in those who commit suicide, ranging from an impulsive desire for escape from an unbearable reality to a fully premeditated act, they have particularly romanticized the latter, as seen in a popular expression, *kakugo no jisatsu*, or suicide of resolve. The term has often been used in newspapers and popular literature from at least the 1870s, particularly in relation to the suicides of intellectuals such as Mishima Yukio.[3] Suicide of resolve signifies the sense of *free will* with which individuals have taken their own lives, as a way of actively creating meaning through their own death. Depending on the circumstances, the meaning of a suicidal act can vary considerably. Notably, in some cases it is a way of taking responsibility; in other cases it is a protest against social injustice and an attestation by the socially weak of their own victimhood. Partly because of this cultural valuation of suicide, Japanese psychiatrists, unlike their Western counterparts, who were able to emerge as 'liberating' agents by asserting that suicide is not a religious sin or a crime but the product of an illness to be treated, have largely failed to have a similarly significant influence on Japanese thinking about suicide.

This situation seems to be changing, however, as Japanese have seen suicide rates skyrocket since 1998. More than 30,000 victims have been recorded annually for ten consecutive years. That number is three to five times greater than those who die in traffic accidents. As the suicide victims have included a large number of middle-aged workers severely hit by the economic recession, a new term has emerged in the media as a national concern: *karô jisatsu*, or overwork suicide, refers to the suicide of the people who are driven to take their own lives after excessive overwork.[4] The concern about overwork suicide heightened in 2000, when the Supreme Court ordered Dentsû Inc., Japan's biggest advertising agency, to compensate the family of a deceased employee, Ôshima Ichirô,[5] with the largest amount ever to be paid for a worker's death in Japan. While Dentsû argued that Ichirô's suicide was intentional, the Supreme Court determined that it was impulsive and accidental, triggered by clinical depression, which had been caused by long and excessive overwork. After the precedent-setting verdict, a number of similar legal victories followed. The alarmed Ministry of Labour (integrated into the Ministry of Health, Welfare, and Labour in 2001) began to implement important policy changes, beginning with the treatment of the mentally ill in the workplace in 1999 and culminating in the Basic Law on Suicide Countermeasures in 2006. Psychiatrists have played a pivotal role in these developments. While this outcome has often been discussed as a triumph of the workers' movement, this chapter calls attention to the fact that it may also signal the beginning of broad-scale medicalization of suicide in Japan. Psychiatrists, through the overwork-suicide disputes, seem to be persuading Japanese that those who take their own lives under tremendous social pressure may also be victims of depression.

As an anthropologist, I am concerned about, first of all, how Japanese psychiatrists have come to successfully challenge the cultural notion of suicide and, secondly, how psychiatry has come to be used to assert that suicide is socially produced. Social scientists have long shown that medicalization is a process whereby a problem of living comes to be redefined as a pathology of individual biology. Indeed, it was in part against French psychiatrist Étienne Esquirol that Émile Durkheim established his sociological theory, demonstrating that suicide is not caused by the individual diseased brain (as Esquirol had claimed) but rather by forces of society.[6] Psychiatry has since been criticized as an apparatus of depoliticization that serves to conceal social contradictions by locating problems within individual biology.[7] However, Japanese psychiatry, which had similarly been critiqued for its biological individual reductionism in the past, was instead used to establish a social cause for suicide in the Dentsû case. While this new, 'socializing' form of medicalization can be found, for instance, in the PTSD discourse in North America,[8] what may be distinctive about the Japanese situation is the extent to which the psychiatric argument has also destabilized the cultural aestheticization of suicide by way of emphasizing these workers' social – and *biological* – victimhood.

In order to examine how this form of medicalization of suicide has become possible in Japan, this chapter first sketches the history of the medicalization of suicide in that country – and the lack thereof – and demonstrates how psychiatrists have engaged with the cultural notion of suicide of resolve. Second, the chapter examines the current medico-legal discourse about overwork suicide to show how some psychiatrists, in order to establish the social causality of suicide, have employed a distinctive theory of melancholic pre-morbid personality as a pathology of the Japanese work ethic. Third, the chapter examines the subsequent changes in governmental regulations and their impact on psychiatry. This unfolding history involves different ideas about biology, personality, social stress, psychopathology, and free will, all of which have become contested through the debates about what causes suicide.[9] The chapter asks in the end what the consequences are of advancing the idea of social causality of suicide by way of psychiatry and what implications this process may have for the way Japanese think about those who are driven to take their own lives.

Suicide as Seen through the History of Japanese Psychiatry

Since the first academic department of psychiatry was established at Tokyo Imperial University in 1886, Japanese psychiatry has had a rather ambiguous relationship with the cultural notion of suicide. The history of Japanese psychiatry may be divided into three phases in terms of its predominant approaches to suicide: early medicalization (1880s-1930s), tension between the forces of medicalization and de-medicalization (1940s–80s), and re-medicalization (1990s to present). Pre–Second World War psychiatrists tried to advance – with some success – the biological view of suicide against the cultural idea by arguing that it resulted from neurasthenia. Postwar suicide experts began to explore the relationship between biology and socio-cultural forces on suicide, while left-wing psychiatrists from the 1960s moved to de-medicalize and existentialize the idea of suicide of resolve. From the 1990s, psychiatrists again began to challenge this notion by arguing that suicide is caused by depression. Yet the ways in which 'depression' is now increasingly discussed not only in terms of biology but also in its social causality are notable.

The cultural notion of suicide has never been a static entity but has been interpreted and reinvented in modernity. This shift was reflected in the debates about suicide that occurred in 1903, when, amidst a heightened sense of social unrest before the Russo-Japanese War (1904–5), Japan's first so-called modern suicide took place. An elite student, Fujimura Misao, jumped over a waterfall in scenic Nikko, north of Tokyo, after inscribing on a tree trunk what became a famous suicide note: '(life is) incomprehensible.' As similar suicides increased, disputes about the meaning of suicide erupted in the media. Some intellectuals, reappropriating the premodern idea of suicide from the Edo Era as a protest of the oppressed against the social order, further elaborated the theme that suicide is an act of expressing individual free will against the impossible demands of modernity. Others increasingly began to discuss it in terms of an illness called neurasthenia (*shinkei suijaku*). Neurasthenia, referred to as a 'national disease' by the 1910s, became a customary label that the media employed to explain suicide.[10] The rise of neurasthenia discourse thus signalled the first instance of medicalization of suicide in Japan.

What caused neurasthenia, however, was a point of heated debate between those who believed it to be social pressure and those who asserted it to be biological, individual weakness. For many Japanese writers of the time, neurasthenia was, as George Beard's well-known conceptualization suggested, a quintessential product of *overwork*. It was said to most affect the men of prime working years, especially those engaged in the new modern professions of 'brain labor.'[11] Natsume Sôseki, one the most important writers in modern Japanese history (who claimed to be neurasthenic himself), asserted in 1911 that neurasthenia was a pathology of the peculiar modernity that Japanese suffered from. As a result of the external threat of colonialism, Japanese were thoroughly overworked from having to achieve industrialization and urbanization in less than half the time it had taken Westerners. 'Unnaturally accelerated' development, particularly for the overworked elites at the forefront of modernity, brought on neurasthenia.[12]

State administrators and politicians, however, tended to regard neurasthenia as a sign of individual weakness. A highly influential statesman, Ôkuma Shigenobu, delivered a speech that exemplified this perspective to a gathering of lawyers and psychiatrists in 1906: 'These days, young students talk about such stuff as the 'philosophy of life' (applause from the floor). They confront important and profound problems of life, are defeated, and develop neurasthenia. Those who jump off a waterfall or throw themselves in front of a train are weak-minded. They do not have a strong mental constitution and develop mental illness, dying in the end. How useless they are! Such weak-minded people would only cause harm even if they remained alive (applause).'[13]

What provided the scientific basis for these politicians' view was psychiatrists' notions of neurasthenia and suicide. Some psychiatrists, particularly those trained in American psychiatry, adhered to the view of neurasthenia as a product of overwork. However, most academic psychiatrists, who had become steeped in German, Kraepelinian neuropsychiatry and degeneration theory, increasingly came to assert that neurasthenia was a matter of individual biological vulnerability, and suicide the 'self-destruction of the inherently weak.'[14] Katayama Kuniyoshi, an authority in forensic medicine and former acting chair of psychiatry at Tokyo Imperial University, wrote in the newspaper *Tokyo Asahi Shimbun* in 1907 that suicidal individuals were 'dispersing poison in society' and that the nation must 'strengthen its body and mind so that it can eliminate such pathological molecules.'[15] Kure Shûzô, the professor at Tokyo Imperial University heralded as the 'father of Japanese psychiatry,' wrote in the *Yomiuri Shimbun* in 1917 that the recent increase in suicide rates among prostitutes must be understood, not in terms of the hardships these women faced, as 'amateurs would presuppose,' but rather in terms of their 'inherent, mental abnormality,' which would also explain why they turned to such an immoral profession in the first place.[16] Psychiatrists continued to look for a possible cause of suicide through anatomical dissections of brains, suggesting that it might be linked, for instance, to an 'unusual accumulation of fat in the cerebral cortex.'[17] They reasoned, as Nakamura of Tohoku University did in 1940, that because 'there are many people placed in similar (stressful) situations who do not commit suicide,' those who do 'must have an exceptional condition in their mental state.' For these psychiatrists, the 'true cause' of suicide was to be located in individual brains.[18]

Psychiatrists increasingly rejected the 'overwork' theory of neurasthenia and suicide, but they could not afford to dismiss entirely the cultural notion of suicide, which was, as the nation geared up to the Second World War, becoming insidiously romanticized as an honourable act of self-sacrifice. In this political climate, while some clinicians ardently investigated parent-child suicides as a distinctively 'Japanese' phenomenon,[19] even biological psychiatrists such as Nakamura saw the need to insist that suicide of courage and dignity might well be possible by a 'few great persons.' He added that 'it is an exception' which would be hard to achieve even 'for most people of culture today.'[20] Pre-war academic psychiatrists, however, continued to maintain their belief in genetic, biological determinism, even though the political influence of their view – as well as the effect of medicalization – gradually waned.

In the late 1950s, during the first 'suicide boom' of the post–Second World War era, Japanese began to grapple with the question of why so many people were choosing to take their own lives, especially after they had just survived a devastating war. This time some young psychiatrists such as Katô Masaaki and Ôhara Kenshiro started to criticize psychiatry's lingering genetic determinism and to assert instead that Japanese suicide behaviour needed to be understood as a product not only of biology but of culture as well.[21] While they helped to establish the new field of suicidology by emphasizing socio-cultural factors, there emerged another strand of more radical social psychiatrists during the anti-psychiatry movement from the 1960s on. They attempted to further de-biologize – and existentialize – suicide.

The anti-psychiatry movement was especially vehement and long-lasting in Japan, as the Psychiatry Department of Tokyo University was occupied by left-wing students in 1968 and run under their management for the following decades. Most psychiatric societies remained paralysed well into the 1980s.[22] Since the movement had begun as a criticism of the use of lobotomy, biological reductionism of any sort was questioned, as was the case with suicide.

Some anti-psychiatrists began to argue that to dismiss the suicides of psychotic patients as the result of impulsively driven biological symptoms was not only to fail to recognize the existential nature of their attempt but to do further harm to their human dignity.[23] Following this line of thought, Takemura and Shimura conducted a survey of suicides among institutionalized psychiatric patients. They concluded that in a significant number of these cases (about one-third), there were 'comprehensible reasons' behind patients' suicidal acts.[24] Other psychiatrists, as they began to experiment with an open-ward policy, were asking how far their psychiatric jurisdiction should extend over the suicidal. In a 1973 symposium on the Mental Hygiene Law held by the Japanese Society of Psychiatry and Neurology, psychiatrists fiercely debated whether they should respect patients' free will even if their refusing psychiatric treatment might result in their suicide.[25] During this turbulent period, suicide of resolve became a symbolic label for psychiatrists with existentialist leanings who were committed to bringing agency back to patients by granting them the possibility of normalcy and intentionality in their suicide attempts.

Ironically, the existential, humanistic argument for suicide of resolve also exposed its contradictions when it came to be used to protect psychiatrists from being held legally responsible for patients' deaths. Amidst the move towards deinstitutionalization and rising consciousness about human rights, psychiatrists from the 1970s were increasingly facing lawsuits by the families of patients who had committed or attempted suicide in hospitals. In a highly controversial verdict, some psychotherapeutically oriented psychiatrists were acquitted of the charge of therapeutic negligence with the argument that the psychiatrists' humanistic care, as it promotes patients' autonomy and freedom, might well be incompatible with suicide prevention.[26] The existential perspective, by privileging individual intentionality and free will, downplayed patients' victimhood, reducing suicide of resolve to a convenient label for attributing the blame to individuals' 'free will.'

Perhaps intimidated by lawsuits and certainly by the rising public sentiment against psychiatric intrusion into private life, most psychiatrists during the 1980s remained reluctant to get involved in suicide prevention. At the same time, there began a series of attempts by social psychiatrists to help those active in the workers' movement to establish the social cause of mental illness on the job. An important decision was made by the Labour Standards Inspection Office in 1984 when a man who had attempted suicide received workers' compensation. Working against a strict deadline and given a diagnosis of 'neurosis or reactive depression,' this high-speed train designer threw himself in front of a train, only to be saved.[27] His depression was determined to have been caused by excessive work stress. The case marked a triumph for social psychiatrists in that it was the first time that workers' compensation had been awarded on the basis of reactive depression caused by work stress, but it failed to set a precedent. Subsequent similar claims for compensation for mentally ill workers were often dismissed both in court and by the bureaux of the Labour Standards Inspection Office. This was particularly the case when the workers in question had committed suicide, because the legal definition of suicide had been construed on the idea of free will. Suicide was judged to be by definition an intentional act of self-killing.[28] The rare cases in which workers' compensation was granted involved suicides that had evidently occurred as 'accidents' on the job. The deceased were judged to have been in such an acute psychotic state that they were driven to the suicidal act without fully comprehending its consequences.[29] Thus the Dentsû case (whose initial verdict came in 1996) was significant in the sense that not only was the blame for a worker's voluntary death attributed to the company but also a psychiatric diagnosis of depression had successfully been used to help to establish that suicide was not a 'private' problem but a 'social' one. Indeed, this understanding of suicide was incorporated into the Basic Law on Suicide Countermeasures in 2006.

Yet the use of psychiatry to establish the social cause of suicide was in no way a straightforward matter. As the principal attorney for the plaintiff in the Dentsû case later confessed in his book, when he initially turned to psychiatry to prove what seemed to him like a commonsensical idea – that excessive work stress can cause a mental breakdown and even suicide – this turned out to be a rather difficult argument to make.[30]

Psychiatry and the Social Cause of Suicide

In the epoch-defining Dentsû case, Ôshima Ichirô, a twenty-four-year-old employee, killed himself after working for a year and a half at Dentsû. Ichirô died after habitually working long hours, often staying all night in the office and going home in the morning, only to leave again after a few hours. According to the plaintiff, in the eight-month period leading up to his death, his work time averaged a little short of three hundred hours per month, meaning that he spent almost double the number of regular working hours in the office. Ichirô received positive evaluations from his bosses because of his high motivation, and his responsibility gradually increased. In his second year he began to show signs of despondency, lack of energy, and insomnia. He himself confessed to his boss that he felt a loss of confidence, but no serious measures were taken to decrease his workload. In the weeks prior to his death, Ichirô was spending even longer hours at work in preparation for a big summer public relations event, pulling all-nighters every three days. He was then making pessimistic statements such as 'I'm no use' and 'I'm no good as a human being.' On the way to the PR event, he exhibited strange behaviour such as weaving while driving and talking about a 'spirit' possessing him. Following the event, Ichirô left the site to head back to Tokyo, reaching home at 6:00 in the morning. He called in sick around 9:00 a.m. Within an hour, he had hanged himself in the bathroom.[31]

The defence initially claimed that Ichirô's death was intentional. Later the company's counsel came to accept that he may have been depressed but argued that it was endogenous depression, for which the company should not be held responsible. The basis of its argument was that Ichirô had what Japanese psychiatrists call a 'melancholic pre-morbid personality,' a distinctive and rather peculiar theory of depression that has long been influential in Japanese psychiatry. Thus the subsequent legal debates about the nature of Ichirô's suicide came to reflect the historical arguments in twentieth-century Japanese psychiatry about this theory of depression. In particular, the case revived discussions about whether depression was a product of individual biology or of society.

Originally, the concept of depression as an expression of personality had developed in the aftermath of the conceptual confusion surrounding neurasthenia as an illness of overwork. In the 1910s, as neurasthenia gradually became psychologized in the West, Japanese academic psychiatrists began to assert that neurasthenics who were victims of overwork were extremely rare and that most self-claiming neurasthenics merely suffered from an inherent personality weakness.[32] Just as neurasthenia was increasingly delegitimized in this way, another concept emerged as an illness of overwork *and* personality; this was the distinctive Japanese psychiatric concept of melancholic pre-morbid personality.

In the early 1930s Shimoda Mitsuzô, professor of psychiatry at Kyûshû Imperial University, noticed a group of patients seeking medical care for their neurasthenic symptoms, such as despondency and sleep disturbance, but who did not seem to recover even after a period of rest. Diagnosing them to be suffering from unipolar (presenile) depression, Shimoda emphasized that these patients were not feeble degenerates, as the Kraepelinian conception of the mentally ill might suggest, but rather socially adaptive people ('many from the upper class') who had developed depressive symptoms only later in their otherwise successful lives. Shimoda's group also noted that 20 per cent of their patients were doctors. Drawing upon the work of Ernest Kretschmer, who in 1921 proposed that manic-depressives have a constitution called cyclothymia, Shimoda argued that his own patients possessed what he called immodithymic personality (shûchaku kishitsu). He explained that patients with this personality had an 'abnormal emotional process,' in which an emotion would persist with intensity until the patients developed depression at the height of their exhaustion. Depression was thus a 'biological response for self-preservation.'[33] Shimoda suggested that this pathogenic personality was also what made these people successful in their work in the first place. 'People with this abnormal personality are enthusiastic about work, meticulous, thorough, honest, punctual, with a strong sense of justice, duty, and responsibility ... They are the kind of people who gain the trust of others by being reliable, who are praised as model youths, model employees, and model officers.'[34]

Shimoda's theory was largely ignored in the pre-war era, but it was rediscovered and further developed from the 1950s, particularly after the advent of antidepressants.[35] At the time, psychiatrists were beginning to treat a much wider range of depressed patients in the community and finding that many of them were in fact 'diligent, serious, meticulous, and responsible,' as Shimoda had described them.[36] Since then, this theory has become standard textbook knowledge in Japanese psychiatry and has continued to be aired on and off in the media, long after similar personality theories such as Type A personality in the United States lost their scientific credibility.[37] Particularly from the late 1990s, the theory of melancholic pre-morbid personality has again been disseminated in psychiatric and pharmaceutical campaigns for antidepressants, while few Japanese – including many clinicians – seem to recognize that this is hardly universal scientific knowledge outside Japan. As the theory became widespread, however, two opposing, yet complementary, interpretations emerged as to what was the true cause for this depression-prone personality.

These two interpretations stem from different psychiatric understandings of 'personality.' The first was based on the traditional psychiatric idea of personality as genetically determined *constitution*. As Shimoda himself envisioned his theory to account for why some people, placed in similar situations, seem more vulnerable to depression than others, psychiatrists began to use patients' personality as the marker for endogenous depression (with a strong genetic basis), to be differentiated from reactive depression (predominantly caused by social factors). The second interpretation of personality emerged in the mid-1960s as depression experts were beginning to realize that antidepressants – treatment according to the biologically oriented view – alone did not seem to cure depression. Psychotherapeutically oriented psychiatrists were then asking why they were seeing so many depressed men, particularly among those who would usually be regarded as ideal normative workers.[38] Reflecting on Shimoda's famous dictum that the depressed are 'model employees,' they began to argue that melancholic personality is not simply a matter of constitution but rather a kind of social personality, even a specific *historical* product of the Japanese work ethic.

This social theme was further developed during a series of workshops on manic depression held at the height of the anti-psychiatry movement. Tracing the historical rise of melancholic pre-morbid personality, the participants explored how Japanese society came to reproduce and reward melancholic types, with their self-sacrificing devotion to the collective, such that they begin to take their responsibility too much to heart.[39] Others noted how the rise of industrialization and the nuclearization of families caused alienation in melancholics, whose strong desire for a sense of belonging made them particularly vulnerable to depression.[40] For these psychiatrists, conceptualizing depression only at the level of individual biology missed the point. The alarming depression rate required that psychiatry – and Japanese society as a whole – start thinking about depression in social terms.[41]

These dual – biological and social – interpretive traditions were played out against each other in the legal disputes during the Dentsû case. At the Tokyo District Court the dispute focused on establishing the amount of overwork that Ichirô had endured, as the official record itself did not show the actual hours. Underreporting work hours is a routine practice in Japanese workplaces and is referred to as 'service overwork.' Once the facts about the overwhelming number of hours of overwork were established, the court granted, without too much conceptual debate, the verdict of 'fatigue depression.'[42] However, in the subsequent proceeding at the Tokyo High Court, the defendant aggressively rebutted the plaintiff by questioning the exact nature of Ichirô's 'depression.' The defence argued his melancholic pre-morbid personality had caused an excessive sense of responsibility and created the condition of chronic overwork, for which the company should not be held responsible. The Tokyo High Court partially accepted this argument and introduced comparative negligence by reducing the amount of compensation by 30 per cent. The 1997 verdict stated:

> Not everyone becomes depressed from being overworked or being in a stressful situation. The individual constitution and personality are also factors involved in causing depression. Ichirô was serious, responsible, thorough, and a perfectionist; he had the tendency to voluntarily take up a task and responsibility for it beyond his capacity. It cannot be denied that his so-called melancholic pre-morbid personality resulted in increasing the amount of his own work, leading to delays and inappropriate methods of managing the work, and creating situations where he worried about the outcome of tasks that were beyond his control.[43]

In the final round of disputes at the Supreme Court, what helped bring about all-out victory for the plaintiff was the social interpretation of depression. The plaintiff succeeded in portraying Ichirô's depression as a not merely a result of his constitution but as an embodiment of the pathology of the Japanese workplace itself, emphasizing how Ichirô came to be so bound, both physically and *psychologically*, by company life that he could no longer think outside it.[44] The judges concluded that he had committed suicide impulsively and accidentally, under the pathological influence of depression. Reflecting the psychiatric, existential framing of fatigue depression, the verdict even ventured to explain the psychological state of mind that Ichirô was in right before his death. It stated: 'Having completed the work [for the summer event], he came to be in a psychological state in which he felt the weight lifted from his shoulders. But at the same time, he came to feel empty that he would continue to face the same kind of long working hours as before, and under a deepening depression, committed suicide impulsively and accidentally.'[45]

The Dentsû case overturned the long-held legal assumption about suicide as an act of free will and instead established its social causality by way of a psychiatric argument of depression. Ironically, perhaps, the term 'suicide of resolve' was now used in the context of a legal discourse to indicate merely individual responsibility, stripped of the culturally evocative meaning of the social, existential angst behind such an act.

Policy Changes and the Impact on Psychiatry

While these overwork-suicide litigations have enlarged a space for medicalizing suicide, they have also served to destabilize – even discredit – traditional Japanese psychiatric knowledge. In response to these verdicts – and no doubt to psychiatry's conceptual confusion, which became apparent during the Dentsû proceedings – the Ministry of Labour introduced drastic changes in its mental health policies. It abolished the traditional psychiatric diagnoses from its criteria for determining workers' compensation, replacing them with ICD-10 criteria, which have served to significantly broaden the notion of 'mental illness.'[46] In so doing, the ministry abandoned the traditional psychiatric assumption about endogeneity, challenging ideas that there exists a qualitative (and not just quantitative) difference between the normal and the abnormal and that some mental illnesses, such as schizophrenia and manic depression, are genetically determined. Instead, the ministry introduced the 'stress-diathesis model' of mental illness, thereby conceptualizing psychopathology clearly as a product of interactions between individual biology and society. Though such conceptual changes had been gradually taking place within Japanese psychiatry, especially after the advent of the DSM-III in 1980, the ministry's decisions nonetheless astonished Japanese psychiatrists, as they opened up possibilities for almost all forms of psychopathology to be legally examined in terms of social causes.

The ministry had turned social stress into something quantifiable. In order to examine how much psychological stress the worker was exposed to in a particular work environment, the ministry created the Stress Evaluation Table.[47] This table consists of thirty-one items for both work- and non-work-related stressful events. These potentially stressful events, such as trouble with a client, a change of boss, promotion as well as a death in the family, divorce, even a child's school-entrance examination, are each given a predetermined number of points. Experts can simply extract stressful events from a worker's record, add up the points, and see which stress – either at work or at home – was the greater contributing factor to the worker's mental breakdown and/or suicide. If it is then determined that work stress outweighed that of home and that the worker suffered a mental illness and/or suicide as a consequence, then the case is approved for workers' compensation. By predetermining these points, the ministry emphasized that stress evaluation has to be *objective*: that is to say, examiners should not base their judgment on how the particular worker *subjectively* responded to the event but determine *objectively* how the same event would be experienced by any average worker. This process is meant to avoid the multiple and often competing interpretations that psychiatrists tend to make and to speed up the diagnostic process by *standardizing* how to measure stress.

However, the juridical world immediately challenged this standardization of human suffering. In 2001, in another landmark case, this time involving a Toyota employee who had killed himself, judges accepted an even broader range of social causes for suicide. In this case the worker, who had committed suicide at the age of thirty-five, was, by all accounts, an ideal 'Toyota man' – hard-working, serious, yet cheerful. He maintained good relationships with everyone while exhibiting strong leadership. Under Toyota's 'Just-in-Time System,' where a delay in one section could halt the whole production process, he was working with strict deadlines. While he normally thrived on challenges, he became increasingly distressed when the number of subordinates he had to oversee quickly doubled. He had to draw up a plan that he knew would be hard to meet. At this time, he received additional orders to go on an overseas business trip and to serve as the chairperson of the labour union. His wife noticed that he began to wake up suddenly in the middle of the night to jot down ideas for work. The night before his death, he came home and told his wife that he could no longer 'keep up with the Toyota way' and confessed that he had gone up to the company rooftop that day to jump off, only stopping himself when his children's faces came to mind. That night, as his wife saw him bathing with their one-month-old daughter and weeping quietly in the tub, she made him promise to see a doctor the following morning. He left home before dawn and threw himself to his death from a nearby building.[48]

In the Toyota case the corporate – and the governmental – assertion of 'objective stress' became the focus of debate. The defence argued that it was a suicide of resolve, as his workload was no heavier than that of his peers. In fact, because the company was implementing a new policy for reducing overwork at the time, the worker's time sheets did not show excessively long hours of overwork (though disputes remained as to the actual hours of 'service overtime'). The plaintiff instead emphasized how work intensified under the company's new policy and that it was not the quantity but rather the *quality* of work that should be considered. The judges accepted that what mattered was not how each stress was 'objectively' scored, as in the Stress Evaluation Table, but how the worker subjectively experienced the stress. Furthermore, in response to the defence's argument that the worker's alleged depression was caused by his own vulnerability (i.e., 'melancholic pre-morbid personality'), the verdict at the Nagoya District Court stated that the work conditions should be set to accommodate, not the 'average' worker, as the ministry's guidelines state, but rather those who are 'most vulnerable to stress' as long as their personalities remain within an acceptable range found among workers doing the same kind of jobs. In arguing for this radically 'subjective' approach, the judges stated that the causal mechanism of depression was yet to be scientifically proven and that the government's guidelines – and, by implication, psychiatrists – fell short of providing a clear and sufficient standard for 'objectively' diagnosing mental illness at work.[49]

The Ministry of Health, Welfare, and Labour reacted strongly against this verdict, and psychiatrists have had to confront the uncertainty of their own professional knowledge. As is often the case when psychiatrists become involved in legal disputes, the psychiatric diagnoses became sharply polarized. Some psychiatrists I interviewed lamented that their own profession may have sacrificed scientific rigour in order to demand social justice and, to quote one expert, 'retreated to the realm of storytelling.' As this expert put it, the diagnosis of overwork suicide risks becoming a process in which they already have a conclusion. Then they are left to piece together the information and build up a case to establish either the genetic story or a social story. They know that they have little on which to go in terms of 'hard science' in making either argument. They are thus all the more confounded by how the ongoing medicalization, spurred on by a workers' movement, has served to open up the aetiology of depression and suicide to legal, public decisions beyond the control of psychiatrists themselves. The debates have created highly *moral*, rather than *scientific*, arguments about the nature of workers' psychiatric suffering.

Psychiatrists have had to ask themselves how far they are willing to go with the argument that mental illness and suicide are socially produced. Many psychiatrists I interviewed seemed to find some justice in demanding corporate responsibility for depressed workers' suicides by using a psychiatric argument, as they regard the depressed as typically hard-working men victimized by the inhumane conditions of Japanese workplaces. Yet psychiatrists have appeared far more ambivalent when they have been asked to determine if workers' schizophrenia, or even personality disorder, has been caused by overwork.[50] Few psychiatrists would believe in a simple model of direct cause and effect between work stress and psychopathology, as they have been trained to pay close attention to individual differences and individuals' specific vulnerabilities. Yet on the question of how to conceptualize individual vulnerability, they are far from having a satisfactory model beyond often crude genetic determinism that is sometimes coupled with the notion of melancholic pre-morbid personality. In trying to determine who are the vulnerable, what causes such vulnerability, and who should be held responsible for it, psychiatrists are made to confront their own scientific, as well as moral, orderings of the mentally ill, which are implicitly built into their diagnostic system.[51] This conceptual tension was exemplified in an unforgettable scene I encountered in 2004 at an international conference on depression in Japan. After a series of typical talks on depression by Japanese psychiatrists emphasizing how hard-working salarymen are often the victims of depression, a French psychiatrist stood up and asked with a dramatic gesture, 'Can a homeless person become depressed in Japan?' Despite the laughter that followed, his comment effectively drew out the implicit morality embedded in the Japanese psychiatric representation of depression, where certain kinds of suffering – by certain *kinds* of people – may have been more readily recognized and legitimized.

Questioning the Suicide of Resolve

MacDonald and Murphy argue that the medicalization of suicide in early modern England occurred, not as a process of top-down domination by medical experts, but rather as a complex interplay of various actors who promoted medicalization for different reasons.[52] A similar process seems to be at work today in Japan, where psychiatrists are becoming implicated in the bottom-up medicalization of suicide as part of a social movement that seeks to legitimize workers' suffering by way of a psychiatric diagnosis. Through this process, psychiatrists, some of whom hold a deep-seated ambivalence about such medicalization, are succeeding in finally overcoming the long-held Japanese resistance to psychiatry and undermining the manner in which suicide has been culturally sanctioned as an act of free will. This change is clearly reflected in the Ministry of Labour's 1999 guidelines, which state that the kinds of suicides that would have been previously regarded as 'suicides of resolve' can now be examined as potentially resulting from psychopathology. An illuminating example from the guidelines, one much emphasized by media commentators, is that of a hypothetical case in which a worker commits suicide after leaving a suicide note. In the context of granting workers' compensation in years past, this would automatically have been assumed to be a sign of intentionality and thus make the case ineligible for workers' compensation; today, however, even cases such as this are open to psychiatric scrutiny. Also, as the guidelines have significantly expanded the notion of mental illness to include milder forms of depression, a worker who appeared on the surface to be acting normally can now be regarded as potential victim of psychopathology. The psychiatric argument has thus dismantled the rigid and rather 'archaic' assumption about free will embedded in the legal definition of suicide[53] and highlighted the idea that those who kill themselves from work stress are not agents of their own deaths but rather *victims*, and that society has to take responsibility for their deaths.

While this development signals an important shift in the discourse about suicide in Japan, whether it will also bring about a conceptual transformation in the way ordinary Japanese privately think about what constitutes normality and agency in the act of killing oneself is open to question. Despite the previous resistance to medicalization, there seems to have been little debate about the serious implications of accepting the psychiatric framing of suicide as a manifestation of psychopathology. This may be because a certain level of ambiguity and duality remains in talking about suicide as pathologically driven. A quick glance at the testimonies of the families who have sued companies to hold them responsible for the suicides of their loved ones attests to the implicit duality. They talk about the deceased as having been so ill that they were unable to understand what they were doing, while suggesting at the same time that their loved ones had been 'making a protest' against the companies that had done them an injustice.[54] Such accounts also indicate the possibility that these families see their loved ones as having performed a meaningful social act with a certain degree of intentionality. This interpretation raises questions about the extent to which people 'truly believe' the psychiatric explanation, as opposed to using it as a means of getting public recognition for suicidal individuals' suffering.

While psychiatrists remain largely silent about these contradictions, there are two key possibilities for the future of the medicalization of suicide in Japan. On the one hand, the 'socializing' form of medicalization may well be part of a transitional period before a move towards the re-biologization of suicide sets in. There are already signs of this pattern. With Japan's gradual economic recovery, suicide today is being talked about less as explicitly linked to the specific historical conditions of economic depression and more in terms of individual clinical depression, which itself is increasingly portrayed as an isolated biological state. This shift is being accelerated by the global medicalization and pharmaceuticalization of depression, even though the new nexus of 'depression-suicide' is what helped to create the unusual liaison whereby social and biological psychiatrists have come together in challenging the cultural notion of suicide. With the increasingly aggressive campaign by the pharmaceutical industry to promote a much broader notion of depression, psychiatrists have far more incentive than ever to explain suicide in terms of depression and to treat the suicidal by biological means. Some in the government have already been discussing the possibility of introducing routine mental health examinations at workplaces with the aim of screening out the potentially 'vulnerable.' There thus is a possibility that such medicalization will create attempts to establish a more thorough biological management of suicide in the future.

On the other hand, while psychiatry is transforming the cultural notion of suicide in Japan, it may be that Japanese psychiatry itself is being transformed via the discourse on overwork suicide to bring about a more flexible, dynamic understanding of suicide. The Supreme Court decision in the Dentsû case and many subsequent legal disputes about overwork suicide have depicted suicide and depression, not as manifestations of stark insanity, but as a state between normality and abnormality. The overwork suicide discourse has thus 'normalized' depression in a significant departure from the genetic determinism of the past and the popularly held assumptions about the biological deficiencies of the mentally ill. Coupled with the global rise of depression discourse, the psychiatric discourse about overwork suicide may thus be indicative of a more fundamental conceptual shift that Japanese psychiatry has been going through, as it tries to overcome its rigid dichotomy between biological and social approaches to diagnosis and treatment and move towards a more complex, nuanced understanding of how people are driven to take their own lives.

NOTES

I would like to thank Professors Margaret Lock, Allan Young, Katô Satoshi, Takahashi Yoshitomo, Suzuki Akihito, and Chris Oliver for their inspiring comments. The dissertation research on which this chapter is based was generously funded by McGill University, the Wenner-Gren Foundation for Anthropological Research (Grant no. 6682), and the Japan Foundation.

1 'Suicide,' *Encyclopedia Britannica*, 11th ed. (1910–1911), 50; written by Henry Harvey Littlejohn, professor of forensic medicine at the University of Edinburgh.
2 Maurice Pinguet, *Voluntary Death in Japan*, translated by Rosemary Morris (Cambridge: Polity Press, 1993); Takahashi Yoshitomo, 'Jisatsu Keikô [Suicidal Tendencies],' *Rinshô Seishin Igaku* [Journal of Clinical Psychiatry] 23, no. 1 (1994).
3 Japanese names are written in the order of family name followed by given name.
4 The term was coined by lawyer Kawahito; see Kawahito Hiroshi, *Karô Jisatsu* [Overwork Suicide].(Tokyo: Iwanami Shoten, 1998). A Japanese suicide expert pointed out to me that overwork suicide accounts for only a small segment of the total suicides in Japan. Nevertheless, it has been disproportionately represented in the media and has played an important

role, symbolically and politically, in changing the way Japanese deal with suicide.

5 Hereafter referred to as Ichirô. It is customary in such legal documents to use the first name so as to avoid confusion with other family members with the same last name.

6 Émile Durkheim, *Le suicide* (Paris: Alcan, 1897); translated by J.A. Spaulding and G. Simpson as *Suicide: A Study in Sociology*. (London: Routledge & Kegan Paul, 1952).

7 Ivan Illich, *Medical Memesis: the Expropriation of Health* (London: Calder & Boyars, 1975); Irving K. Zola, 'Medicine as an Institution of Social Control' *Sociological Review* 20, no. 4 (1972).

8 Allan Young, *The Harmony of Illusions: Inventing Post-Traumatic Stress Disorder* (Princeton: Princeton University Press, 1995).

9 For this purpose, I conducted archival research using the *Japanese Journal of Psychiatry and Neurology* from its first issue in 1902 to the present and examining a few popular journals and a number of newspapers from the 1870s to the 2000s. I also conducted anthropological fieldwork around Tokyo for two years, interviewing numerous depression and suicide experts, joining a closed seminar on overwork suicide with psychiatrists and lawyers, and sitting in on an overwork suicide legal proceeding at the Tokyo District Court.

10 See Kitanaka Junko, '"Shinkei Suijaku" Seisuishi: "Karô no Yamai" wa ikani "Jinkaku no Yamai" eto Stigumaka saretaka [The Rise and Fall of Neurasthenia: How the "Illness of Overwork" Became Stigmatized as the "Illness of Personality" in Japan],' *Eureka*, May 2004.

11 XYZ, 'Shinkeisuijakushô: Sôjûshi, Bunshi, Kanri, Gakusei Shokun no Ichidoku o Yôsu [Neurasthenia: Operators, Writers, Government Officials, and Students, Read This],' *Taiyô* 8, no. 7 (1902).

12 Natsume Sôseki, *Sôseki Bunmeiron Shû* [Sôseki's Ideas on Civilization] (Tokyo: Iwanami Shoten, 1986).

13 Ironically, Okuma, as he discussed later in this speech, had a brother who suffered from mental illness; the fact that even the family of the mentally ill came to speak of them in such a disparaging tone shows the extent to which the degeneration paradigm permeated the intellectuals' ways of thinking at the time. See Ôkuma Shigenobu, 'Seishinbyô ni Taisuru Zakkan [Impressions on Mental Illness],' *Shinkeigaku Zasshi* (Journal of Neurology) 4, no. 12 (1906): 616.

14 On these debates, see Tsubouchi Shôyô, 'Jisatsu Zehi [Pros and Cons of Suicide],' *Taiyô* 9, no. 9 (1903).

15 Katayama Kunika, 'Jisatsu to Shakai [Suicide and Society],' *Tokyo Asahi*

Shimbun, 22 October 1907; 'Jisatsu no hôigakuteki yobôhô [Prevention of Suicide from the Perspective of Forensic Medicine],' *Shinkeigaku Zasshi* 10 (1911).

16 Kure Shûzô, 'Jôshi Kenkyû: Shôgi ni Shinjû no Ooi Riyû [Study on the Love Pact: the Reason Why So Many Prostitutes Commit Dual Suicide],' *Yomiuri Shimbun*, 19 July 1917.

17 Ihara Shigehiko, 'Ichijisatsurei no Kôsatsu [A Case of Suicide],' *Seishin Shinkeigaku Zasshi* (Journal of Psychiatry and Neurology) 29, no. 6 (1928): 549.

18 Nakamura Ryûji, 'Jisatsu to Seishinbyôri [Suicide and Psychopathology],' *Seishin Shinkeigaku Zasshi* 44, no. 7 (1940): 484.

19 Komine Shigeyuki, 'Oyako Shinjû no Seiin ni tsuite no Kôsatsu [On the Causes of Parent-Child Suicides],' *Seishin Shinkeigaku Zasshi* 42, no. 3 (1938).

20 Nakamura, 'Jisatsu,' 484.

21 Katô Masaaki, *Jisatsu* [Suicide] (Tokyo: Misuzu Shobô, 1954); Ôhara Kenshirô, *Nihon no Jisatsu* [Suicide in Japan] (Tokyo: Seishin Shobô, 1965).

22 Akimoto Haruo, *Seishin Igaku to Han Seishin Igaku* [Psychiatry and Antipsychiatry] (Tokyo: Kongô Shuppan, 1976); David Healy, *The Creation of Psychopharmacology* (Cambridge: Harvard University Press, 2002).

23 Katô Masaaki, Moriyama Kimio, et al., 'Jisatsugaku ni Tsuite [Suicidology],' *Seishin Igaku* [Clinical Psychiatry],' 12, no. 10 (1970).

24 Takemura Kenji and Shimura Hiroshi, 'Kaihô Ryôhô no Jissen no Moto De Okita Jisatsu no Keiken [Experience of Suicide Cases That Occurred under Open-Ward Therapy],' in *Seishin Byôin ni Okeru Jisatsu* [Suicides in Mental Hospitals], ed. Seishin Byôin Kyôkai [Association of Mental Hospitals] (Tokyo: Makino Shuppan, 1977; *Jisatsu no Sain* [Signs of Suicide] (Osaka: Shinryô Shinsha, 1987).

25 Kanazawa Akira et al., 'Seishin Eiseihô [Mental Hygiene Law],' *Seishin Shinkeigaku Zasshi* 76. no. 12 (1974): 830.

26 Okada Yasuo, 'Seishinka Kanja no Jisatsu Jiken: I no tachiba kara [Suicide Cases of Psychiatric Patients: From a Medical Perspective],' *Jurist Suppl.* (1989), 91; Nishizono Masahisa, 'Seishin Ryôhô,' *Seishinka Mook* 13 (1986).

27 Kaneko Tsuguo, 'Rôsai Nintei o uketa Jisatsurei [Cases of Suicide That Have Been Granted Workers' Compensation],' *Shakai Seishin Igaku* [Social Psychiatry] 13, no. 4 (1990).

28 Okamura Chikanobu, *Karôshi Karôjisatsu Kyûsai no Riron to Jitsumu* [Theory and Practice of Providing Relief to Overwork Death and Overwork Suicide] (Tokyo: Junpôsha, 2002).

29 Kuroki Nobuo, 'Jisatsu to Seishin Shikkan ni Kansuru Rôsai Hoshô no

Dôkô [Recent Trends in Work-Related Compensation Involving Job-Related Suicide and Mental Disease],' *Seishin Shinkeigaku Zasshi* 104, no. 12 (2002).

30 Fujimoto Tadashi, *'Jisatsu Karôshi' Saiban 24 Sai Natsu Adoman no Ket-subetsu* ['Overwork Suicide' Lawsuit: 24-Year-Old Advertisement Man's Departure] (Tokyo: Daiamond Sha, 1996).

31 Kawahito, *Karô Jisatsu*, 19–28.

32 Uematsu Shichikurô, 'Toshi Seikatsu to Shinkeisuijaku [Urban Life and Neurasthenia],' in *Sankôkanhô Seishin Eisei Tenrankai Gô* [News on Mental Hygiene Exhibition], ed. Nihon Sekijûji Sha (Japan Red Cross) (Tokyo: Nihon Sekijûji Sha, 1929).

33 Shimoda Mitsuzô, *Seishin Eisei Kôwa* [Lectures on Mental Hygiene] (Tokyo: Iwanami Shoten, 1942); also see Naka Shûzô, 'Shorôki Utsuyûshô [Senile Depression],' *Shikeigaku Zasshi* 34, no. 6 (1932).

34 Shimoda Mitsuzô, 'Sôutsubyô ni Tsuite [On Manic Depression],' *Yonago Igaku Zasshi* [Yonago Medical Journal] 2, no. 1 (1950): 3.

35 Shinfuku Naotake, 'Rôjin no Seishinbyôri [Psychopathology of the Elderly],' *Seishin Shinkeigaku Zasshi* [Journal of Psychiatry and Neurology] 57, no. 4 (1955); Kasahara Yomishi, 'Utsubyô no Byôzen Seikaku ni Tsuite [On Pre-morbid Personality of Depression],' in *Sôutsubyô no Seishin Byôri I* [Psychopathology of Depression I], ed. Yomishi Kasahara (Tokyo: Kôbundô, 1976).

36 Hirasawa Hajime, *Keishô Utsubyô no Rinshô to Yogo* [Clinical Practice and Prognosis of Mild Depression] (Tokyo: Igaku Shoin, 1966); Shimazaki Toshiki and Taeko Yazaki, Review of Hubert Tellenbach, *Melancholie*, *Seishin Igaku* 5, no. 1 (1963). These psychiatrists illuminated the similarities between Shimoda's personality concept and Tellenbach's notion of 'typus melancholicus,' in *Melancholy: History of the Problem, Endogeneity, Typology, Pathogenesis, Clinical Considerations* (1961; Pittsburgh: Duquesne University Press, 1980).

37 Shiba Shintaro, *Nihonjin to Iu Utsubyô* [Depression Called 'Japanese'] (Kyoto: Jinbun Shoin, 1999).

38 Doi Takeo, 'Utsubyô no Seishin Rikigaku [Psychodynamics of Depression],' *Seishin Igaku* 8, no. 12 (1966); Iida Shin, ed., 'Sôutsubyô,' *Gendai no Esprit* 88 (1974).

39 Nakai Hisao, 'Saiken no Rinri to Shite no Kinben to Kufû [Industriousness and Ingenuity as the Ethics of Reconstruction],' in *Sôutsubyô no Seishinbyôri I* [Psychopathology of Manic Depression], ed. Yomishi Kasahara (Tokyo: Kôbundô, 1976).

40 Iida Shin,' Sôutsubyô no Jôkyôron to Kongo no Kadai [Situational Cause of Depression and New Issues],' *Seishin Shinkeigaku Zasshi* 75 (1973).

41 This emerging discourse about depression as a product of the Japanese work ethic may also have prepared a suitable 'narrative' for the rising profession of occupational psychiatrists, many of whom were beginning to practise within corporations and for whom work seemed to be a central cause underlying their patients' depression.

42 This diagnosis was submitted by Dr Kaneko Tsuguo, then director of the prestigious Matsuzawa Hospital, who had a social leaning and had also introduced Ivan Illich's *Limits to Medicine* in 1979.

43 Tokyo Kôsai (Tokyo High Court), 1997, Songai Baishô Seikyû Kôso Jiken (Appeal for Compensation For Damage), 1647.

44 The Supreme Court criticized the previous verdict by stating that using individual personality, when it remains within the normal range, for comparative negligence is an incorrect interpretation of the law.

45 Saikôsaibansho (Supreme Court), 2000; Songai Baishô Seikyû Jiken, 1647.

46 Katô Satoshi, 'Gendai Nihon ni okeru Utsubyô no Jisatsu to Sono Yobô [Suicide Caused by Depression and Its Prevention in Contemporary Japan],' *Seishin Shinkeigaku Zasshi* 107, no. 10 (2005).

47 Rôdôshô (Ministry of Labour), *Shinriteki Fuka ni yoru Seishin Shôgaitô ni Kakawaru Gyômujôgai no Handan Shishin ni tsuite* [Standards for Determining Work-Related Mental Disorders Caused by Psychological Stress], 14 September 1999.

48 Asahi Shimbun, 'Shokuba no "Jakusha" ni Hikari, Karô Jisatsu ni Rôsai Nintei Hanketsu [Light on the "Weak" in Workplaces: Workers' Compensation Granted in Overwork Suicide Lawsuit],' 18 June 2001; also see the Nagoya Chihô Saibansho (Nagoya District Court)'s verdict issued on 18 June 2001 (no. 814).

49 Watanabe Kinuko, 'Karô Jisatsu no Gyômu Kiinsei [Work as the Cause for Overwork Suicide],' *Jurist* no. 1223 (1 June 2002): 102–5.

50 Nomura Yoshihiro, Naoki Kinomoto, Takaharu Hiranuma, Masahiko Sugita, Nobuo Kuroki, Masaharu Katô, Fumio Itô, Yasuji Kodama, and Yôkichi Ôno, 'Karôshi to Kigyô no Songai Biashô Sekinin: Dentsû Karôshi Jisatsu Jiken [Overwork Death and Corporate Liability: Dentsû Overwork Suicide Case],' *Baishô Kagaku* (Journal of Compensation Science), no. 30 (2003).

51 Kuroki Nobuo, 'Kigyô ni Okeru Jisatsu to Rôsai Hoshô [Suicide in Workplace and Worker's Compensation],' *Nihon Shokugyô Saigai Igaku Kaishi* [Japanese Journal of Traumatology and Occupational Medicine] 48, no. 3

(2000): 227–33; Kashimi Yumiko, 'Minpô 7: Chôjikan Zangyô ni Yoru Karô Jisatsu to Shiyôsha Sekinin [Civil Law 7: Overwork Suicide From Long Hours of Overtime and Employer's Responsibility],' *Jurist* no. 1202, (10 June 2001).

52 Michael MacDonald and Terence R. Murphy, *Sleepless Souls: Suicide in Early Modern England* (Oxford and New York: Oxford University Press, 1990).

53 Okamura, *Karôshi*, 399.

54 Kawahito, *Karô Jisatsu*, 26; Kawahito Hiroshi, *Karôshi to Kigyô no Sekinin* [Overwork Death and Corporate Responsibilities] (Tokyo: Shakai Shisôsha, 1996; Kamata Satoshi, *Kazoku ga Jisatsu ni Oikomarerutoki* [When a Family Member Is Driven to Suicide] (Tokyo: Kôdansha 1999); Shinbun Akahata Kokumin Undôbu (Akahata Newspaper), *Shigoto ga Owaranai Kokuhatsu Karôshi* [I Cannot Finish Work: Overwork Death] (Tokyo: Shin Nihon Shuppan, 2003).

12 Twentieth-Century Trends in Homicide Followed by Suicide in Four North American Cities

ROSEMARY GARTNER AND BILL MCCARTHY

Shortly after 7 a.m. on 1 December 2004 Toronto police received a telephone call from forty-seven-year-old Brian Langer that sent them rushing to the home he shared with his twenty-seven-year-old wife, Andrea Labbe, and their three children. Dozens of firefighters, paramedics, and police officers converged on the house, where they found Labbe's slashed, bloodied, and lifeless body in the dining room. Langer lay in an upstairs bedroom, unconscious from stab wounds to the stomach. Their daughters – Zoe, age three, and Brigitte, two – were in another bedroom also suffering from stab wounds. Only seven-month-old Margot escaped injury; she was found unharmed, crying in her crib. News reports contrasted the horrific scene, including blood splattered walls and other evidence of a frenzied attack, with the picture painted by neighbors, relatives, and friends of a happy, loving family. That afternoon Brian Langer and Zoe died in hospital from their wounds, while investigators tried to reconstruct the events that had led to their and Labbe's deaths. By the end of the day, police announced they were not looking for any suspects, and they characterized the killings as a multiple murder-suicide arising from a domestic dispute.

Those who study homicide use the term 'familicide' to describe events such as these; that is, cases in which a person slays a spouse and one or more of their children.[1] Familicides are relatively rare, but within this class of events, cases that include the perpetrator's suicide are common. For example, in about half of all familicides in Canada and England between the mid-1970s and 1990, the killer committed suicide.[2] The Langer-Labbe case is distinctive among familicides, not because the killer committed suicide, but because the killer was a woman. Forensic evidence indicated that Andrea Labbe fatally wounded her husband and her oldest daughter and seriously injured another daughter, before killing herself. Although highly unusual in the statistical sense, this case exemplifies other common characteristics of homicide-suicides, such as the nature of the relationships between the killers and their victims.

In this chapter we analyse the characteristics of homicides followed by suicide to examine a set of issues raised in the literature on these deaths. In particular, we explore the relationship between trends in homicide-suicide and its component behaviours, homicide and suicide. The data we use to address these issues span the period 1900 through 1990 and are drawn from four cities, two in Canada (Toronto and Vancouver) and two in the United States (Buffalo and Seattle). Over nine decades of data from four urban areas in two countries enhance the generalizability of our findings, relative to studies of homicide-suicide that rely on smaller numbers of cases, more limited time periods, or single jurisdictions.

In our first set of analyses we combine the data from these cities largely because the number of homicide-suicides in each city is relatively small. We compare key characteristics of our cases of homicide-suicide with those from other research to increase our confidence that the patterns we observe are not idiosyncratic. We then turn to an analysis of city-specific as well as city-aggregated data to compare trends in homicide-suicide with the separate trends for homicide and suicide. In that analysis we examine whether our data follow commonly observed patterns in the epidemiology of homicide-suicide. In our final analysis we investigate whether the types of victim-offender relationships that characterize homicide-suicides have remained stable or have changed over time.

Characteristics of Homicide-Suicide in Four Cities, 1900–90

Our data on homicide-suicide are from our larger study of patterns in homicide over the twentieth century. Drawing from police, coroners', and medical examiners' records, newspapers, and jail and court records, we have compiled information and case narratives on 7,582 homicides in Buffalo, Seattle, Toronto, and Vancouver between 1900 and 1990.[3] For these homicides, we have information on 6,184 persons identified by the authorities as the primary offenders.[4] Of these, 451, or 7 per cent, were known to have committed suicide within the first day or two after the killing and before they were in custody; the vast majority of them did so at the scene of the crime. The percentage of killers who committed suicide in these four cities is similar to that observed in other studies of homicide-suicide in urban areas in Canada and the United States during the twentieth century.[5] These 451 offenders killed 552 victims. Averaged over time and across cities and based on the population aged fifteen and older, the annual rate of homicide-suicide was .36 per 100,000 population, compared to an overall average annual homicide rate of 4.9 per 100,000 population.

Among the most well-established findings in the literature on homicide-suicide are the predominance of male offenders and of female victims.[6] The former is not surprising, since males are overrepresented both among homicide offenders and among victims of suicide. The sex distribution of homicide-suicide offenders in the four cities we study mirrors previous research. Approximately 88 per cent (395) of the 451 homicide-suicide offenders were males; 12 per cent (56) were females.[7] Moreover, the sex distribution of homicide-suicide offenders is not distinctive from the sex distribution of other homicide offenders in these four cities: 87 per cent of offenders who did not commit suicide were male.

Consistent with previous research, the sex distribution of victims of homicide-suicide in these four cities differs dramatically from that of other homicides: females are overrepresented among victims of homicide-suicide (72 per cent), whereas male victims predominate in other killings (73 per cent). Thus, while the sex distributions of homicide offenders and homicide-suicide offenders are almost identical, the sex distributions of homicide victims and homicide-suicide victims are quite different.

According to our and others' data, the overrepresentation of females among victims of homicide-suicide reflects the much greater number of male homicide-suicide offenders and the nature of the relationships between these offenders and their victims. When men commit homicide-suicide, their victims are usually their intimate female partners.[8] In these four cities, 61 per cent of the homicide-suicides by males targeted only the offender's intimate partner, and in another 8 per cent of cases the offender killed his intimate partner and another person (table 12.1).[9] Kent Stow, twenty-four years old and a scion of one of Buffalo's wealthiest families, was such an offender. He had been forced to resign from an executive position with the Lackawanna Steel Plant in 1902 because of 'melancholia' linked to a physical illness. He, his twenty-year-old wife, and their six-month-old baby lived with his parents,

Table 12.1
Relationships between male and female homicide-suicide offenders and their victims in Buffalo, Seattle, Toronto, and Vancouver, 1900–90

Offender's relationship to victim	Male offenders (total N=395)[1]	Female offenders (total N=56)
Intimate partner	239 (61%)	11 (20%)
Intimate partner and parent, or familicide	23 (6%)	2 (3%)
Intimate partner and other[2]	9 (2%)	–
Parent	26 (7%)	36 (68%)
Other kin	14 (3%)	–
Unrelated victim	83[3] (21%)	4[4] (7%)

1 In one case of male-perpetrated homicide-suicide, information on the relationship between the victim and offender was missing.
2 The other victims in these cases included parents, other kin, or lovers of the killers' intimate partners.
3 As noted in the text, 30 of these 83 males killed women with whom they were infatuated but who did not return the men's attentions. Of the remaining 53 men, 23 killed friends or acquaintances; 13 killed housemates, roommates, or neighbours; 8 killed business relations or co-workers; 4 killed strangers; 3 killed rivals in love triangles; and 2 killed police officers.
4 Three of these women killed friends or acquaintances, and one killed a house mate.

who had heard him threatening to kill his wife and commit suicide because he believed (incorrectly) that she was receiving attentions from other men. On the morning of 10 August 1903 he shot his wife in what was described by newspapers as a jealous frenzy and then shot himself. Rita Tomeczek suffered a similar fate in Toronto in 1966. She had separated from her common-law husband of ten years, Ivan Sabelnikoff, because of his heavy drinking and his threats to kill her. Sabelnikoff showed up at her apartment on 23 August begging her to return to him. She refused and called her mother to say goodbye; Sabelnikoff shot her while she was on the telephone and then turned the gun on himself.

The predominance of female intimate partners among the victims of male homicide-suicides replicates earlier research. However, in contrast to other studies, our initial examination of victim-offender relationships indicated that a relatively large percentage of male homicide-suicide offenders – 21 per cent, or 83 of 395 offenders – killed victims who were neither intimate partners nor kin (the next largest group of homicide-suicide victims). We therefore examined the narratives of these 83 cases and found that at least 30 involved men killing women – often landladies, neighbours, or co-workers – whom they were infatuated with or had pursued, but who were uninterested in or had rejected them. When the women rebuffed their solicitations, the men killed them and committed suicide. For example, in 1926 T.H. Seymour, the sixty-two-year-old night clerk of the Seattle Sheldon Hotel, killed Ada Marrenger, the hotel's fifty-year-old proprietress, before taking his own life. A police investigation revealed that Seymour had shot Marrenger in the hotel lobby in a moment of jealous hatred because she had refused his attentions. Classifying cases such as this as a variant of intimate-partner homicide raises the percentage of male homicide-suicides that targeted actual or desired intimate partners to 76 per cent.

Familicides are another variant of intimate partner-homicide-suicides but are less common than other types. They are also the type of homicide that is most likely to end in the suicide of the offender.[10] There were 36 familicides in the four cities we studied: men committed 34 of these, and 23 (68 per cent) of these men ended their own lives. Approximately 6 per cent of the cases in which men committed suicide after killing others were incidents of familicide. One such case occurred on 20 November 1950 in Buffalo. Police were called to 610 Fulton Street, where they found the bodies of Mary Tama and her sixteen-year-old daughter, Gloria, in their home. Nearby lay Stanley Tama, forty-two, who had stabbed himself to death after stabbing and killing his wife and daughter. A second daughter, Katherine, was found on the street, unconscious from head injuries inflicted by her father with a whetstone. Stanley Tama had been unemployed for some time because of injuries he had sustained while working at the Bethlehem Steel Plant and was said to be deeply depressed.

A smaller proportion of male killers who committed suicide, about 7 per cent, targeted only their children. For example, Paul Wach, a fifty-five-year-old Vancouver taxi driver, had carried on an argument with his ex-wife, who had custody of their three children, for a number of years. On Father's Day in 1981, he picked up the children – Wayne, age nine, Linda, seven, and Gloria, five – and took them to his apartment, where he shot all three and then himself.

The relationships between the 56 female homicide-suicide offenders and their victims differ substantially from cases involving male offenders. Over two-thirds (70 per cent) of female offenders took their own lives after killing only their children. A case in Toronto in 1947 is illustrative. Margaret Stages, who had been in and out of psychiatric hospitals for three years, took her six-year-old son, Bobby, to her bedroom, turned on the gas jets, and killed them both. Her suicide note offered some insights into her actions: 'The devil is in all of us. Bobby's body is full of trouble. He is with me.' Another 20 per cent of females – such as Vivien Breitner – committed suicide after killing only an intimate male partner. Breitner, age twenty-seven and a clerk at Boeing in Seattle, had been living with Paul Adams, a twenty-nine-year-old naval officer, for a few months. In March 1945 both were found dead in their apartment; Breitner's last communication indicated that she was 'fed up' and so had turned on the gas while Adams slept. Only two women killed intimate male partners and at least one of their own children: Fumiyo Takabe strangled her two children and stabbed her husband before hanging herself in Vancouver in 1989, and Mildred Biddeman used her police-officer husband's gun to kill him and their two children before turning the gun on herself in Buffalo in 1958. These two women, like most of the women who committed homicide-suicide, had histories of treatment for psychiatric problems and/or psychiatric hospitalization. In the cases in which mothers killed their children and themselves, over 65 per cent of the women were known to have been hospitalized for mental illnesses and/or to have attempted or threatened suicide in the past. In another 25 per cent of these cases, records stated the women had been suffering from depression before the killings.

Gender and Typologies of Homicide-Suicide

Several scholars have used the differences between male and female homicide-suicides to develop gender typologies of these events. These typologies highlight three major types of *male* intimate-partner homicide followed by suicide, categorizations that are consistent with patterns in our data.[11] In the first and most common type, a woman is killed by an intimate male partner who can be characterized as morbidly jealous, overly possessive, psychologically dependent, and/or enraged over what he perceives as her rejection of him. A second type, which often involves the killing of both the man's intimate partner and their children, is typically motivated by shame and guilt over financial or some other sort of public failure or is due to some form of mental illness. The third type, sometimes labelled 'altruistic' homicide-suicide, is characterized by older offenders and victims, one or both of whom suffer from ill health.[12] In a relatively small proportion of these cases, the older men who kill their wives and then themselves have histories of mental illness.

The dominant type of *female*-perpetrated homicide-suicide involves the killing of children by mothers who are described as suffering from some sort of mental disorder, typically depression, psychosis, or a personality disorder. In their review of research, Felthous and Hempel describe two common scenarios in murder-suicides by mothers, both of which imply that the mother's suicide is the primary goal.[13] In one scenario, a woman suffering from health or marital problems becomes suicidal; seeing her children (or child) as an extension of herself, she kills them as part of her suicidal act. In the other scenario, a mother wants to spare her children (or child) from some perceived terrible fate – mental illness, an intolerably harsh world, and so on – and so kills them and herself. A third category of homicide-suicide by mothers often discussed in the literature concerns women experiencing postpartum depression. In these cases the women kill their infants within a few weeks or months of their births. This type of homicide-suicide occurs infrequently in our data. Of the 59 children killed by mothers in these four cities, only 3 were under the age of one and only 10 were under the age of two.[14]

Overall, the patterns we document in homicide-suicide in Buffalo, Seattle, Toronto, and Vancouver between 1900 and 1990 closely resemble those described in other research on homicide-suicide. Specifically, the proportion of homicides followed by suicides, the sex distributions of victims and offenders, and the relationships among offenders and their victims look much the same as in other times and places. As a result, we have some confidence that our subsequent findings are generalizable beyond the four cities in our analysis.

Prior Research on the Epidemiology of Homicide-Suicide

Much research on homicide-suicide has been epidemiological and describes aggregate patterns and trends in the incidence of homicide-suicide. Some of this research draws on concepts derived from the work of Freud, Durkheim, Menninger, and others, but most is atheoretical and descriptive. One commonly discussed issue in this research is whether homicide-suicides are more similar to homicide or to suicide. A number of analyses have found that trends in homicide-suicide rates more closely follow trends in suicides.[15] On this basis, some researchers conclude that homicide-suicides are a sort of extended suicide. That is, they view the primary motivation of the killer to be self-destruction.[16] In contrast, other scholars argue that homicide-suicides more closely resemble homicides. In their view, the primary motivation is the killing of another person, with suicide resulting from the remorse, guilt, and/or fear of apprehension and punishment that arise after the homicide.[17] Finally, some judge the evidence as showing that homicide-suicide, while combining elements of both of its component parts, is a distinctive phenomenon that cannot be reduced to those parts.[18]

Coid draws on this comparative literature and, in particular, patterns in homicide to suggest three 'epidemiological laws' of homicide-suicide.[19] The first of these states that 'the higher the rate of homicide in a population, the lower the percentage of offenders who ... commit suicide.' The second states that the rate at which homicide offenders commit suicide 'appears to remain the same in different countries, despite considerable differences in the overall rates of homicide.' And the third states that, over time, the rate at which homicide offenders commit suicide 'remains the same, despite a fluctuation in the overall [homicide] rate.' Findings from several studies support the first two of these laws: in locales with high homicide rates, the proportion of homicide offenders who commit suicide tends to be relatively low, and rates of homicide-suicide tend to vary less across locales than do total homicide rates.[20]

Coid's third law has received less support because few studies have analysed data for time periods long enough to establish trends; however, two studies support the third law. Milroy, in his research on homicide-suicide in England from 1946 through 1996, and Kivivuori and Lehti, in their analysis of homicide-suicide in Finland between 1960 and 2000, conclude that the rate of homicide-suicide was relatively stable over time, whereas the proportion of homicide offenders who committed suicide declined substantially.[21] Three other studies that examine trends in homicide-suicide over many years – Adler's research on Chicago cases between 1875 and 1910, Gillespie and colleagues' study of Canadian data from 1961 through 1983, and Stack's analysis of Chicago cases from 1965 through 1990 – do not present their data in ways that allow tests of Coid's third law.[22] However, Gillespie and colleagues document a substantial decline in the likelihood of suicide following homicide, and data provided by Adler

Table 12.2
Homicides and homicide-suicides in Buffalo, Seattle, Toronto, and Vancouver, 1900–90

	Average annual homicide rate	Average annual homicide-suicide rate	Percentage of homicides that were homicide-suicides
Seattle	7.34	.72	9
Buffalo	6.97	.30	5
Vancouver	3.79	.26	6
Toronto	1.62	.17	9

suggest that the proportion of homicides in Chicago which ended in suicides decreased substantially after 1910.

In the analysis that follows, we examine how well Coid's laws describe homicide-suicide in four North American cities in the twentieth century. In addition, we consider whether the trends in the total homicide-suicide rate parallel those in the homicide rate, the suicide rate, and the rates of the major types of homicide-suicide. This analysis allows us to speak to the issues of whether homicide-suicide more closely matches homicide or suicide in its temporal patterning and whether different types of homicide-suicide follow disparate trends over time.

Coid's Laws of Homicide-Suicide and Patterns in Homicide-Suicide in Four Cities, 1900–90

To test the applicability of Coid's three laws, we first present data separately for each city and then combine the data across the cities to show trends over time. Table 12.2 synthesizes data on the average annual homicide rate, the annual average homicide-suicide rate, and the percentage of homicides that were homicide-suicides in each of the four cities over the ninety-one years of this study. In these cities, higher homicide rates are not associated with a lower percentage of homicides that were homicide-suicides. Indeed, in the cities with the lowest and highest homicide rates – Toronto and Seattle, respectively – a similar proportion of offenders committed suicide. Thus Coid's first law is not supported by these data.

There is also considerable and comparable variation in the homicide and homicide-suicide rates for these cities, according to table 12.2. For example, Seattle has the highest homicide and homicide-suicide rates;

in that city, rates there were more than four times greater than those in Toronto, the city with the lowest rates. The cross-city variation is inconsistent with Coid's second law of relative cross-national stability in the offender suicide rate. It is possible that the data in table 12.2 do not support Coid's first two laws because they come from cities in two countries with relatively similar rates of homicide and suicide, or because by aggregating the data over ninety-one years, they average out some of the inter-city variation. Here it is important to note that the research cited earlier which finds support for Coid's first two laws covers a wider range of countries. Thus we cannot reject his first two laws as invalid. However, the cross-sectional data in table 12.2 raise questions about the generality of those laws.

Coid's first and third laws can also be assessed with data on trends over time in homicide-suicide. Those trends can be described in two ways. One can track trends in the *rate of homicide-suicide*, or, alternatively, one can track trends in the *percentage of homicides that are homicide-suicides*. Each method tells a somewhat different but equally important story. The rate of homicide-suicide indicates the absolute risk of homicide-suicide in a population, whereas the percentage of homicides that are homicide-suicides shows the risk of suicide by the offender, given that a homicide has been committed. Theoretically, the two measures are independent of each other. In other words, upward or downward trends in the rate of homicide-suicide do not necessarily tell us anything about trends in the percentage of homicides that are homicide-suicides.

The average rate of homicide-suicide in these four cities peaked at .65 in 1910 and declined to its lowest point (.17) in the 1960s; it then rose slightly and levelled off in the 1970s and 1980s (figure 12.1).[23] This trend was mirrored by the trend in the overall homicide rate through the 1950s. In the 1960s, however, the two trends diverged: the homicide rate increased from the 1950s to the 1970s and levelled off thereafter, whereas the homicide-suicide rate dropped from the 1950s to the 1960s, increased slightly to 1970, and then levelled off. The different trends in the homicide and homicide-suicide rates are reflected in the trend in the percentage of homicides that were homicide-suicides (figure 12.2). From 1900 through the 1950s, this ranged between 9 per cent and 13 per cent, but from the 1960s onward, the percentage of homicides that were homicide-suicides declined to between 4 per cent and 6 per cent.

These trends speak to Coid's first and third laws of homicide-suicide. Recall his first law, which states that the higher the homicide

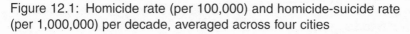

Figure 12.1: Homicide rate (per 100,000) and homicide-suicide rate (per 1,000,000) per decade, averaged across four cities

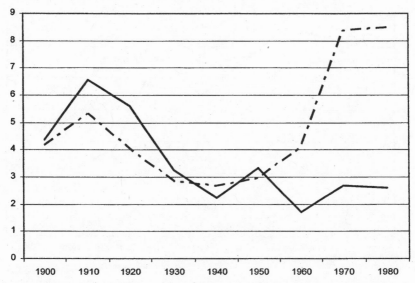

Note: The dashed line represents the homicide rate; the solid line represents the homicide-suicide rate. The homicide-suicide rate is expressed per 1,000,000 population so that it can be shown on the same scale as the homicide rate.

rate, the lower the percentage of homicides that are homicide-suicides. For the latter part of the twentieth century, this law is supported by our data. In the 1970s and 1980s, homicide rates were at their highest levels, while the percentage of homicides that were followed by the offender's suicide was lower than at any other point in the century. However, through the 1920s the homicide rate was relatively high, and the percentage of homicides that involved suicides was at its highest level; after this point both rates declined through the 1940s. Thus the pattern for the earlier part of the century is less consistent with Coid's first law.

His third law states that the rate of homicide-suicide remains stable over time, despite a fluctuation in the total homicide rate. Measuring stability or fluctuation in rates over time can be done in a number of ways, the simplest being the difference between the lowest and highest points in a time series. Measured this way, the homicide rate

Figure 12.2: Percentage of homicides that were homicide-suicides, averaged across four cities

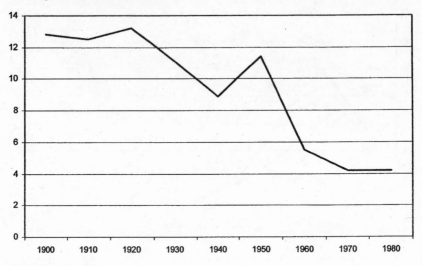

at its peak (8.49 per 100,000 in the 1980s) was just over three times greater than the homicide rate at its lowest point (2.71 per 100,000 in the 1940s), whereas the homicide-suicide rate at its peak (.66 per 100,000 in the 1910s) was almost four times that of the homicide-suicide rate at its lowest point (.17 per 100,000 in the 1960s). An alternative way to compare the variability of the two rates is by juxtaposing the mean of each rate with its standard deviation. The standard deviation of the homicide rate is 53 per cent of its mean, whereas the standard deviation of the homicide-suicide rate is 59 per cent of its mean. In other words, the variability of these two rates, according to this measure, is very similar. These results are inconsistent with Coid's third law.

Whether they are measured according to rates or ratios, there is clear evidence that homicide-suicides decreased over the twentieth century in these four cities. The downward trend in the rate was particularly marked from 1910 to 1930 (figure 12.1), whereas the downward trend in the percentage of homicides that were homicide-suicides was more notable after the 1950s (figure 12.2). For both measures, however, the lowest levels occurred during the post-1950s decades. Regardless of which measures we consider, it is not the case that the rate of homicide-

Figure 12.3: Average annual city/provincial suicide rate (per 100,000)

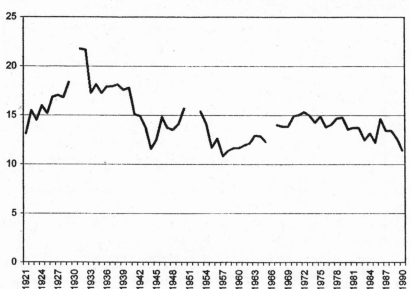

suicide was stable while the homicide rate fluctuated. Thus Coid's third law is again not supported by this analysis.

If, as some people have speculated, homicide-suicides are more similar to suicides than to homicides, it may be that this decline in homicide-suicide reflects a decline in the suicide rate. Although we were not able to gather data on suicide rates for each city over the ninety-one-year period, we did find data on suicide rates in Buffalo and Seattle and in Ontario and British Columbia[24] for the period 1921 through 1990.[25] The suicide rates fluctuated a good deal from year to year, but rates from the mid-1950s onward are lower on average than those prior to the 1950s (figure 12.3). We calculated Pearson correlation coefficients between the homicide-suicide, suicide, and homicide rates using annual data from 1921 to 1990 to determine how closely the homicide-suicide rate tracks the suicide rate, as compared to the homicide rate. The homicide-suicide rate is positively and significantly correlated with the suicide rate ($r = .274$, $p = .026$) but not with the homicide rate ($r = -.095$, $p = .435$). The significant association between the suicide and homicide-suicide rates suggests that the factors which drive trends in the former may also affect trends in the latter; however,

Figure 12.4: Homicide-suicide rate by males who killed intimate partners, averaged across four cities (per 100,000 males)

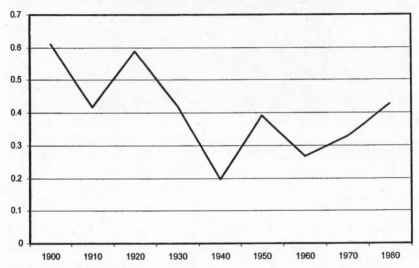

this correlation is relatively small. In other words, the trends in the homicide-suicide rate are far from a simple reflection of the trends in the suicide rate. Thus neither of the trends in the component elements of the homicide-suicide rate adequately accounts for the trends in homicide-suicides.

As noted earlier, explaining the trends in homicide-suicide is beyond the scope of our analysis. However, we might gain a better understanding of them by determining whether the decline is specific to a particular type of homicide-suicide. The two main types of homicide-suicide in our data set are homicide-suicides in which the homicide victim is (1) a male offender's intimate partner or (2) the offender's child (or children).

Trends in Intimate-Partner Homicide-Suicides by Males

Of the 939 men who killed intimate partners in these four cities, 271 (29 per cent) committed suicide at the scene or soon thereafter.[26] This proportion decreased steadily over time from a peak of 58 per cent in the first decade of the century to less than 20 per cent in the 1970s and 1980s. Moreover, while the rate of intimate-partner homicide-suicides by males fluctuated substantially over time, the overall trend was downward (figure 12.4). Thus, like the overall homicide-suicide rate, rates of intimate-partner homicide-suicides by males were highest early in the century and lower in most of the remaining decades. As with total homicide-suicides, homicide-suicides by males who killed intimate partners became less common over time.

We examined the narratives for the 271 cases of male-perpetrated intimate-partner homicide followed by suicide to determine if the decline in these killings was restricted to a particular type of intimate-partner relationship. Recall that prior research suggested three types of cases: morbid jealousy or rage over the partner's rejection (real or perceived), familicides arising from shame or mental illness, and altruistic killings involving older offenders and victims. Caution must be used in interpreting analyses based on these categories because of difficulties in identifying motives in homicide-suicides, but in 74 per cent of the cases there was sufficient information to make a 'best guess' as to motive (e.g., from suicide notes or from persons who had spoken to the offenders before the killings). The predominant type of intimate-partner homicide-suicide by males in our data is the morbidly jealous/possessive/spurned attention category. This type accounted for almost 75 per cent of the cases with sufficient information to categorize. Familicides and so-called altruistic homicide-suicides constitute the remainder of the cases in about equal proportions. There were no major changes over time in the distribution of these types, although the proportion of cases that were altruistic homicide-suicides did increase slightly over time. On the whole, however, the decline in the rate of intimate-partner homicide-suicides by males occurred across each of the major types of intimate-partner homicide-suicide.

Trends in Homicide-Suicides by Parents Who Killed Their Children

Of the 245 people known to have killed one or more of their children (but no one else), 65 (27 per cent) committed suicide at the scene or shortly thereafter. Mothers constituted 62 per cent of parents who killed only their children. However, mothers were no more likely than fathers to kill themselves after killing (only) their own children; 25 per cent of mothers (39 of 153) committed suicide compared to 28 per cent of fathers (26 of 92).

We examined trends over time in homicide-suicides committed by

Figure 12.5: Homicide-suicide rate by parents who killed their children, averaged across four cities (per 100,000 adults)

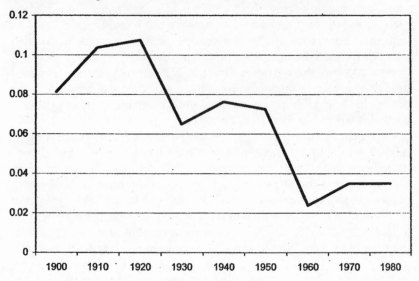

parents by combining the data for fathers and mothers. The *rate* at which parents killed themselves after killing their children declined over time, with particularly dramatic drops between the 1920s and the 1930s and between the 1950s and the 1960s (figure 12.5). The *percentage* of parents who took their own lives after killing their children also fell substantially over the century, from 36% prior to the 1960s to only 19% from 1960 onward. Thus, whether measured as a rate or a percentage, homicide-suicides by parents killing their children reached their lowest levels after 1960, and this was true for both fathers and mothers. Like trends in homicide-suicides generally, homicide-suicides by parents who killed their children became less common over time.

Was this decline in suicide by parents killing their children specific to particular types of filicide? It is difficult to track trends reliably over time because we are dealing with small numbers. However, our reading of these 64 cases indicates that the motivations and circumstances of these killings varied little over time. In all decades, records indicate that the vast majority of mothers who killed children and themselves suffered from some form of mental illness, and many faced problems with their physical health, marriages, or financial situations.

The main motivations were also similar for fathers over time: depression and despondency or anger over marital problems or financial troubles, severe psychological disorders, and apparently altruistic motives.[27] Thus the decline over time in the rate and proportion of homicide-suicides by parents who killed children was not accompanied by a change in the nature of these killings.

Discussion and Conclusion

Our goals in this chapter were to document characteristics of and trends in homicide-suicides in four North American cities for the years 1900 through 1990. With regard to the characteristics of homicide-suicides, our findings are largely consistent with other research. We found that most offenders were males and most victims were females; men's victims were usually their intimate female partners, whereas women's victims were typically their children; and the cases with the highest proportion of homicide-suicides were familicides, which were almost always committed by males.

Some of our findings, however, raise questions about conclusions drawn by other researchers. For example, we found only partial support for and some evidence to challenge Coid's epidemiological laws of homicide-suicide. As his first law predicts, the proportion of homicides that were homicide-suicides was lower in the decades with the highest homicide rates. However, in contrast to this first law, some decades had both relatively high homicide rates and high homicide-suicide rates, and the proportion of homicides that were homicide-suicides was not necessarily smaller in cities with higher homicide rates. Our analysis also raises questions about Coid's second and third laws and the predicted associations between homicide-suicide rates and homicide rates across space and time. We found that the variability in homicide rates is not any greater than the variability in homicide-suicide rates in these four cities.

With regard to trends over time in homicide-suicide, we found that both the rate of homicide-suicide and the proportion of homicide offenders who committed suicide were lower after the 1950s, compared to earlier decades. This decline also characterized the two most common types of homicide-suicide: those in which males killed intimate female partners and then themselves and those in which parents killed their children before taking their own lives. Yet, while the rate and proportion of these homicide-suicides fell, the motivations for and circumstances surrounding them appeared not to change over time.

We have also demonstrated that the trend in homicide-suicide rates is independent of the trend in the total homicide rate. In other words, whatever factors drive trends in homicides do not appear to exert much influence over homicide-suicides. In contrast, trends in homicide-suicides are to some degree associated with trends in suicides. Thus understanding the factors responsible for changes in the suicide rate over the twentieth century might shed some light on changes in the rate of homicide-suicides. However, we must use caution in generalizing findings from research on trends in suicides to trends in homicide-suicides; the two are only moderately correlated, even though homicide-suicide rates can be thought of as a variant of suicide rates. Instead, future research should explore the effects of changes in social, cultural, and economic conditions that may independently influence homicide-suicides. In the cities we study, child killings, familicides, and spousal homicides represent a smaller proportion of cases in the post-1950 period, compared with the century's first five decades. This decline likely contributed substantially to the drop in homicide-suicides, in a period that saw increases in other types of homicides that are rarely followed by suicide (e.g., killings involving young males in public places).

Changes that may have contributed to the decline in child and partner homicides include growing availability of contraceptives, smaller families, greater access to and social acceptance of divorce, increased social and economic support for single-parent families, improved access to counselling, and advances in diagnosing and treating mental health problems. Some of these factors also may have contributed to the post-1950s decrease in suicides by people who killed spouses and/or children. As well, the decrease in suicides after spouse and child killings perhaps reflects an increasing individualization whereby people were able more easily to separate themselves – psychologically and emotionally – from other members of their family, as the family's power as a 'master status' or cornerstone of identity diminished over time. Gender-role strictures also relaxed after mid-century, altering expectations about what it meant to be a husband and provider or a mother and nurturer. These sorts of changes may have weakened feelings of remorse and guilt over the killing of an intimate partner or a child and/or attenuated the belief that one's spouse or children are extensions of one's self and thus should not be left behind when one decides to commit suicide. Regardless of their origins, our findings with regard to trends in homicide-suicides are consistent with the claims of Marzuk and colleagues, who argue that 'murder-suicide occupies a distinct epidemiological domain,' and with Milroy, who maintains that 'homicide-suicide represents a distinct sub-category of homicide.'[28] As such, this particularly tragic form of violence deserves more study in its own right by scholars from a range of disciplines.

NOTES

1 See, e.g., M. Daly and M. Wilson, *Homicide* (Hawthorne, NY: Aldine de Gruyter, 1988).

2 M. Wilson, M. Daly, and D. Antonietta, 'Familicide: The Killing of Spouse and Children,' Aggress Behav, 1995, 21, 275–91.

3 In cross-checking our annual count of homicides in each city with counts obtained from various sources (e.g., police department or medical examiners' annual reports, FBI statistics, etc.), we discovered almost no discrepancies. In some cities for some years, the total number of cases for which we have data is slightly more than the number reported in other sources. But in no year is the discrepancy between counts more than two.

4 We use the term 'primary offender' to denote the person deemed primarily responsible for the killing by the authorities. In approximately 10 per cent of homicide incidents, more than one person was considered to have been directly involved in the killing. None of the homicide-suicides involved more than one offender.

5 See J. Adler, '"If We Can't Live in Peace, We Might as Well Die": Homicide-suicide in Chicago, 1875–1910,' *J Urban Hist*, 1999, 26, 3–21; J. Boudouris, 'A Classification of Homicides,' *Criminology*, 1974, 11, 525–56; R. Cavan, *Suicide* (Chicago: University of Chicago Press, 1928); L. Danson and K. Soothill, 'Murder Followed by Suicide: A Study of the Reporting of Murder Followed by Suicide in *The Times*, 1887–1990,' J Forensic Psychiatry, 1996, 7, 310–322; B. Danto, 'Suicide among Murderers,' *Int J Offender Ther Comp Crim*, 1978, 22, 140–8; L.I. Dublin and B. Bunzel, 'Thou Shalt Not Kill: A Study of Homicide in the U.S.,' *Survey Graphic*, 1935, 24, 127–31; M. Gillespie, V. Hearn, and R.A. Silverman, 'Suicide Following Homicide in Canada,' *Hom Stud*, 1998, 2, 46–63; M. Hillbrand, 'Homicide-suicide and Other Forms of Co-occurring Aggression against the Self and against Others,' *Prof Psychol Res Prac*, 2001, 32, 626–35; P.M. Marzuk, K. Tardiff, and C.S. Hirsch, 'The Epidemiology of Murder-suicide,' *JAMA*,

1992, 267, 3179–83; D.J. West, *Murder Followed by Suicide* (Cambridge: Harvard University Press, 1966); M. Wolfgang, 'An Analysis of Homicide-suicide,' *J Clin Exp Psychopath Q Rev Psy and Neur*, 1958, 19, 208–21. Estimates of the percentage of homicides that are homicide-suicides vary in whether they use the number of victims or the number of offenders as the denominator; using victims as the denominator yields a lower percentage. The percentage of homicides in which the offender commits suicide varies more across other countries, in large part because the number and nature of homicides varies a good deal cross-nationally.

6 See Adler, '"If We Can't Live in Peace"'; N. Allen, 'Homicide Followed by Suicide: Los Angeles, 1970–1979,' *Suicide Life Threat Behav*, 1983, 13, 155–65; J. Barnes, 'Murder Followed by Suicide in Australia, 1973–1992: A Research Note,' *J Sociology*, 2000, 36, 1–11; B. Barraclough and E. C. Harris, 'Suicide Preceded by Murder: The Epidemiology of Homicide-Suicide in England and Wales, 1988–1992,' *Psychol Med*, 2002, 32, 577–84; C.Y. Chan, S.L. Beh, and R.G. Broadhurst, 'Homicide-suicide in Hong Kong, 1989–1998,' *Forensic Sci Int*, 2004, 140, 261–7; A.R. Felthous and A.H. Hempel, 'Combined Homicide-Suicides: A Review,' *J Forensic Sci*, 1995, 40, 846–57; Gillespie et al., 'Suicide Following Homicide'; Hillbrand, 'Homicide-suicide and Other Forms'; J. Kivivuori and M. Lehti, 'Homicide Followed by Suicide in Finland: Trend and Social Locus,' *J Scand Stud Crim Crime Prevent*, 2003, 4, 223–30; C.M. Milroy, 'The Epidemiology of Homicide-suicide (Dyadic Death),' *Forensic Sci Int*, 1995, 71, 117–22; S. Stack, 'Homicide Followed by Suicide: An Analysis of Chicago Data,' *Criminology*, 1997, 35, 435–53; West, *Murder Followed by Suicide*; Wolfgang, 'An Analysis of Homicide-Suicide.'

7 There were a small number of transgendered and transsexual offenders in our data set, but none of them committed suicide.

8 See Adler, '"If We Can't Live in Peace"'; Allen, 'Homicide Followed by Suicide'; Barnes, 'Murder Followed by Suicide'; Barraclough and Harris, 'Suicide Preceded by Murder'; R.W. Byard, 'Murder-Suicide: An Overview,' *Forensic Path Rev*, 2005, 12, 337–47; C. Carcash and P.N. Grabowsky, 'Murder-Suicide in Australia,' in *Trends and Issues in Crime and Criminal Justice* (Canberra: Australian Institute of Criminology, 1998); West, *Murder Followed by Suicide*; Wolfgang, 'An Analysis of Homicide-Suicide'; M. Cooper and D. Eaves, 'Suicide Following Homicide in the Family,' *Violence Vict*, 1996, 11, 99–112; P. Easteal, 'Homicide-Suicides between Adult Sexual Intimates: An Australian Study,' *Suicide Life Threat Behav*, 1994, 24, 140–57; Gillespie et al., 'Suicide Following Homicide'; Hillbrand, 'Homicide-suicide and Other Forms'; Marzuk et al., 'Epidemi-

ology of Murder-Suicide'; E. Morton, C. Runyan, and K.E. Moracco, 'Partner Homicide-Suicide Involving Female Homicide Victims: A Population Based Study in North Carolina, 1988–1992,' *Violence Vict*, 1998, 13, 91–106; G.B. Palermo, 'Murder-Suicide: An Extended Suicide,' *Int J Off Ther Comp Crim*, 1994, 38, 205–16; West, *Murder Followed by Suicide*.

9 In our data, three men killed intimate male partners and then committed suicide.

10 See Daly and Wilson, *Homicide*; Wilson et al., 'Familicide'; D. Bourget, P. Gagne, and J. Maomai, 'Spousal Homicide and Suicide in Quebec,' *J Am Acad Psychiatry Law*, 2000, 28, 179–82; Cooper and Eaves, 'Suicide Following'; Easteal, 'Homicide-Suicides between Adult Sexual Intimates'; Morton et al., 'Partner Homicide-Suicide'; M. Rosenbaum, 'The Role of Depression in Couples Involved in Murder-Suicide,' *Am J Psychiatry*, 1990, 147, 1036–9; A. Starzomski and D. Nussbaum. 'The Self and the Psychology of Domestic Homicide-Suicide,' *Int J Off Ther Comp Crim*, 2000, 44, 468–79.

11 S. Palmer and J. A. Humphrey, 'Offender-Victim Relationship in Criminal Homicide Followed by Offender's Suicide: North Carolina, 1972–1977,' *Suicide Life Threat Behav*, 1980, 10, 106–18; A. Berman, 'Dyadic Death: Murder-Suicide,' *Suicide Life Threat Behav*, 1996, 26, 342–50; Rosenbaum, 'The Role of Depression'; Felthous and Hempel, 'Combined Homicide-Suicides'; West, *Murder Followed by Suicide*; Easteal, 'Homicide-Suicides between Adult Sexual Intimates'; Starzomski and Nussbaum, 'Self and the Psychology.'

12 For an alternative perspective on such homicide-suicides, see Cavan, *Suicide*, which describes such cases as having 'superficially altruistic motivation, in which the suicide kills someone because he believes them to be completely dependent upon him and liable to suffer without his continued protection'; and see M. Dawson, 'Intimate Femicide Followed by Suicide: Examining the Role of Premeditation,' *Suicide Life Threat Behav*, 2005, 35, 76–90.

13 Felthous and Hempel, 'Combined Homicide-Suicides.' See also S.H. Friedman, D.R. Hrouda, C. Holden, S.G. Noffsinger, and P. Resnick, 'Filicide-Suicide: Common Factors in Parents Who Kill Their Children and Themselves,' *J Am Acad Psychiatry Law*, 2005, 33, 496–504; T.K. Shackleford, V. Weekes-Shackleford, and S. Beasley, 'An Exploratory Analysis of the Contexts and Circumstances of Filicide-Suicide in Chicago, 1965–1994,' *Aggress Behav*, 2005, 31, 399–406; and Marzuk et al., 'Epidemiology of Murder-Suicide.' Friedman et al. conclude that the motives of fathers and mothers who kill their children and themselves are typically altruistic and acutely psychotic; this finding is consistent with Marzuk et

al.'s conclusion that clinical depression and maternal salvation fantasies are common among women who kill their children and themselves.

14 West, in *Murder Followed by Suicide*, finds a similar pattern. He notes that the traditional belief is that women kill their children during the puerperium; but he found only 11 of 45 children under the age of five killed by their mothers were less than a year old.

15 See Adler, '"If We Can't Live in Peace"'; West, *Murder Followed by Suicide*; J. Butea, A.D. Lesage, and M.C. Kiely, 'Homicide Followed by Suicide: A Quebec Case Series, 1988–1990,' *Can J Psychiatry*, 1993, 38, 552–6; Kivivuori and Lehti, 'Homicide followed by Suicide.'

16 See Adler, '"If We Can't Live in Peace"'; West, *Murder Followed by Suicide*; Butea et al., 'Homicide Followed by Suicide'; Kivivuori and Lehti, 'Homicide Followed by Suicide'; C.M. Milroy, 'Homicide Followed by Suicide: Remorse or Revenge,' *J Clin Forensic Med*, 1998, 5, 61–4; Hillbrand, 'Homicide-Suicide and Other Forms'; Marzuk et al., 'Epidemiology of Murder-Suicide.'

17 See Easteal, 'Homicide-Suicides between Adult Sexual Intimates'; A. Henry and J. Short, *Suicide and Homicide* (New York: Free Press, 1954); Stack, 'Homicide Followed by Suicide'; Berman, 'Dyadic Death'; Allen, 'Homicide Followed by Suicide'; A. Wallace, *Homicide: The Social Reality* (Sydney: New South Wales Bureau of Crime Statistics and Research, 1986).

18 Starzomski and Nussbaum, 'Self and the Psychology'; Marzuk et al., 'Epidemiology of Murder-Suicide'; Adler, '"If We Can't Live in Peace"'; C. Campanelli and T. Gilson, 'Murder-Suicide in New Hampshire, 1995–2000,' *Am J Forensic Med Path*, 2002, 23, 248–51; Milroy, 'Homicide Followed by Suicide'; Cooper and Eaves, 'Suicide Following Homicide.'

19 J. Coid, 'The Epidemiology of Abnormal Homicide and Murder Followed by Suicide,' *Psychol Med*, 1983, 13, 855–60, 857.

20 Carlos Carcach and P.N. Grabosky, *Murder-Suicide in Australia* (Canberra: Australian Institute of Criminology, 1998); Hillbrand, 'Homicide-Suicide and Other Forms'; Kiviuori and Lehti, 'Homicide Followed by Suicide'; Marzuk et al., 'Epidemiology of Murder-Suicide'; Milroy, 'Epidemiology of Homicide-Suicide'; Starzomski and Nussbaum, 'Self and the Psychology.'

21 Milroy, 'Homicide Followed by Suicide'; Kivivuori and Lehti, 'Homicide Followed by Suicide.'

22 Adler, '"If We Can't Live in Peace"'; Gillespie et al., 'Suicide Following Homicide'; Stack, 'Homicide Followed by Suicide.'

23 Unless otherwise noted, rates are expressed per 100,000 population aged

fifteen and older. For each city, rates were calculated using the population at the mid-point of the decade as the denominator. The numerator was the total number of homicide-suicides during the decade.

24 Suicide rates in Toronto and Vancouver are available for the years 1921–49 from the Dominion Bureau of Statistics, *Vital Statistics* (Ottawa: Dominion Bureau of Statistics, 1921–49). To determine whether the respective provincial rates tracked their corresponding city rates, we calculated Pearson correlation coefficients between these rates. The trends in the Toronto and Ontario suicide rates are positively and significantly correlated (.84), as are the trends in the Vancouver and British Columbia suicide rates (.66). Trends in the provincial rates therefore appear to be reasonable proxies for trends in the city rates.

25 Data on suicide rates for British Columbia and Ontario come from Dominion Bureau of Statistics, *Mortality from Suicide* (Ottawa: Health and Welfare Division, 1960), and Health Canada, *Suicide in Canada: Update of the Report of the Task Force on Suicide in Canada* (Ottawa: Health Statistics Directorate, 1994). Data on suicides in Buffalo and Seattle come from U.S. Department of Commerce, *Vital Statistics of the United States* (Washington, DC: Bureau of the Census, 1921–44); Federal Security Agency, *Vital Statistics of the United States* (Washington, DC: Public Health Service, 1945–49); U.S. Department of Health, Education, and Welfare, *Vital Statistics of the United States* (Washington, DC: Public Health Service, 1950–75); and U.S. Department of Health and Human Services, *Vital Statistics of the United States* (Washington, DC: National Center for Health Statistics, 1976–90).

26 This analysis includes males who committed familicide.

27 Three fathers killed children who suffered from serious physical or mental health problems, as did two mothers.

28 Marzuk et al., 'Epidemiology of Murder-Suicide,' 1395; Milroy, 'Homicide Followed by Suicide,' 63. Kivivuori and Lehti reiterate these conclusions in 'Homicide Followed by Suicide.' They argue that homicide-suicide 'is a distinct type of homicide, and not merely a function of differential offender reactions to homicide' (232).

13 'I may as well die as go to the gallows': Murder-Suicide in Queensland, 1890–1940

JONATHAN RICHARDS AND JOHN WEAVER

Anything we can learn about murder-suicides that can aid comprehension of these rare occurrences is worthwhile. As Rosemary Gartner and Bill McCarthy demonstrate in their contribution to this volume, abundant research initiatives have applied quantitative methods and assembled remarkable data sets to make sense of these disturbing cases, which so often involve attacks of men on women. There are certainly patterns in the gender of assailants and victims that remain consistent across a number of English-speaking jurisdictions. However, the act of forming data sets from scratch, in order to study a notoriously difficult topic such as murder-suicide, can lead to scepticism about the depth of understanding that is achievable through quantification. Faith in numbers has had a good run, but we should occasionally look deeper and, as Gartner and McCarthy have done, read the documents and newspaper stories that supplied the numbers. When cases must be assigned to categories for analysis, problems intervene. Silences in the primary sources may frustrate efforts to reach understanding, although challenging too is the task of sorting through layers within a well-documented incident. With the complication of multiplicity especially in mind, this probe of murder-suicides emphasizes the value of qualitative information and appeals for a decomposition of categories and more discussion of cases within quantified studies. This entreaty originates from a respectful understanding of quantification, since statistics have produced the subject's important core observations, some of which are repeated and affirmed in this account.

Our study originates in a project on suicide in Queensland, northeastern Australia. Several Australian researchers have tackled murder-suicide from the perspective of criminology. In 1998 Carcach and Gra-

Table 13.1
The gender of perpetrators and victims

Gender of perpetrators	Number (percentage) of perpetrators	Female victims	Male victims	Number (percentage) of child victims
Male	74 (89.1%)	52 (64.2%)	15 (18.5%)	14 (17.3%)
Female	9 (10.9%)	0	0	22 (100.0%)

bosky, examining crime statistics in Australia, noted that 'the most common situation surrounding a murder-suicide relates to disputes over the termination of a relationship.'[1] They recommended a typology of murder-suicides based on relationships. Forty-three per cent of offenders in their 144 cases were partners or former partners of the victim. Most murder-suicides in Australia allegedly involved persons in intimate or parent-child relationships. Jo Barnes revisited the topic in 2000 and argued that murder-suicide is both a familial and a gendered activity. In her study of 405 incidents in Australia between 1973 and 1992, 90 per cent of offenders were male, and 70 per cent of victims were female.[2]

In Queensland we found 83 murder-suicides subjected to inquests between 1890 and 1940. For most of this period, the state's magistrates investigated every suicide brought to their attention, and during the 1920s, when they relaxed their procedures for suicides, they still convened inquests into all murder-suicides. In general outline, the Queensland murder-suicides conform to patterns found elsewhere. Eighty-nine per cent of perpetrators were male, and 64 per cent of their adult victims were female (table 13.1). As Gartner and McCarthy observe in their four-city study, perpetrators have been predominantly male and victims mainly female. The presence of men as offenders in murder-suicides is consistent with their prominence as offenders in homicides generally; however, the prominence of women as victims in these types of homicides is notable because homicides committed by men generally have other male victims. The relationships in many murder-suicides led Jo Barnes to claim that it was 'essentially a domestic event.' Mental or physical illness 'did not appear to be prevalent in the majority of cases.' While we concur with Barnes's observation about gender, the contentions about murder-suicides as domestic events and the comments about a relative absence of mental illnesses are more problematic. First, with respect to domestic events, the conclusion fails to take

Table 13.2
Contributing factors mentioned by witnesses

Contributory factors	Men	Women
Jealously	10	
Termination of a relationship or imagined relationship	17	1
Alcohol abuse	5	1
Dispute	11	
Mental Illness	12	8
Bad Temper	3	
Poverty or unemployed	9	3
Japanese male	5	
Returned soldier	7	
Prostitute was victim	5	
Criminal action pending	4	
Low self-esteem	4	
Defence of reputation	2	

into account the obsessions that some men developed for women with whom they shared *no* domestic relationship. Second, in Queensland, when witnesses' statements about mental illness, alcohol abuse, violent tempers, and feelings of inadequacy are brought together, we have half the cases in which men were perpetrators. Judging from witnesses' depositions, the majority of women who killed their children had symptoms of a mental illness, and in several instances their domestic circumstances contributed to their mental state.[3]

Barnes contended that 'the patriarchal nature of our society provides a fertile context for an individual to kill a loved one and then commit suicide.' Queensland society was certainly patriarchal, and the majority of violent actors were male, but the Queensland cases from 1890 to 1940 indicate that patriarchy – significant context though it was – cannot explain why very few possessive, jealous males committed these terrible acts and hundreds of thousands of others did not. Male jealousy is not an uncommon emotion. The Queensland inquest files indicate potential contributory factors or circumstances; sometimes several complicating circumstances surfaced in one case, and for that reason there are more contributing factors than cases (table 13.2). Without question, the number of plausible contributing factors was even greater. Witnesses could be remarkably forthcoming; however, some surely withheld information.

Women's Burdens

The overall suicide data for Queensland show that a substantial proportion of women took their own lives on account of romantic disappointments (69 cases out of 406, or 17 per cent). This motive was rare for murder-suicides perpetrated by women, but it did occur. Widow Annie Merchant drowned herself and her three-year-old son near Southport on 22 March 1891. She was involved in a love triangle, but her lover had returned to his wife. A final meeting on 20 March was acrimonious: 'Annie Merchant struck me with an umbrella. Mrs Merchant was in a passion. She might have said I was deceiving her. I said the best thing I can do is to clear out.' The life of a poor widow was not easy, and Merchant had been let down by a man who had trifled with her.[4]

Other women were let down by men in their lives. Twenty-year-old Emily Sainsbury drowned her one-year-old son and herself in the Brisbane River in early July 1906. Sainsbury had lived at home until fifteen years of age, when she went into domestic service; she continued in service up to July 1905, when she had a male child. She received no support from the father. While trying to raise her son, she was giving her own father money, and he could not abide her infant and wanted the child out of the house. In these desperate circumstances, she went to the Salvation Army Maternity Home but soon left with her son.[5] Marion Spence was one month from giving birth when she poisoned her four children at Maryborough in June 1894. The doctor who conducted the post-mortem claimed that 'women will often take strange ideas into their head which cannot reasonably be accounted for.' But there were concrete reasons for her distress. Her husband had told her that he was going to quit work. Spence asked him to wait until the baby was born, but he would not answer. In the past, he said, she had threatened to kill herself when he got drunk and was locked up: 'Since our marriage when talking generally she has said she would like to take all her youngsters with her when she was dead.' The strain of raising four children, the prospect of a fifth, and dealing an irresponsible husband were not strange ideas in her head.[6]

Some women were mentally unbalanced, and the close identification of younger mothers with their young children meant the children's involvement in their mothers' distress. Sarah Owens, an alcoholic servant, drowned herself and her four-year-old daughter at Rockhampton in October 1902. She had been staying with a friend, who asked her to go to bed. Owens took offence and left the house with Jessie saying, 'You will have to bury me for stink if not for love.' That same witness recalled a previous conversation: 'One hole will do for the two of us.'[7] Margaret Finnan put a shotgun to her head after killing her only child at Ravenswood in December 1904; she had recently been treated for 'womb and ovary troubles.'[8] She left several notes that suggest she suffered from a mental illness.

> Mary was only seven weeks old when she said the words Jesus, Mary and Joseph. Oh! How soon I let them die away from her and wandered away from God, when she was only ten months old; now I can see it all too late. God expected me to look after myself, too, in order that I might be able to perform his will. Well! If I only had, my husband. I could have, for we should do that together, but now I have let my soul go to the devil; and poor man! I am not doing him justice to live with him although he is satisfied. If only I could have said Well! Let them do what they like. I will have no say, but I said all along and now I got no say.

Finnan's daughter was not a normal healthy child. She blamed herself: 'She is not right. I would like to kill her and then she would not live to be a scourge but I have not nerve. I was going to axe her yesterday. She cannot be any good, after what I gave her in my milk, and you are not the same man since I came back.'

Men seldom killed their children, but in one rare instance the explanation offered by the perpetrator resembled that presented in the Finnan case. The self-exculpatory motive was to save a child from suffering. Debates on this case alone could occupy a volume, although from a certain analytical perspective, it amounts to a familial murder-suicide. Richard Croker shot himself in the head after killing his eight-year-old son at Brisbane in November 1932.[9] He left a note:

> The extreme step which I contemplate taking is the result of careful consideration. Enid [his nine-year-old daughter] has a chance in life, but Bob is so backward that I realise he has but a very poor chance. Indeed, rather than allow him to go through life with such a handicap, I will end it all. I realise that my action is going to be very hard on all those who are left behind, but Enid is young and will forget to a certain extent and I hope that all others will try to realise that I have tried to act in the interests of my backward child. If I am to be held responsible before any higher tribunal I am prepared to accept the responsibility.[10]

Mental illness compounded by isolation affected twenty-one-year-old Amy Tobler, who drowned her three children in the Burnett River in June 1920. Her husband said that 'she appeared to be worried over not receiving letters from her mother. My wife was usually in good health but at times became depressed.' Tobler's mother-in-law testified. 'She complained of a bad headache and refused to see a doctor. She seemed to recover from that, and a few days before her death in a conversation I had with her, I asked her to prepare my child for school during my absence. She said she would if she was fit, as she had a bad head again.'[11] Mental illness was the verdict in the case of Bernice Sommers, who drowned her four-year-old son and herself in Gladstone Harbour in March 1922. The family was 'always on the lookout every night to see that she did not get away and kept the doors locked at night.' The police magistrate concluded that 'the deceased had been practically insane for a considerable time past and had made several attempts to put an end to her life.' She had been treated by doctors without success.[12]

Gertrude Ott died at Brisbane in September 1926 after killing her eight-year-old son.[13] She was being treated for goitre, headaches, and womb trouble.[14] Vera McLaurin killed her four-year-old daughter, Mary, and herself at Babinda on 8 November 1927. Her husband, Douglas, said they had been married for six years. The family lived at various places in town. His work took him away five days a week. 'My wife was not of a very robust nature, she often complained of pains in her back which necessitated her having to go to bed at times. She was very high strung and of a very nervous disposition and often complained to me of not being able to sleep at night. She would not go to the Doctor for treatment. Recently she complained of failing eyesight.'[15] Similarly, witness William Martin described Gertrude Ott as 'an extremely nervous woman, especially when alone.' Mental illness was a factor in that instance, as in several others, but the specific nature of the affliction and pain is unknown. The origins of the suffering, too, may be obscure, but often they seem entangled with domestic fatigue, stress, and abuse. Suicide, as a means of escape, was the intention for most of these women, and perhaps through some form of reasoning – passing to a better life after death – they believed they had to take their children with them. Or else they reasoned that they could not leave their children to face such troubles as they had endured.

The Complexities of Spousal Assault Cases

Patricia Easteal, who used Australian data from 1990, concluded that 'more than one-fifth of the offenders in homicides between adult sexual intimates took their own lives.'[16] She identified two subgroups of murder-suicide, namely, elderly partners facing deteriorating health conditions and males estranged from female partners and pathologically possessive. Easteal further proposed that self-destruction 'would seem to be the principal object' in some cases, but in others 'the principal motivator appeared to be the killing of the partner who either abandoned the offender or was perceived as unfaithful.'[17] The Queensland inquests disclosed no evidence of elderly partners, but they did show abundant variations on a theme of outrageous possessiveness. Jealousy is no excuse for violence, although it can have real as well as imagined roots, and in terms of a mental disorder leading to a murder-suicide, delusions of infidelity do not have to be intrinsically absurd. The morbid mental process is expressed by impaired reasoning, the extravagance of the allegations, the consuming attention given to the subject, and aggressive action.[18] In murder-suicide cases involving delusions of infidelity, the termination of a relationship arrives as an especially dangerous moment. Hugh Lawrence killed his wife, May, at Barcaldine in January 1920. Separated three weeks after they married, they had lived apart. He accused her of 'misconduct with other men.' 'I have heard he was of a very jealous disposition and had a very passionate and vindictive nature,' said one witness.[19] Harry Lett killed his wife at Cairns in April 1922. He had claimed that she was planning to go away with another man. The man in question said she was tired of her husband and wanted to go to Sydney 'to take up dancing on the stage.'[20] Jealousy, poverty, and a sense of hopelessness could have contributed to destabilizing Patrick McLoughlin, who shot his wife, Mary, at their home in Roma on 28 January 1901. McLoughlin was an older man and a hawker. They were poor and 'had periodical rows ever since they were married.' A neighbour testified, 'I think McLoughlin was jealous of his wife.'

Mary McLoughlin had left her husband to stay with a neighbour, to whom she 'complained her husband was threatening to kill her and himself, and abusing her. She said she was frightened to live with him in the house. She asked me to go down and speak to him.' 'I said "Paddy, what is up with the little woman?" He told me all about it. He got very excited and he said to me "Has she been to you?" I told him

I had met her casually. He said she was going about the town trying to ruin him. He said she had been unfaithful to him.' He was told to see Father Lee but could not find him. 'He said I am done for. I am ruined.' Fifteen minutes later, McLoughlin shot his wife and himself.[21]

If a main motive in murder-suicides involving a murderous husband was jealousy, then it is worth pointing out that it may not have been a single emotion but one entangled with saving face, alcohol abuse, and a history of violence. Market gardener Charlie Wassell, a Melanesian, murdered his wife, Agnes, and their neighbour Ida Pratt at Moore's Creek in November 1913. Agnes and Charlie had been married for seventeen months. They were all drinking prior to death; Charlie and Agnes were both seriously addicted to alcohol. 'Wassell and his wife lived very unhappily. She was continually clearing out, she generally used to go to other kanaka boys [South Sea Island labourers] and stay with them for some days.' Charlie had been arrested in the previous year for assaulting her. 'He was a bad and violent tempered man,' said a neighbour.[22] Not many witnesses remarked frankly and at length on the temperament of jealous men, but some mentioned bad tempers. The bodies of an estranged couple, Florence and Fritz Skau, were found at Townsville on 14 February 1930. Their son said they had separated about eighteen months earlier 'on account of his threats to my mother. He was a very bad tempered man and often threatened to take my mother's life.'[23]

Excessive drinking was involved in a number of incidents. The murder-suicide of John and Maria Lewis at Gympie in February 1923 was the fatal outcome of a drunken brawl. Addicted to drink, impoverished, and raising seven children, they fought that day over two bottles of beer.[24] James Corday shot his estranged wife, Maria, at Charters Towers on 7 May 1901. Maria Corday had fled from her husband and boarded with Mrs Mundey. On the night of 6 May, Corday invited his wife and Mrs Mundey to a concert. They stopped for drinks at several hotels on their way home. 'Corday and his wife were quarrelling all the time in the Theatre.' The next morning he appeared outside the Mundey house and asked to see his wife. He said, 'I will walk down with you as far as the Royal Hotel and bid her [his wife] goodbye. When near the Royal Hotel, he said "Come in and have a parting drink."' 'We went into a parlour,' reported Mrs Mundey. He shot his wife there. In a note he blamed her: 'Dear friends, when you find me don't think it was cowardice that I have done but my life is wrecked through the wife I have had. I done it for revenge.' Postscripts added, 'Revenge is sweet' and 'Jealousy.'[25] In this and in several other cases, the flight of the spouse to another house triggered outrage. The fact that the wife's new location was known and was unprotected put her at risk.

The themes of alcohol abuse, low self-esteem, and the flight of a spouse merged in the Trevethan case. On the evening of 28 February 1893, twenty-four-year old William Trevethan, a post and telegraph master, shot his wife and committed suicide near Georgetown.[26] He had been 'addicted to drink for many months, but lately became worse, until he appeared to be thoroughly sodden with drink.' Trevethan 'had been recently suffering from perineuritis (nerve damage) causing paralysis of one arm.' He could not work effectively and required his wife to help him sort mail. Feeling inadequate, he contemplated suicide: 'My Dear Kate, I suppose this will be the last line you will receive through (or by me) as I have been determined to commit suicide and tonight will most probably be the last of me. I intended doing it before but it is up a tree now. I have told a lot of (last sentence crossed out).' He may not have intended to kill his wife, but when she fled to avoid his drinking, he flew into a rage and demanded she come home, make breakfast, and assist him with the mail.[27] This case appears to have been an exception to a generalization that the intentions of males in murder-suicides are primarily murder and secondarily suicide.

Jealousy could be mixed with a returned soldier's instability. Patricia Prestwich noted in her contribution to this collection that French veterans of the First World War suffered disproportionately from mental illnesses and want of steady employment. That was the case, too, in Queensland. In May 1931 unemployed farm labourer George Moore, an orphan and returned soldier, committed suicide at Pinnacle after shooting his three-year-old daughter while she slept. George and Elsie Moore separated in early January 1931 because of his violent fits of jealousy. He tried several times to take their three children away from her. Elsie recalled a conversation in December 1930: 'My late husband came in from his work and said to me I will finish you. I said Oh, what has gone wrong with you? He said I know all about you. Randall [his employer] has told me the lot. I said What has Randall told you? He said Randall told me that you have been out with all of the mob and that Farlow [a boarder with the family] and you were no good ... He caught me by the hair and threw me across the bed. He struck me several times and tried to choke me. I lost consciousness.'

George claimed he knew of 'seven young men who had a do with her.' It was believed that his mother died in an asylum. Interestingly, after the separation, he lived with his mother-in-law, who hoped they would reunite. She believed that the tragedy had been brought about through his worry as a result of unemployment and gossip concerning his wife's sexual exploits.[28]

Another complicated, multiple-factor murder-suicide involved wharf labourer and returned soldier William Griffiths, who killed his wife, Alice, at Townsville on 1 November 1935. Their daughter, Daphne, declared that her parents only argued 'when Daddy was drunk. Then he used to hit and punch my mother.' In March 1935 Alice and Daphne left the family home. When Alice returned to get her sewing machine, announcing that it was in her name, William erupted. He hit her with his closed fist and said to his daughter, 'Don't touch her. Get out or I will cut your throat with a razor.' A neighbour testified that 'their home life was very unhappy with frequent quarrels.' He provided details: 'I would say at times he appeared to me to be mentally unbalanced, mostly when he was drinking. He would then seem to be always wanting to fight and he would come home at three or four in the morning and play his gramophone or lift his windows up to annoy people.' Griffiths's daughter added that 'sometimes we thought father was not right in the head. When Father was very drunk he would race up and down the verandah at home sometimes and knock his head on the wall. Father was a returned soldier, and in receipt of a pension. Father was getting the pension because of wounds he had received in the head. He used to complain of vile headaches.'[29] William Wade committed suicide at Maxwelton after shooting Emily Steward in January 1932. She and Wade had previously lived at Julia Creek; their relationship was not clearly spelled out, but they could have been on intimate terms. He tried to get money from her, but when she refused, he smashed the hotel up and shot her dead. Police said he 'was said to have gained great distinction at the late Great War.' The case leaves undeveloped their previous relationship but raises again the phenomenon of poorly adjusted returned soldiers. The presence of seven returned soldiers among the seventy-four male cases is worth noting.[30]

Attacks on a spouse might centrally be about relationships, but the nature of the relationships could be elusive, as the previous case indicates, or so involved that the words 'family' and 'relationship' fail to do justice to the sources of trouble and the mental state of the offender.

On 23 August 1902 farmer Albert May shot his sleeping wife, Bertha, at their home near Nanango.[31] Before he took his own life, he killed their four children. Police noted that Albert appeared to sleep in a separate room, while Bertha slept with the children. In Albert's room they found a note: 'Thank Mrs Labudda for it,' a reference to his mother-in-law. The precipitating factor seems to have been a court case. Albert May had sued Mrs Labudda for defamation of character. The exact trajectory of the feud can never be known, but conflict extended beyond husband and wife.[32] Sources of family friction occasionally appear with straightforward clarity, putting the worst of male conduct on full display, but other circumstances may intrude that could have contributed to an individual placing little value on his life. In an especially violent incident, farmer Norman Wallis committed suicide after killing his wife and their four young children at Yandina in July 1931. He had told a neighbour that his wife refused to 'have connection' with him as often as he would have liked, but he had been having sex with a young girl he employed on the farm until she told him she was pregnant. But Wallis also had serious financial worries.[33] A fusion of suicidal despair and homicidal rage seems possible on this occasion, and once we allow such complexity into the discussion, the possibility of theorizing fades. The effort to class murder-suicide as either a subcategory of suicide or a subcategory of homicide imposes a polarity on an array of motives, some known and others not.

Escape from economic distress and a perverse desire to take a spouse with one formed a combination in several instances. The murder-suicide of Ferdinand and Phyllis Boie occurred near Atherton in March 1920. They had boarded at the Peeramon Hotel with their two sons. Ferdinand could not get regular work and appeared despondent. Witnesses said he was attentive and helped Phyllis on wash days even when he was working.[34] William Lum Wan, a storekeeper at Proserpine, fatally wounded himself after killing his wife in August 1930. They had six children. Lum, a witness said, was 'worried over the depression.'[35] Finances were part of James Crisp's problems. He shot his wife, Muriel, at the Gresham Hotel, Brisbane, on 3 August 1927, only two weeks after their marriage in Sydney.[36] Crisp lived at the hotel, where his wife-to-be worked. Her mother took her in tow to Sydney in July, to get her away from him, but he followed. When Muriel and James returned to Brisbane, it was as a married couple. He was undoubtedly obsessed with her, but also swamped by financial difficulties. He had drawn five cheques totalling over £500 from an account with a balance of £3. Criminal charges were pending.[37] A criminal aspect surfaced in another case. Richard Arnold fatally wounded his de facto wife, Maggie Zoeller, and then shot himself at a boarding house in Brisbane on the evening of 24 July 1929. Maggie and Richard had lived together but had separated. Somehow he persuaded her to go with him to a boarding house, and there he shot her. He was no ordinary jealous male; this was no mere relationship. She had charged him with theft, and he was out on bail on a cattle-stealing charge. Moreover, Richard was exceedingly jealous and had once followed Maggie and another man.[38]

Some spousal attacks remain largely mysterious if we press beyond the obvious. What can be analysed, let alone concluded, if little is known about the details and dynamics of the relationship that is at the centre of hypotheses about murder-suicides? To put that a different way, does the concept of a relationship achieve anything more than crudely situating an event when witnesses offer nothing that suggests a history of abuse? Storekeeper William Jobling murdered his wife, Bridie, and committed suicide at North Rockhampton during the night of 13 December 1918. Their daughter testified that 'my mother and father had differences sometimes, but my father never used any violence towards my mother.' His body was found next morning. Police found a note: 'My dearest children, in a fit of melancholy last night I murdered your poor mother, who was one of the best and truest wives that ever breathed.'[39] We should be sceptical about both the statement of the witness and the note, but on what grounds can we presume to know more than the parties involved? If we claim that the case fits the pattern of relationship suicides and leave it at that, then our reasoning not only seems circular but fails to engage with the available evidence – admittedly vague – which suggests depression, an uncharacteristic assault, and remorse.

Obsessions with Girlfriends and Fantasy Sweethearts

A study by Danson and Soothill that collected one hundred years of reports of murder-suicides in the London *Times* maintained that these were mainly family affairs. Overwhelmingly, the women who took their own lives had killed their children, while men had usually killed spouses or partners.[40] The Queensland inquests reveal that most of that state's murder-suicides were family affairs, but there were also variant relationships. Samuel Nelson, a tram conductor, shot Edith

Willowdean at East Brisbane on 28 September 1918.[41] Willowdean's husband had not returned to live with her at the end of the war. Nelson had moved in, and she needed his financial support. He became both a border and a male companion. When he learned that she had another male friend, he left her. They were reconciled, but her association with the other man continued.[42] 'My mother used to meet a man named Tom in Queen Street and in Edward Street. My mother told me that Tom was just a friend. My mother told Sam about him. I heard my mother say something about Tom at the table one night. I never heard Nelson say anything about Tom.' Nelson was unhappy, said her son. 'Since my mother told Sam about Tom he was sick. He said his nerves were bad and he could not sleep at night. After that he drank and smoked.' Harold James was a young man who committed suicide after killing his girlfriend, Phyllis Busby, and her mother in July 1934 near Gympie. Her mother had tried to end the romance. He left a note: 'I can't get a crack at the old woman so we will go the two of us.'[43]

A number of men turned violent when women rejected a sexual pass. The noteworthy complication once more is the character of the relationship. Some women were not girlfriends but targets of rape and objects of men's fantasies. There was no romantic relationship between Vincenzo Oriti and Catena Guiffre, whom he killed near Ingham. He was friends with her husband but threatened her 'because she refused to consent to his wishes to be intimate with her.'[44] Asthma patient Charlie Fahl fatally wounded nurse Elsie Newton and killed himself in 1924. She did not encourage him or give him her address, but he found her anyway. When she rejected his advances, he said, 'You have got very uppish and beastly sarcastic.' A suicide note, dated 2 May 1924, indicated that he had become obsessed. He was married and deranged. Elsie was, he wrote, his 'only true love': 'My wife thinks no more of me than medicine. God knows I have repeatedly tried to be a good husband but she was never satisfied with what I did. God forgive me for what I am about to do but I think it will be my only way to gain happiness and that is for Dear Elsie and I to go to other worlds together. A better living girl I have never come in contact with.'[45] Infatuation with a landlady, a nurse, a neighbour, or a prostitute, as we will see, could transmute into a morbid obsession. The reasons for this shift, the essential problem of analysis, are not apparent beyond the guess of mental derangement.

Farmhand Norman McDowell, an impoverished young man with few prosects, killed his former girlfriend, Bernice Skuse, near Goombungee in October 1938 after she ended their engagement. He left a note: 'No doubt you will think what I have done is an awful thing, but there isn't anyone in this world who realizes what Bernice meant to me.' It continued: 'No one understands just what an orphan has to go through ... I just can't go on living this life and thinking of Bernice in someone else's arms.' Although this was a relationship case, McDowell's allusion to his hardships as an orphan intimates why he found lost affection difficult.[46]

There were relationships forced by a man with wavering on the girl's part. Albert Horne, a tanner, died at Brisbane in January 1914. Widowed four years earlier, he had met domestic servant Elizabeth Johnstone for a walk. Albert cut Elizabeth's throat and his own. He left a note: 'Goodbye to all from Elizabeth and Albert. We have had some trouble for some time which is better off not talked about. We have both decided to take our own lives, it is for the best. We wish to be buried together in Lutwyche cemetery.' The police magistrate decided that they had quarrelled; Horne's note was a clumsy attempt to cover his culpability.[47] The murder-suicide of Charles Bayldon and his girlfriend took place on 13 November 1924. Bayldon, a returned soldier, had fought in Egypt and France. 'He was suffering from shell shock,' said one witness. Bayldon was told by the girl's mother that she did not want to marry him. She was sixteen. He was thirty-seven and 'unattractive.'[48]

A similar case involving a returned soldier and a fixation on a woman who spurned him occurred at Longreach. Stanley Weight, a railway yardman, shot cook Elizabeth Zanetti in March 1926. He entered her room and asked, 'are you going to be different to me now?' She answered, 'don't be coming to the quarters.' An acquaintance had talked with Weight that morning. 'He said "I had a row with the girl last night." I said "You do not want to take this to heart, forget all about it." I said "You will probably be with her again tonight." He replied "No, you will never see us in the street again."' Another witness recalled a conversation. 'He said to me "Things do not look too bright for me. I have had a tiff with Liz." I said "Don't worry, let her go. You have your car – get out of the district – you will soon forget about it." He said "That is the trouble. I cannot seem to leave her. She is the only woman I have ever taken a fancy to and I seem mad over her."'[49]

Clarence Walter Ney's unshakable possessiveness toward a young girl worried those familiar with him until he and Isobel Arnold were found dead in her backyard at Nebo on 27 March 1939.[50] Isobel's mother, Elizabeth, testified: 'About twelve months ago Clarence Ney asked me if he could marry Isobel when she became eighteen years of age. I said, No. Not until she is twenty or twenty-one years of age. He said. I will wait until she is twenty-five if I can have her. He used to visit the house two or three times a day when he was in Nebo and came every night ... He seemed to be very fond of her. He was also very jealous of her.' Ney claimed unconvincingly that he had tired of Isobel Arnold and broken off their association. His mother testified: 'On the 23rd March I said to him "How is Bella?" He replied "She is alright, she is down there for anybody. I have finished with her now." I said "Don't be silly boy." He replied "You will see." I said "Walter, always remember if there was good, there is always better."'[51]

As we have suggested at several points, some murder-suicides involved relationships outside the family, and witnesses disclosed information about the perpetrators' background that may have had a bearing on the incident. The next four cases present further complexities. Robert Carey, a jockey, cab driver, and horse trainer, shot shopkeeper Lena Carter at Childers on 16 May 1913 and then committed suicide. They had once been friendly, but he alleged that Carter had robbed him, and so he went looking for her and demanded money. He told a witness he would get his money or shoot her. She refused.[52] Denniston Nettlefield, a twenty-two-year-old clerk living at the Empire Hotel in Fortitude Valley, committed suicide after shooting nineteen-year-old Norah Campbell in a car in the early hours of 16 May 1929. A letter to Nettlefield's mother read, 'Most of my time is spent with a girl who I have been very friendly with in the last few months. She is a girl called Campbell, Norah Campbell, and she is down in Brisbane studying for pharmacy. She is an awfully nice girl and very good company to be with.' Other letters revealed that he owed money. His books at work were irregular. Campbell may have rejected Nettlefield because he had financial troubles; she was the daughter of a doctor. According to Netterfield's employer, she jilted him. He phoned her on the evening of 15 May, asking her to go out 'one last time as he was leaving for Sydney the next morning.' His defalcations were a contributing problem that he sought to escape.[53]

The murder of twenty-five-year-old Amee Harris and the suicide of her forty-year-old brother-in-law, Robert McDowall, took place at

Abingdon Downs in September 1929. Harris had been employed as his bookkeeper since 1924. The relationships were complicated. Alcohol abuse was involved. McDowall's wife fled the station and her husband's drinking in 1926 and again in 1928. She denied estrangement, but he and Harris had an odd relationship. He was very jealous of her, and she was protective of him. On a recent trip, she threw a whiskey bottle from the car; on the day of the murder, McDowall pleaded with her for the key to the liquor cupboard. McDowall's wife insisted there was 'nothing to notice between my husband and sister.' She continued: 'My husband was quick tempered; he often said we had hair trigger tempers.'[54] Like many alcoholics, he was malnourished, and that condition may have contributed to his mental instability.

Returned soldier Ernest Frederick Rook committed suicide after killing his sister-in-law Ida Rook, at Dalby on 30 March 1931. His estranged wife lived in London. He received a war pension for a head wound and had lived with his brother's wife off and on for about six months. Her daughter testified that 'my mother told me on one occasion that she was afraid of my uncle as he had grabbed at her several times when passing her.' She found her mother's attire unusual: 'I have never known my mother to do her work about the house without having bloomers on.' The examination of the body failed to show scientific evidence of intercourse but everything pointed to it. A witness said that Ernest Rook had told her he did not like his brother's wife because she turned Roman Catholic. 'I went to the War and I fought for the British, not for those Catholics.' He added that 'if Arthur's wife was mine I'd kill her.' A mate of Rook's said he had heard him, when under the influence of drink speak, about cutting his throat. Mental illness cannot be dismissed as a contributing factor. It would be true, but also not illuminating, to portray these last four cases as involving a relationship.[55]

A broken romance or thwarted dalliance could affect a third party. Kathleen Bennett was fatally wounded by labourer William Haynes at Rockhampton in October 1921. The perpetrator and victim knew each other only by sight.[56] Haynes, who had been working out of town and 'drinking pretty heavily,' arrived at his brother's house asking for his brother-in-law. When Bennett, a lodger, answered the door and said, 'You know he does not live here,' Haynes fired at her. He likely suffered from mental illness; he had been wounded three times at the front. A witness remarked that 'when the deceased came back from the war he told me he had been wounded, gassed and had heart trouble. He said that he had a silver plate in his head.' Another witness remarked that a girl had recently left him. That started him drinking. He was 'a regular madman when he was drunk.' In December 1923 station hand Thomas Fitzgerald killed overseer Stanley Humble at Eddington station. Humble had warned Fitzgerald away from the jackeroos' quarters, where he had abused housekeeper Mrs Downey.[57] One witness recalled saying to Fitzgerald that 'you can never have the woman,' to which he replied that 'as sure as the stars are shining, there are three bullets. One for Mrs Downey, one for Humble and putting his finger on his forehead said one for me straight up there and it won't miss.'[58]

Additional Circumstances and Complications

To explore murder-suicides, it is advantageous to consider relationships as fully as possible. Some were inherently dangerous. Prostitutes work in a trade where they might meet on intimate terms possessive clients or work for controlling pimps. At least five of the fifty-two women murdered were prostitutes. In late December 1896 a Japanese ship's carpenter shot a woman in a brothel on Thursday Island and killed himself. They had once lived together at Cooktown.[58] Fred Johnson, a labourer, died on 9 September 1898 in Brisbane.[60] He was found with his throat cut. He had probably killed Mary Gray. A neighbour said that Johnson and Gray once had lived together until Johnson had gone to Bundaberg. She then stayed with another man, who was with her when Johnson arrived. Johnson stayed the night. The next morning the three drank beer together; the other man went out and returned to find the two dead.[61]

Japanese pearl diver Katsuma Okomoto fatally wounded prostitute Yoshiye Omori with a revolver, fired at two other women, and killed himself on Thursday Island on 7 March 1907. Okomoto 'had been previously sentenced to ten years' imprisonment for killing a man by stabbing him at Port Darwin.'[62] German marine engineer Karl Eberhardt fatally shot Lilian Jewett, a Brisbane prostitute, and committed suicide on 31 May 1909. Eberhardt murdered her after spending several hours in her company. They were old friends, but 'the discovery by him of the life she was leading so wrought on his feelings that in a fit of frenzy he determined to take her life and end his own existence.'[63] If we allow for a degree of editorial moralizing, the incident still suggests that a particular group of women were at considerable risk. Iwajiro Okawa, a Japanese laundryman, shot himself after killing prostitute Ada Williams at Winton in March 1928. He was jealous of her seeing other men.[64]

Another sub-population deserves attention. There are reasons to consider Queensland's Asian men separately. They were discriminated against and not permitted to bring wives to join them. Suicide was not absolutely condemned in Japan, where the double suicide of lovers was an established literary and artistic trope. Some men could not persuade a woman to join them voluntarily. Japanese diver Yoosuke Yosuke fatally wounded widow Shina Nakogawa and boarding-house keeper Fugita Tatsu before turning his revolver on himself on Thursday Island on the night of 26 October 1895.[65] Before she died, Shina Nakogawa gave a statement. He had broken into her bedroom and demanded that she go outside with him. 'I do not know why he shot me. He never asked me to marry him.' Police said that Yosuke 'was at this time under bond to keep the peace.' Tatsu's widow said he owed her husband sixteen pounds, and 'he had obtained a judgement in court for that amount.'[66] In the confines of the mostly male pearl-diving community on tiny Thursday Island, jealousies, gambling, and debts led to numerous assaults and a few murders. Some men who shed blood accepted their fate but wanted to save honour by taking their own lives. The island's peculiar society had little in common with mainland communities, and that observation reminds us of the importance of context. The records of a jurisdiction may enable us to look for changes in the patterns of a phenomenon over many years; however, a jurisdiction is only an administrative entity, not a society. To fathom circumstances it is important to situate cases.

The murder-suicides by Japanese men were not confined just to Thursday Island. Tomosabro Shintani, a cook at a Townsville hotel, shot himself after killing waitress Margaret Gallagher in July 1908. His brother testified that the deceased had deserted from the Japanese army. Another witness said Shintani had recently received a letter prompting him to say that 'he did not care what he did now and that he would kill two or three before he died.' According to a third witness, the letter from Japan advised that he would be shot as a deserter if he returned. He said, 'I don't care now. I want to die. I will kill all you girls before I die.' He had previously threatened girls working at the hotel with murder and was jealous if they spoke to other men.[67] Another Japanese male, Hayashi, killed his countryman

Tokozo Takaki and committed suicide at Mackay on 26 June 1915. Hayashi suffered from tuberculosis. He held a grudge against Takaki who had complained about his spitting habits. According to police, he went to a house planning to kill other Japanese men.[68] Iwamatsu Kohara, a laundryman, died in January 1914. He and his wife had recently resumed living together in Ingham. They quarrelled. He shot and stabbed her, set the house on fire, and then killed himself.[69] A witness said that Mrs Kohara was afraid of her husband and until recently had been living with another Japanese man on Thursday Island. That lover had written a letter to Mrs Kohara saying he was coming to get her. It was assumed that her husband read it.[70] The case of Iwajiro Okawa, who shot himself after killing a prostitute, has already been mentioned in the discussion of prostitutes.

Several Chinese males who committed murder-suicide appear to have been involved in feuds over money and possessions in their largely male communities. At Boulia, Chinese cook Loo He Kong fatally stabbed Jimmy Foo Jah on 3 December 1900. Then he took strychnine. Foo Jah had a sleeping mat made of two rice bags. This mat disappeared, and he accused Loo He Kong of theft. Day after day, Foo Jah shouted so that Loo He Kong could hear him: 'That fellow thief steal my mat.' Loo He Kong had had enough.[71] Ah Yok stabbed Yong Chong to death before hanging himself at Cloncurry in December 1922. Yong left a note: 'I honest man and am satisfied to die. I am hard up and I die for my money. Ah Yok is spiteful and thinks he is a smarter man than all other Cloncurry Chinamen. He say I can do nothing to him. Ah Yok says Yong Chong got no money and nobody help him. God said me to kill Ah Yok. I know if I kill Ah Yok my penalty will be to die and I will go to heaven.'[72]

Several men either faced serious criminal sanctions or had been to prison and wanted to defend that secret. Reputation meant something even to the disreputable and unstable. Charles Young, a wood carter at Silverspur, shot himself in the head after fatally wounding his wife's brother in July 1908. Evidence was presented of quarrels between their families. Young's brother-in-law threatened to tell police that the deceased had raped his daughter several times. The girl told her aunt and uncle about his abusing her. Young told his wife that 'those bastards' would not 'give him a second chance.' Other witnesses said he was bad-tempered and often threatened to kill his whole family.[73] Labourer Robert Donnelly fatally wounded cook Terence McDonald and then killed himself at a work camp at Saltwater Creek on the morning of 16 March 1909. Donnelly came to breakfast with a rifle in his hands. 'He said "Teasdale, Henzel and Johnston, keep your seats. I won't molest you. I am going to shoot the rest of the bastards."' McDonald said, 'don't be a bloody fool, Bob.' Donnelly turned towards him. 'You are always pulling me to pieces. I will give it to you first.' He left a note: 'I here leave a few lines about the way my life has be slandered away by the low degraded people of Queensland.' A pouch contained 'A Notice to Offender upon his Discharge,' showing that Donnelly, who had been sentenced to seven years in prison for manslaughter, had been placed on a seven-year good behaviour bond.[74] There was at least one more 'paranoid,' explosive man. Michael Hayes, a labourer, died at Maryvale from shotgun wounds to the head after killing James King in July 1916. Hayes had fired shots at a group of men. One witness said he heard him say that 'you have been looking for it and you have got it. You are all against me.'[75]

A few inquests unearthed biographical details that leave us in a quandary about how to classify them on account of multiple motives and unfathomable turns. Alexander Bennett had been adopted through the State Children Department at the age of two. At the age of sixteen, on the evening of 30 June 1937, he shot his adoptive mother, Annie Bennett, and killed his adoptive father, William Bennett.[76] He then committed suicide. In the second week of June, Alex had been fired from his job. His employer found him very hostile. A neighbour who knew Alex testified that 'as a little chap the boy was very loveable. He altered after he left school. He got very wilful.' In fact, he had been ejected in 1934 as a problem child. Things worsened when he started keeping company with a fourteen-year-old girl he met in early 1937. He ignored his mother's orders not to stay out at night, punched her, and left home on 1 May. According to Mrs Bennett, 'he punched me on more than one occasion. He said to me "If you throw your weight around I'll flatten you out." I was always chastising him. I sometimes smacked him when he was a very naughty boy.' She recalled speaking to him a fortnight before the tragedy. 'He called me everything he could lay his tongue to. He said What the Hell do you want here?' She said she and her husband were kind parents: 'We did everything that was humanly possible for him. We purchased a piano for him and had him taught for six years. We also gave him a camera and a bicycle. There was nothing that the boy wished for that he did not get. He knew that if he had come and spoken kindly to us we would have given him anything willingly ... Often we thought there was just a bit of a kink in deceased's makeup. He often had fits of violent temper.'[77]

Queensland's inquests into murder-suicides have disclosed details that reinforce the conclusions of other Australian and international studies. Male-female relationships and, more especially, their dissolution, are critically important. However, qualitative evidence elaborates upon and complicates this pattern. A few remaining cases involve relationships, but the lived experience of the relationship is glimpsed fleetingly; the obscure events and their reception by a troubled mind were crucial. The murder-suicide of Helena Bauer and her son William near Kingaroy was discovered on 21 October 1920.[78] William had been living on the farm for the past twelve years. He was a single man. His mother was on a visit and about to leave when he shot her. There was no apparent motive, and the police considered him a 'very steady sober man.' In July 1926 selector Frank Henderson took strychnine after he shot his eighteen-year-old daughter, Annie, and his mother-in-law, Harriett Hollist, at Boxwood station.[79] After his first wife passed away twenty years earlier, he had married her sister, who had also since died. Henderson left a note saying, 'Grannie and myself have had a row over Annie.' He had threatened to send his daughter to the Warwick Convent 'if she was not careful' and added, 'I am having my revenge on the old woman ... I think I done the best thing by killing them out of the bloody rode [sic].' While perplexing, these cases involved mentally unbalanced men likely affected respectively by isolation and loss. Sixty-five-year-old retired shearer Thomas Burke shot thirty-seven-year-old housekeeper Jane Tarkalson in the head, wounded fellow employee George O'Brien, and then killed himself at Nanyah station on 25 May 1929.[80] His conduct prior to the shootings suggests he was mentally ill. Nicholas Dawson took strychnine at Strathfield Station near MacKinlay (Cloncurry) after killing Andrew Marsden in October 1910.[81] Apparently, the two workmates had argued over a dog.

Conclusions

Many studies show that murder-suicides predominately concern relationships, often family relationships, and frequently occur at the end of a relationship. Successive quantitative analyses have strengthened the trustworthiness of these generalizations, but data alone may never provide complete explanations. The eighty-three inquests into murder-suicides in Queensland between 1890 and 1940 add details and disclose mysteries. Fields such as criminology and suicide studies that dwell on motives are bound to encounter the impenetrable, but that obstacle is no reason to abandon the struggle for knowledge or, for example, to dismiss suicide notes and witnesses' statements because they may be loaded with self-justification. The words of perpetrators and witnesses even in that frame of mind are connected to motives. Quoting Jean Baechler, Victor Bailey noted that 'it is not necessary to be able to explain *everything* in order to try to understand something.'[82] It would take knowledge in several fields of analysis – history, psychiatry, sociology – to piece together the psychodynamics from the shards of testimony about mental illness, alcohol abuse, poverty, isolation, war trauma, prostitution, and national cultures. However, the fact that these additional considerations featured in witnesses' testimony both extends knowledge and deepens questioning.

NOTES

1 Carlos Carcach and P.N. Grabosky, *Murder-Suicide in Australia* (Canberra: Australian Institute of Criminology, 1998), 3.
2 Jo Barnes, 'Murder Followed by Suicide in Australia, 1973–1992: A Research Note,' *Journal of Sociology* 36, 1 (2000), 3
3 For similar conclusions, see D.J. West, *Murder Followed by Suicide* (London: Heinemann, 1965), 143–4.
4 'A Mysterious Affair,' *Queenslander*, 28 March 1901, 592; file 120, Department of Justice, Inquests, bundle 188 (or JUS/N188, which will be the form of citation hereafter), Queensland State Archives. Most cases will require only one citation and will appear at the end of the narrative for that case.
5 File 315, JUS/N357.
6 File 233, JUS/N224.
7 File 337, JUS/N309.
8 File 351, JUS/N327.
9 'City Tragedy,' *Brisbane Courier*, 4 November 1932, 14.
10 File 895, JUS/N956.
11 File 455, JUS/N710.
12 File 277, JUS/N738.
13 'Shocking Tragedy,' *Brisbane Courier*, 13 September 1926, 7.
14 File 1010, JUS/N831.

15 File 1139, JUS/N858.
16 Patricia Weiser Easteal, *Killing the Beloved: Homicide between Adult Sexual Intimates* (Canberra: Australian Institute of Criminology, 1993), 94.
17 Ibid., 108
18 Ronald Rae Mowat, *Morbid Jealousy and Murder: A Psychiatric Study of Morbidly Jealous Murderers at Broadmoor* (London: Tavistock, 1966), 114–15.
19 File 57, JUS/N702.
20 File 558, JUS/N744.
21 File 66, JUS/N293.
22 File 4, JUS/N543.
23 File 184, JUS/N905.
24 File 161, JUS/N756.
25 File 261, JUS/N297.
26 'A Deplorable Tragedy,' *Queenslander*, 4 March 1893, 426.
27 File 160, JUS/N211.
28 File 490, JUS/N930.
29 File 71, JUS/N1006.
30 File 222, JUS/N943.
31 'Tragedy at Wooroolin,' *Queenslander*, 30 August 1902, 503.
32 File 262, JUS/N307.
33 File 895, JUS/N956.
34 File 269, JUS/N706.
35 File 687, JUS/N915.
36 'A City Tragedy,' *Brisbane Courier*, 4 August 1927, 17.
37 File 1160, JUS/N859.
38 File 794, JUS/N897.
39 File 66, JUS/N293.
40 L. Danson and K. Soothill, 'Murder Followed by Suicide: A Study of the Reporting of Murder Followed by Suicide in *The Times*, 1887–1990,' *Journal of Forensic Psychiatry* 7, 2 (1996), 310–22.
41 'Tragedy at East Brisbane,' *Brisbane Courier*, 30 September 1918, 8.
42 File 107, JUS/N684.
43 File 460, JUS/N983.
44 File 454, JUS/N869.
45 File 334, JUS/N781.
46 File 810, JUS/N1055.
47 File 71, JUS/N545; 'Sensation at Lutwyche,' *Brisbane Courier*, 21 January 1914, 5.
48 File 775, JUS/N788.
49 File 438, JUS/N819.

50 File 252, JUS/N1063.

51 File 252, JUS/N1063.

52 File 329, JUS/N527.

53 'Two Dead: New Farm Park Tragedy,' *Brisbane Courier*, 17 May 1929, 15; file 24, JUS/N896.

54 File 755, JUS/N897.

55 File 298, JUS/N926.

56 File 651, JUS/N729.

57 File 55, JUS/N774.

58 File 56, JUS/N774.

59 File 22, JUS/N248.

60 'Murder and Suicide at Petrie Terrace,' *Brisbane Courier*, 10 September 1898, 8.

61 File 430, JUS/N267.

62 File 162, JUS/N372.

63 'Murder and Suicide,' *Brisbane Courier*, 1 June 1909, 5.

64 File 330, JUS/N866.

65 'Tragedy at Thursday Island,' *Queenslander*, 2 November 1895, 893. It is impossible to be certain that the names were transliterated correctly by journalists or officials.

66 File 360, JUS/N237.

67 File 336, JUS/N401.

68 File 345, JUS/N584.

69 'Murder and suicide,' *Brisbane Courier*, 22 January 1914, 7.

70 File 150, JUS/N548.

71 File 510, JUS/N291.

72 File 33, JUS/N753.

73 File 301, JUS/N400.

74 File 176, JUS/N418.

75 File 507, JUS/N615.

76 'Triple Shooting: Two Dead,' *Courier Mail*, 1 July 1937, 13.

77 File 492, JUS/N1032.

78 File 653, JUS/N714.

79 File 829, JUS/N827.

80 File 735, JUS/N896.

81 File 569, JUS/N457.

82 Victor Bailey, *This Rash Act: Suicide across the Life Cycle in the Victorian City* (Stanford: Stanford University Press, 1998), 33.

Contributors

Paulo Drinot is lecturer in history at the University of Manchester and a social historian who works on modern Peruvian history. He did his BSc at the London School of Economics (1994) and his MPhil (1996) and DPhil (2000) at the University of Oxford. He has published articles in various academic journals and recently co-edited a volume entitled *Beyond Domination and Resistance: Studies in Peruvian History, Sixteenth to Twentieth Centuries* published by the Institute of Peruvian Studies, Lima.

Andrew M. Fearnley is a PhD candidate in history at the University of Cambridge. He is currently writing his doctoral dissertation on 'Ideas of Race and Insanity in the Post-Bellum US,' a broad consideration of how shifting modes of racialized thought have shaped understandings of mental illness. He has published a lengthy consideration of this research in *Reviews in American History*; he also has articles forthcoming in *Gender & History* and the journal *Social History of Medicine* on the topic of suicide and race.

Rosemary Gartner is a professor of criminology and sociology at the University of Toronto. Her research interests include historical and comparative patterns in lethal violence. Recent books include *Murdering Holiness: The Trials of Franz Creffield and George Mitchell* (2003; co-authored with Jim Phillips) and *Marking Time in the Golden State: Women's Imprisonment in California* (2005; co-authored with Candace Kruttschnitt).

Rab Houston is professor of modern history at the University of St Andrews, Scotland. He is the author of several books, including *Madness and Society in Eighteenth-Century Scotland* (2000), and co-author (with Uta Frith) of *Autism in History: The Case of Hugh Blair of Borgue* (2000). His current project is a comparison of patterns and understandings of suicide in Scotland and England between 1500 and 1850.

Junko Kitanaka is a medical anthropologist and associate professor in the Department of Human Sciences, Keio University, Tokyo. Her McGill University doctoral dissertation was titled 'Society in Distress: The Psychiatric Production of Depression in Contemporary Japan,' for which she received the 2006 Margaret Lock Prize in Social Studies of Medicine and the 2007 Dissertation Award from the American Anthropological Association. A revised version of her chapter will appear in her forthcoming book from Princeton University Press.

Howard I. Kushner is the Nat C. Robertson Distinguished Professor of Science and Society at Emory University. A graduate of Rutgers University (AB) and Cornell University (MA, PhD), Kushner has focused recent research on historical and clinical aspects of Gilles de la Tourette syndrome and associated neuropsychiatric disorders. He is author of four books and numerous articles, including *American Suicide: A Psychocultural Exploration* (1991) and *A Cursing Brain? The Histories of Tourette Syndrome* (1999).

Bill McCarthy works in the Department of Sociology at the University of California, Davis. He is the author (with John Hagan) of *Mean Streets: Youth Crime and Homelessness* (1997) and recent articles in the journals *Annual Review of Sociology, Social Forces,* and *Criminology.* His current research interests are adolescent crime, homicide and stigma.

Jeffrey Merrick is professor of history at the University of Wisconsin-Milwaukee and received his PhD from Yale University. He has published *The Desacralization of the French Monarchy in the Eighteenth Century* (1990), *Order and Disorder under the Ancien Régime* (2007), and many articles on political culture, gender, sexuality, and suicide in early modern France.

Janet Padiak is an assistant professor in the Department of Anthropology, McMaster University. She is a biological anthropologist interested in historical patterns of health and disease gleaned from the records of the British army surgeons' reports. She received her PhD from the University of Toronto in 2004 with a dissertation entitled: 'Morbidity and the 19th Century Decline of Mortality: An Analysis of the Military Population of Gibraltar 1818 to 1899.' She has published work on several aspects of morbidity and mortality during the nineteenth century, including infant mortality, suicide, influenza, and, in progress, tuberculosis, as well as social and medical aspects of army life and medical care.

Julie Parle is a senior lecturer in the Department of History, University of KwaZulu-Natal, South Africa. Her PhD thesis (2004) was on the topic of mental illness in Natal and Zululand in the nineteenth and early twentieth centuries, and it explores therapeutic options along the spectrum from colonial psychiatry to remedies for love sickness and hysteria through to the exorcism of spirits and the detection of witches. Her monograph *States of Mind: Searching for Mental Health in Natal and Zululand, 1868–1918*, was published by UKZN Press in 2007.

Kenneth M. Pinnow is associate professor of history at Allegheny College in Meadville, Pennsylvania. He has published articles on Soviet forensic medicine as well as Soviet suicide. He is currently completing a book, *The Loneliness of the Collective: Suicide and the Social Science State in Bolshevik Russia, 1921–1929* (Cornell University Press). His next project will examine the development of early Soviet criminology and continue his explorations into the individual and society.

Patricia E. Prestwich is professor emerita in the Department of History and Classics, University of Alberta, Edmonton. She is an historian of modern France and has written extensively on the history of alcoholism and psychiatry in France, including *Drink and the Politics of Social Reform: Antialcoholism in France since 1870* (1988). She has also written on the history of women. She is currently completing research on the treatment of mental illness in France from 1914 to 1939.

Jonathan Richards completed his doctorate on the Queensland Native police force in 2005. He researches and teaches Australian history at Griffith University and has worked as a consultant historian for a number of Indigenous groups over the last ten years. He is currently a research fellow at the Centre for Public Culture and Ideas at Griffith University.

Kevin Siena is associate professor of history at Trent University. He is the author of *Venereal Disease, Hospitals and the Urban Poor: London's 'Foul Wards,' 1600–1800* (2004) and editor of *Sins of the Flesh: Responding to Sexual Disease in Early Modern Europe* (2005). He has published articles on early modern medicine and sexuality and is currently working on a book-length project tentatively titled 'Beyond the Hospital: Pauper Illness-Strategies in Eighteenth-Century London.'

John Weaver is Distinguished University Professor of History, McMaster University. He is the author and editor of several books on legal history and the history of land acquisition, including his award-winning *The Great Land Rush and the Making of the Modern World* (2003). He is currently the principal investigator of a major research project on the history of suicide in Queensland (Australia) and New Zealand.

David Wright holds the Hannah Chair in the History of Medicine at McMaster University. He is also an associate professor in the Department of Psychiatry and Behavioural Neurosciences and the Department of History. He is the author and co-editor of six books on the history of mental health and psychiatry, including (with James Moran) *Mental Health and Canadian Society: Historical Perspectives* (2006).

Index

Abadie (psychiatrist), 143–4
Aboriginal communities: suicide within, 3
accidents and accidental deaths, 10–11; among Indians of Natal, 163; murder vs, 98; in newspapers, 105; in Paris, 74–5; of soldiers, 122, 149; suicide vs, 98
acculturation, 241, 242, 248
Ackerman, Nathan, 240, 241
Adams, Paul, 286
Adler, J., 288–9
adolescents. *See* youth
aestheticization. *See* romanticism
African Americans. *See* black Americans
Africans: characteristics of, 170; and citizenship, 169, 172; common mental landscape with Europeans, 172; mental capacity, 168; suicide among, 9, 157, 168, 169, 170–2
age and aging: and interdisciplinarity in suicide studies, 6–7; in soldiers' suicides, 127, 129; suicide rates and, 78, 142, 188, 237, 238

agency: and black American suicides, 246; in overwork suicides, 273; removal of, 194; in Scottish procedure, 94; in unnatural deaths, 98–9; in victim-precipitated homicide, 245
aggression, 244, 245, 246
Ah Yok, 322
alcohol and alcoholism: Africans and, 171; British soldiers and, 124; as cause of madness, 137; in France, 141; French soldiers and, 138, 139, 141–2; hereditary degeneration and, 141; indentured Indians of South Africa and, 166; and murder-suicide, 311–12, 319, 320; soldiers and, 129; and soldiers' suicides, 130; and suicide, 13, 79, 191
Algerian War, 151
alienation: anomic suicide and, 35; industrialization and, 267; of South African Indians, 157; and suicide, 214
alienists, 4, 22, 49n82. *See also* psychiatrists
altruism, 38